Asthma: Clinical Diagnosis and Therapeutics

Asthma: Clinical Diagnosis and Therapeutics

Edited by Brendol Keith

hayle
medical

New York

Hayle Medical,
750 Third Avenue, 9th Floor,
New York, NY 10017, USA

Visit us on the World Wide Web at:
www.haylemedical.com

ISBN: 978-1-63241-757-2

Cataloging-in-Publication Data

Asthma : clinical diagnosis and therapeutics / edited by Brendol Keith.
    p. cm.
Includes bibliographical references and index.
ISBN 978-1-63241-757-2
1. Asthma. 2. Asthma--Diagnosis. 3. Asthma--Treatment. 4. Bronchi--Diseases.
5. Lungs--Diseases, Obstructive. 6. Respiratory allergy. I. Keith, Brendol.
RC591 .A88 2019
616.238--dc23

Table of Contents

Preface

A common pulmonary condition associated with the chronic inflammation of respiratory tubes, tightening of respiratory smooth muscle and episodes of bronchoconstriction is known as asthma. Its symptoms include shortness of breath, chest tightness, wheezing and coughing. Asthma can be caused by a combination of genetic and environmental factors. It is usually diagnosed on the basis of one's pattern of symptoms. Quick-relief medications such as Beta$_2$-adrenergic agonists, anticholinergic medications and selective adrenergic agonists are used to treat acute cases of asthma. Long-term medications include leukotriene receptor antagonists, corticosteroids, mast cell stabilizers, etc. The various advances in the treatment of asthma are glanced at in this book and their applications and ramifications are looked at in detail. Most of the topics introduced herein cover new techniques of diagnosing and managing this condition. Students, researchers and doctors will benefit alike from this book.

After months of intensive research and writing, this book is the end result of all who devoted their time and efforts in the initiation and progress of this book. It will surely be a source of reference in enhancing the required knowledge of the new developments in the area. During the course of developing this book, certain measures such as accuracy, authenticity and research focused analytical studies were given preference in order to produce a comprehensive book in the area of study.

This book would not have been possible without the efforts of the authors and the publisher. I extend my sincere thanks to them. Secondly, I express my gratitude to my family and well-wishers. And most importantly, I thank my students for constantly expressing their willingness and curiosity in enhancing their knowledge in the field, which encourages me to take up further research projects for the advancement of the area.

Editor

Asthma and the microbiome: *defining the critical window in early life*

Leah T. Stiemsma[1,2] and Stuart E. Turvey[2,3,4*]

Abstract

Asthma is a chronic inflammatory immune disorder of the airways affecting one in ten children in westernized countries. The geographical disparity combined with a generational rise in prevalence, emphasizes that changing environmental exposures play a significant role in the etiology of this disease. The microflora hypothesis suggests that early life exposures are disrupting the composition of the microbiota and consequently, promoting immune dysregulation in the form of hypersensitivity disorders. Animal model research supports a role of the microbiota in asthma and atopic disease development. Further, these model systems have identified an early life critical window, during which gut microbial dysbiosis is most influential in promoting hypersensitivity disorders. Until recently this critical window had not been characterized in humans, but now studies suggest that the ideal time to use microbes as preventative treatments or diagnostics for asthma in humans is within the first 100 days of life. This review outlines the major mouse-model and human studies leading to characterization of the early life critical window, emphasizing studies analyzing the intestinal and airway microbiotas in asthma and atopic disease. This research has promising future implications regarding childhood immune health, as ultimately it may be possible to therapeutically administer specific microbes in early life to prevent the development of asthma in children.

Keywords: Microbiota, Asthma, Early life, Critical window, Hygiene hypothesis, Microflora hypothesis

Background

Recent evidence supports a role of the intestinal microbiome in the development of childhood asthma and atopic disease. Animal model studies have made significant advancements in the quest to understand the gut-lung axis; identifying large-scale shifts in gut microbial compositions in asthma and allergy-induced mice and manipulating the intestinal microbiome with antibiotics, which enhanced the severity of these diseases [1–3]. However, with the advancement of DNA and RNA sequencing technologies and the establishment of large longitudinal human birth cohorts, it is becoming clearer that gut microbial dysbiosis in human atopic diseases is characterized not by global changes to the composition of the intestinal microbiota, but by taxa-specific shifts in abundance at the family, genus, and even species' levels [4–6]. Perhaps unsurprisingly, these taxa-specific changes are most prominent within the first 100 days of life, during which the human immune system is most plastic in its development [4–6]. Given these scientific developments, this review aims to provide an overview of the recent advances in human microbiome research in asthma and atopic disease.

The global burden of asthma and atopic disease

Allergic asthma is an immunoglobulin E (IgE)-mediated chronic inflammatory disease of the airways [7]. Other manifestations of IgE-mediated or "atopic" diseases include: atopic dermatitis (also referred to as eczema), allergic rhinitis, and food allergy [8]. These diseases typically manifest in early childhood and can be chronic life-long burdens for many people. However asthma is often viewed as the most burdensome atopic disorder, due to the prevalence (235 million people worldwide) and associated mortality (an estimated nine asthma-related deaths per day in the United States) [9, 10]. Asthma has become the most prevalent childhood disease in recent decades, affecting approximately one in ten children

*Correspondence: sturvey@cw.bc.ca
4 Department of Pediatrics, BC Children's Hospital, 950 West 28th Avenue, Vancouver, BC V5Z 4H4, Canada
Full list of author information is available at the end of the article

worldwide [8]. Aside from the obvious danger associated with asthma, this disease is very disruptive to a normal daily lifestyle for children, and is the leading cause of emergency room visits and absenteeism from school [11].

Some of the most striking data related to asthma prevalence comes from the United States, where it was reported from 1999 to 2009, that the proportion of people diagnosed with asthma increased by 15% [10]. In other Westernized countries (e.g. Canada, Australia, and the UK) the prevalence of this disease was reported to be even higher (up to 30% in some countries), while many countries in Eastern Europe and Asia report a much lower prevalence of this disease (~5%) [8, 12, 13]. This rapid increase in prevalence of asthma (and other atopic diseases) as well as the apparent geographical disparity suggests an etiology that is more complex than population genetic variation.

'The post-industrial epidemic'

The underlying cause of asthma is a complex product of genetic and environmental factors resulting in significant heterogeneity of the disease. Parental history of asthma increases the likelihood of developing this disease, however assessment of this factor alone is not enough to confirm a person's risk of asthma development [14–16]. There is also evidence of a strong link between sex and increased risk of asthma development in children, as boys are more likely to develop childhood asthma than girls [17, 18]. Further, genome-wide-association-studies have identified candidate genes that play a role in asthma susceptibility (ORMDL3 and SMAD3) [19]. Thus it is clear that human genetics contribute to asthma pathogenesis, however the rapid rise in asthma prevalence suggests changing environmental factors are biasing the developing human immune system toward these hypersensitivity diseases [20].

In addition to the within-generation rise in the prevalence of asthma, there is also an inverse relationship between the incidence of infectious diseases and hypersensitivity diseases, where a high incidence of infectious diseases appears to protect against allergic and autoimmune diseases [21]. Further, the geographical disparity of asthma and atopic diseases is shifting, as developing countries become industrialized and their living conditions become more like the Western world [22]. Thus it appears that there may be a link between the development of hypersensitivity diseases and the urbanization or modernization of society [23]. Many urban environments have similar characteristics (lower air quality, higher population density, lower economic status) that predispose populations to asthma; and similar to the geographical disparity of this disease, rural areas with comparable environments do report greater incidences

of hypersensitivity diseases [24, 25]. There is also the possibility that urbanization does not support optimal immune development due to a decrease in exposure to environmental microbes as humans shift from an outdoor lifestyle to a more indoor lifestyle that is characteristic of urban societies [26].

This concept of decreased microbial exposure in modern or more urban societies has become a booming research area in the etiology of immune dysregulation. One particular arm of asthma etiology in particular, focuses on factors associated with improved health and hygiene; for example, increased antibiotic exposure, and household size [23, 27–35]. In particular, David Strachan extensively studied the relationship between household size and atopic disease in the late 1980s, and his initial findings led him to propose the hygiene hypothesis of allergic disease in 1989 [36]. This hypothesis sets the stage for the current analyses assessing the role of microbial exposure in the development of asthma and other hypersensitivity disorders.

External and internal microbes as protectors against asthma

The hygiene hypothesis

The hygiene hypothesis proposes that a lack of early life exposure to microbes alters early life immune system priming and, consequently, increases susceptibility to atopic diseases [20]. Strachan theorized that older siblings promote increased exposure to environmental microbes through inevitable unhygienic contact, which results in decreased likelihood of atopic disease development in younger siblings [36]. He supported his hypothesis by showing that household size was inversely correlated with the development of hay fever (i.e. allergic rhinitis) in a cohort of 11,765 children [37]. Since Strachan's original proposal, the hygiene hypothesis has expanded to include additional environmental factors (such as mode of birth, antibiotic exposure, household pets, etc.), which also alter the microbial exposure of infants [33–35]. Further, with substantial improvements in genetic sequencing technology, the role of indigenous microbes has also been added to the mix.

The microflora hypothesis

The microflora hypothesis extends Strachan's hygiene hypothesis by emphasizing the role of microbes residing in and on the human body (collectively known as the human microbiota) [38]. Originally, these microbes were considered to be commensal, having little effect on human physiology [38]. However they have since been implicated extensively in human health and development, and it is clear that there is a microbial-immune cell interface, in which cross-talk between microbes and immune cells aids in the development of immune tolerance [39–42]. Notably, the focus of this hypothesis is the gastrointestinal tract, one of the most populated zones of the human body [38]. It proposes that perturbations to the colonization and composition of the intestinal microbiota (dysbiosis), disrupts this natural microbe-immune cell interface, biasing the developing infant immune system toward a hyper-sensitive (allergic) state [38, 43]. In support of the microflora hypothesis, a recent study found that uncontacted Amerindians (indigenous peoples of the Americas) exhibited higher levels of bacterial and functional diversity in their skin and fecal microbiota than any other human population previously reported, suggesting that modern societal practices (perturbations) have strong implications in the development of the microbiota [44]. Regarding the role of the intestinal microbiome in asthma, the gut-lung axis attempts to explain the mechanisms guiding gut microbe-lung immune cell cross talk.

The gut-lung axis
Innate immunity microbial crosstalk
The gut-lung axis attempts to mechanistically define how microbes in the gut might influence immune function in the lung [45]. One potential connection is through interactions of the gut microbiota with pattern recognition receptors of the innate immune system [46]. It is well established that pathogen-associated molecular patterns (PAMPs) such as lipopolysaccharide (LPS), CpG, and peptidoglycan can stimulate Toll-like receptor (TLR) signaling, which confers downstream activation of many genes that regulate inflammation and innate immune responses [47]. Similar to the antigen-recognition and IgE-mediated hypersensitivity pathways, dendritic cells (DCs) are also the intermediaries of gut microbiota-immune cell cross talk, as they regularly sample gut microbes in the intestinal lumen or lymphoid tissues [46]. DC sensing of gut microbiota PAMPs promotes immune tolerance in the intestine, but also results in phenotypic changes to DCs and migration to the mesenteric lymph node (MLN) to promote T cell priming [48]. In the MLN, T cells also acquire homing molecules (e.g. CCR4, CCR6), which initiate migration to other parts of the body, including the respiratory mucosa [49].

Thus it is possible that interactions with specific gut microbes, via their corresponding PAMPs, could result in varying phenotypic changes in DCs, with downstream effects on lymphocyte priming/homing and ultimately, shifts in anti-inflammatory responses in the airways [49]. In a house dust mite (HDM) model of allergic inflammation, chronic intranasal exposure to endotoxin (bacterial LPS) has been shown to protect mice from HDM-induced asthma [50]. The proposed mechanism of this protection

is through A20 (ubiquitin modifying enzyme)-mediated inhibition of HDM-induced recruitment of conventional DCs to the lungs and mediastinal lymph nodes [50]. Further, prior 2-week treatment of mice with LPS suppressed proliferation and differentiation of adoptively transferred CD4+ HDM-specific 1-DER T cells in the mediastinal lymph nodes into IL-5 and IL-13—secreting T-helper (Th)-2 cells, highlighting the T cell priming effects of these DCs [50]. Though this is not a gut microbiota mediated pathway, it does highlight the ability of bacterial PAMPs (specifically LPS) to alter DC recruitment to the lungs and protect mice against asthma symptoms.

Role of microbial-derived metabolites—short chain fatty acids
Another area of gut-lung axis research involves microbial-derived metabolites, such as short chain fatty acids (SCFAs). SCFAs are direct by-products of bacterial fermentation of carbohydrates and are key energy sources for many host tissues and gut bacterial species [51]. There are three major SCFAs, acetate, propionate, and butyrate, which are present in a molar ratio of 60:20:20, respectively [51]. These metabolites are known to modify gene expression through inhibition of histone deacetylases (HDACs), cytokine and chemokine production, and cell differentiation, proliferation, and apoptosis [52]. With regard to immune tolerance and inflammatory mechanisms, butyrate and propionate induce extrathymic T-regulatory (T-reg) generation through direct interactions with T cells and indirect interactions through DCs, potentially through the inhibition of HDACs [53]. Clostridial species are prominent SCFA producers, and butyrate production by these particular bacteria was associated with the generation of peripheral T-reg cells in the colon [54]. In a HDM-mouse model of experimental asthma, both acetate and propionate were capable of reducing cellular infiltration into the airways after HDM exposure [55]. Systemic propionate treatment modified bone marrow hematopoiesis and enhanced the generation of DC and macrophage precursors and subsequent recruitment of DCs less effective in promoting Th-2 cell polarization in the lungs [55]. In a later study using the same asthma mouse model, maternal intake of acetate was shown to reduce allergic airways disease in the adult offspring of mice [56]. Notably, both these studies initially assessed the role of a high fiber diet on the production of SCFAs and colonization of intestinal bacteria—highlighting the influence of diet, mediated by gut microbial changes, on the development of the immune system [55, 56]. The latter study, however, emphasizes intrauterine effects on the infant immune system, mediated by maternal diet, suggesting the need to consider prenatal prevention strategies using these gut microbial metabolites [56].

Microbial influences on epigenetics

It is also possible that the intestinal microbiota is linked to lung immunity through microbe-mediated epigenetic modification. Distinct whole blood DNA methylation patterns were associated with two major bacterial phyla, either Firmicutes or Bacteroidetes and pathway analysis revealed differential methylation (associated with a high or low Firmicute/Bacteroidetes ratio) among genes enriched in functional networks such as cardiovascular disease, inflammatory responses, obesity, and lipid metabolism [57]. Further, production of bacterial methyl groups, cofactors (e.g. folate), and enzymes (e.g. methyltransferases) can both directly and indirectly affect host DNA methylation, and consequently may bias cell differentiation toward or against an immune profile that confers tolerance [58, 59]. There is also evidence that early life farm microbial exposures may influence the methylation of genes related to asthma and allergies [60, 61]. Lastly, reinforcing the age-sensitive role of the intestinal microbiota in hypersensitivity diseases, the presence of a conventional gut microbiota in previously germ-free (GF) neonatal (but not adult) mice decreased hypermethylation of CXCL16, which in turn decreased accumulation of invariant natural killer T (iNKT) cells (prominent in the pathogenesis of asthma) in the colon [41]. Thus ultimately, there is much more to learn regarding the mechanisms of the gut-lung axis in asthma and other lung disorders. Current research in asthma and atopic disease centers around how, mechanistically, the intestinal microbiota is linked to these disorders and whether early life changes to the intestinal microbiome can be therapeutically manipulated to promote immune tolerance.

The intestinal microbiota in asthma and atopic disease

Mechanistic studies analyzing how the intestinal microbiome is involved in asthma and atopic disease are typically conducted in mouse models of allergic inflammation. GF mice lacking a microbiota show increased allergic responses, including increased lymphocyte and eosinophil inflammation in the airways, accompanied by increased Th-2 cytokines and elevated IgE production [62]. However many animal studies also focus on roles of distinct bacterial taxa in atopic disease development. In an ovalbumin (OVA)-model of asthma, oral supplementation of mice with two types of Lactobacillus showed that protection from allergic responses is mediated by specific bacterial species [63]. Supplementation with live Lactobacillus reuteri resulted in decreased airway hyper responsiveness, while treatment with Lactobacillus salivarius had no effect on the allergic symptoms of the mice [63]. This species-specific effect was also shown using three bacterial species,

Bifidobacterium longum, Bifidobacterium breve and L. salivarius [1]. L. salivarius had no effect, and both Bifidobacterium species increased Peyer's patch and splenic Foxp3+ T-reg cells in infant mice [1]. However, only B. longum introduced in the perinatal period resulted in T-reg cell induction in adult mice and protected against allergic airway inflammation in OVA-sensitized mice [1]. Notably, the age-sensitive induction of T-regs in adult mice by B. longum suggests the presence of an early life window in which microbial-driven immune changes are most effective.

Antibiotics (which disturb the intestinal microbiota composition) have also been shown to increase airway inflammation in mouse models of experimental asthma [2, 64, 65]. One study showed that combined oral antibiotic treatment of mice resulted in increased allergic inflammation, characterized by increases in serum IgE and circulating basophils [65]. Conventionally raised mice showed decreased proliferation of bone-marrow resident basophil precursors compared to the antibiotic treated mice, suggesting that these shifts in immune cells were mediated by alterations to the microbiota [65]. Thus collectively, these mouse model studies show that gut microbial alterations can result in changes in lung function, but it is becoming clearer through improved mouse-models and longitudinal human cohort research, that these microbe-mediated changes in immune development are most effective in early infancy.

Mouse studies suggest an early life critical window

Age is the main driver of compositional and functional differences in the intestinal microbiota [4, 66]. Thus it is perhaps unsurprising that many mouse studies assessing the role of the gut microbiota in atopic disease, find the results to be time sensitive (Fig. 1a). Cahenzli et al. demonstrate that global shifts in the composition of the intestinal microbiota (increased microbial diversity) in early life is required to regulate IgE production and decrease disease severity in a mouse-model of antigen-induced oral anaphylaxis [67]. In OVA- and HDM-models of allergic airway inflammation, oral infection with CagA-positive Helicobacter pylori resulted in protection against OVA and HDM-induced airway hyper responsiveness [68]. However, this bacterium-mediated protection against asthma was more apparent in mice infected neonatally compared to mice infected as adults [68]. As noted in the previous section (microbial influences on epigenetics), neonatal (but not adult-life) exposure to a conventional microbiota in GF OVA-challenged mice abrogated iNKT cells in the lungs and reduced serum IgE, proinflammatory cytokine levels, and eosinophilia in the bronchoalveolar lavage fluid, protecting mice from developing allergic asthma symptoms [41].

a

Thorburn et al. show that maternal intake of acetate reduces allergic airways disease in adult offspring[56]

Gollwitzer et al. identify shifts in airway micobiota that are associated with decreased responsiveness to aeroallergens[74]

Cahenzli et al. associate increased microbial diversity with decreased IgE production and decreased disease severity in a mouse model of antigen-induced oral anaphylaxis[67]

Birth | 1-week | 2-weeks | 3-weeks | 4-weeks | 5-weeks | 9-weeks

Arnold et al. determine that neonatal (6 days post birth) Cag A-positive Helicobacter pylori infection protects against OVA and HDM-induced airway hyperresponsiveness[68]

Lyons et al. show that perinatal exposure to B. longum induces T-regs and protects against allergic airway inflammation in adult mice[1]

Russell et al. show that perinatal exposure to antibiotics differentially exacerbates lung disease in adult mice[2, 3]

Olszak et al. show that exposure of GF neonatal mice at birth (and continuing until 9-weeks post-birth) protects adult mice from allergic asthma symptoms[41]

b

1-month | 2-months | 3-months

Birth | 1-week | 2-weeks | 3-weeks | 4-weeks | 5-weeks | 6-weeks | 7-weeks | 8-weeks | 9-weeks | 10-weeks | 11-weeks | 12-weeks

Abrahamsson et al. associate decreased gut microbiota diversity at 1-week and 1-month of age with asthma development at 7-years of age[69]

Fujimura et al. identify shifts in neonatal bacterial and fungal taxa that are associated with varying degrees of asthma risk by 4-years of age[6]

Teo et al. associate increased asymptomatic colonization with Streptococcus in the NP microbiome with chronic wheezing at ages 5 and 10 years[79]

Arrieta*, Stiemsma* et al. associate decreased abundance of FLVR taxa and decreased acetate production at 3-months with atopy and wheezing at 1-year of age[4]

Stiemsma et al. identify the L/C ratio as a potential biomarker for identifying children at high risk of being diagnosed with preschool-age asthma.

Fig. 1 Defining the critical window of early life in **a** mice and **b** humans

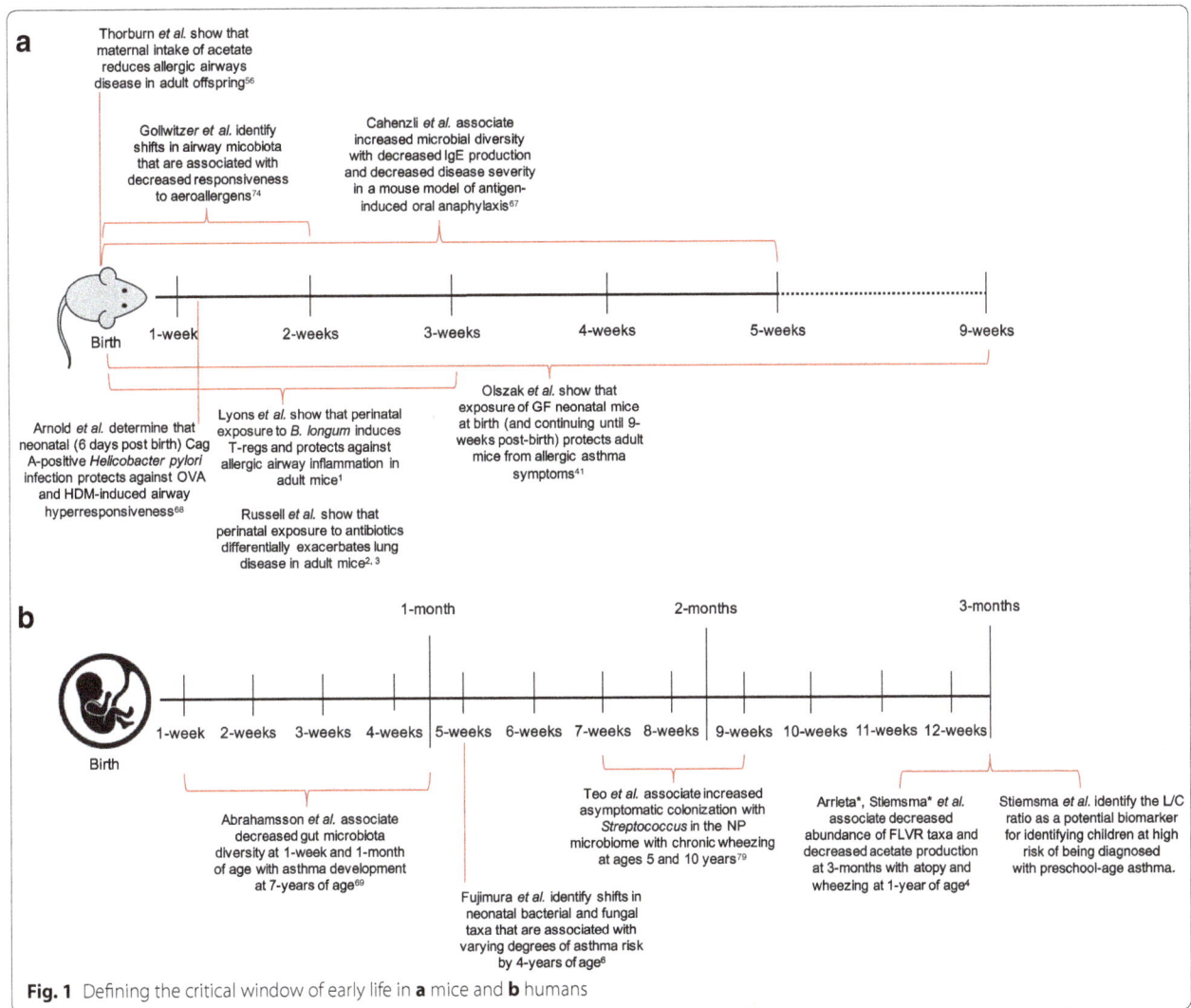

Russell et al. demonstrate the effects of early life antibiotic exposure in mice [2, 3]. This group showed that perinatal (in utero and up to 21 days after birth until weaning) versus strictly prenatal (in utero) vancomycin treatment of OVA-challenged mice exacerbates asthma-related immune responses [2]. Further, perinatal treatment of mice with another antibiotic, streptomycin, exaggerated lung inflammation in a Th-1/Th-17-driven model of hypersensitivity pneumonitis [3]. Notably, each antibiotic promoted expansion of specific bacterial phyla; streptomycin promoted expansion of Bacteroidetes, while vancomycin promoted expansion of Firmicutes [3]. This highlights both the selective effects of antibiotics on gut microbial taxa and the ability of an antibiotic-altered microbiota to differentially enhance disease susceptibility to specific lung diseases [3, 64]. Notably, all of these studies highlight a critical window (from birth to weaning in mice) in which microbial alterations can promote or protect against asthma and atopic diseases. However until recently, this critical window was not characterized in humans.

Longitudinal human studies define the early life critical window

Mouse studies have made substantial mechanistic strides in microbiome-atopic disease research. In parallel, improvements in DNA sequencing technology over the past decade have made analyzing the microbiomes of humans much more feasible. With these sequencing improvements, a similar 'critical window' in which microbial alterations can be associated with the development of asthma and atopic disease is also becoming more apparent in humans (Fig. 1b). Using 454-pyrosequencing, one study associated changes in gut microbial diversity at 1-week and 1-month of age with asthma development at school age [69].

However more recent studies have identified shifts in specific bacterial taxa in early life, rather than global compositional changes, that are associated with increased risk of asthma later in life. In fact, our group identified decreases in the abundances of four bacterial genera, *Faecalibacterium, Lachnospira, Rothia, and Veillonella* (FLVR), in the 3-month fecal microbiota, which were associated with atopy and wheezing at 1-year of age among 319 infants enrolled in the Canadian Healthy Infant Longitudinal Development (CHILD) Study [4]. Atopy and wheezing are clinically used to predict asthma development in children, and subjects positive for both atopy and wheezing were most likely (compared to wheeze only, atopy only, and control subjects) to develop asthma by 3-years of age—suggesting that these early life genera shifts are associated with increased risk of asthma development [4]. Further, these four bacterial taxa ameliorated asthma in an OVA-challenged mouse model, supporting their immune-modulatory roles in protecting against asthma development [4].

Since the CHILD Study is a longitudinal cohort, our group was able to conduct a follow-up study on this same cohort when they reached 4-years of age and could be diagnosed with preschool-age asthma [5]. We found that *Lachnospira* remained decreased in the 3-month fecal microbiota while one particular bacterial species, *Clostridium neonatale*, was increased in asthmatics at this time-point [5]. Demonstrating the diagnostic potential of these particular microbes, we calculated a ratio of *Lachnospira* to *C. neonatale* (L/C) and using quartile analysis, showed that children with the lowest L/C ratio (quartile 1) were 15 times more likely to be diagnosed with preschool-age asthma than children in the other L/C quartiles [5]. Most interestingly, however, both of these studies identified these gut microbial changes in the first 3 months of life only, highlighting this time frame as the early life critical window during which gut microbial dysbiosis is most influential in promoting asthma and atopic disease in humans [4, 5].

Notably however, additional bacterial taxa as well as other microbes (e.g. fungi) have been associated with asthma and atopic disease development in children [6, 70]. In fact, a recent study published in *Nature Medicine* was able to distinguish asthmatic and atopic children by their neonatal (35 days post birth) intestinal microbiome compositions [6]. Children in the highest risk group showed shifts in specific bacterial and fungal taxa, highlighting roles of various gut microbes in human immune development, which are identifiable even earlier than 3-months of age [6]. Thus, even now it is becoming more evident that; (i) there are likely many other gut microbes associated with asthma and atopic disease development in humans; and (ii) that the 'critical window' for

identifying these gut microbial shifts in humans could be even smaller than 100 days post birth. Further, in an effort not to overlook a potentially obvious link between the microbiome and airway inflammation, recent studies have identified associations and mechanistic links between airway microbes and asthma and atopic disease development.

Role of the airway microbiota

Though the intestinal microbiome is one of the most populated regions of the human body, recent research supports a role of the airway microbiome in asthma and atopic disease pathogenesis. In an OVA-induced mouse model of asthma, administration of a common gut pathogen, *E. coli*, to the lung was shown in a TLR4-dependent manner to induce γδ-T cells, decrease activation of lung DCs, and abrogate Th-2 cytokine production to confer protection of mice from allergic airway inflammation [71].

In humans, airway microbial dysbiosis has been associated with increased risk of asthma [72, 73]. 16S rRNA analysis of sputum samples showed higher bacterial diversity and increased abundance of Proteobacteria in asthmatic adults compared to non-asthmatic adults [73]. Another adult study analyzing the bronchial microbiota was able to identify differences in microbial composition associated with asthma severity [72]. When compared to healthy controls, severe asthmatics were enriched in Actinobacteria and *Klebsiella* species [72]. However compared to patients with moderate asthma, patients with severe asthma were enriched in many Actinobacterial taxa and showed decreased abundances of Proteobacteria [72].

Continuing the early life theme, Gollwitzer et al. provide evidence of a 2-week window in which shifts in the airway microbiota are associated with decreased responsiveness to aeroallergens and the induction of Helios⁻ T-regs in a programmed death ligand 1 (PD-L1)-mediated manner [74]. If PD-L1 is blocked only in the first two weeks of life and allergic airway inflammation is induced after 4-weeks of age, the exaggerated allergic airway inflammation in neonatal mice is maintained to adulthood [74]. Further, in a study of 234 human children, researchers associated early (7–9 weeks post-birth) asymptomatic colonization with *Streptococcus* in the nasopharyngeal (NP) microbiome with chronic wheezing at ages 5 and 10 years [75]. Interestingly, they also suggest the NP microbiome as a determinate for the spread of respiratory infections to the lower airways, which are also significant risk factors for asthma development [75]. Thus there may be specific early life non-pathogenic airway microbes associated with asthma, but it is also possible that dysbiosis in the airway microbiota is the mediator between respiratory infections and subsequent development of asthma.

Conclusions and future directions

In conclusion, the current literature suggests a role of the microbiome in asthma and atopic disease development, with particular emphasis on early life dysbiosis. Notably, recent studies have identified shifts in specific bacterial genera and species, which could ultimately be applied as probiotic interventions prior to the development of asthma. These probiotic interventions could be given directly to the baby in early infancy once all safety concerns have been addressed. Another option for colonizing the infant is through maternal exposure to these microbes either before or after delivery. Prior to establishing these probiotic regimens however, shifts in early life gut and airway microbes could also be applied as microbe-based diagnostics to identify children at the highest risk of developing asthma and related allergic diseases.

Before any of these preventative or diagnostic techniques can be applied, future research should focus on validating the current findings in additional longitudinal human cohorts and improving humanized microbiome mouse models of airway and lung inflammation to mechanistically characterize the microbe-immune cell interactions promoting or protecting against asthma and atopic disease. Additionally, targeted-metabolomic and shotgun metagenomic sequencing strategies using stool, urine, and potentially breast-milk samples in human cohorts will better characterize the functional roles of these specific taxa in infant immune development.

Further, to better elucidate this early life critical window in humans, additional longitudinal cohorts should begin stool sample collection beginning at birth and continuing up to age 1 year (with at least bi-weekly collection points within the first 3-months of life). Additionally, the collection of additional biological samples (namely blood and urine) during the first 3-months of life (though this is not often feasible) would be ideal to determine whether these gut microbial alterations occur prior to immune-dysregulation or vice versa.

Moreover, although this review focuses on the bacterial microbiome in asthma, there are many other microbial organisms (fungi and other eukarya, and viruses) that also play key roles in host physiology and immune development [6, 76–79]. Also, with the characterization of other microbiomes within the human body (i.e. placental, blood, breast-milk), it is likely that we will identify even more microbial taxa that are associated with airway diseases. As discussed in the previous sections, there is evidence in mice that asthma is a developmental origin disease, mediated by maternal gut microbial alterations

in utero [56]. Thus it will be important to incorporate multi-biome analyses to potentially identify: (i) how children are being colonized with specific asthma related microbes; and (ii) roles of other microbial taxa in the pathogenesis of asthma and atopic disease. Ultimately however, this literature review presents research with promising future directions, offering an exciting outlook for future microbe-based preventative treatments and diagnostic strategies for asthma and atopic disease in children.

Abbreviations

GF: germ-free; OVA: ovalbumin; HDM: house-dust mite; IgE: immunoglobulin-E; LPS: lipopolysaccharide; PAMP: pathogen-associated molecular pattern; TLR: toll-like receptor; MLN: mesenteric lymph node; SCFA: short chain fatty acid; DC: dendritic cell; iNKT cell: invariant natural killer T cell; CHILD Study: Canadian Healthy Infant Longitudinal Development Study; NP: nasopharyngeal; PD-L1: programmed death ligand-1; Th: T-helper; T-reg: T-regulatory; FLVR: *Faecalibacterium, Lachnospira, Veillonella, Rothia*; L/C: *Lachnospira/C. neonatale*.

Authors' contributions

LTS wrote the manuscript. SET supervised the project and edited the manuscript. Both authors read and approved the final manuscript.

Author details
[1] Department of Microbiology & Immunology, University of British Columbia, Vancouver, BC, Canada. [2] BC Children's Hospital, Vancouver, BC, Canada. [3] Department of Pediatrics, University of British Columbia, Vancouver, BC, Canada. [4] Department of Pediatrics, BC Children's Hospital, 950 West 28th Avenue, Vancouver, BC V5Z 4H4, Canada.

Acknowledgements
Not applicable.

Competing interests
The authors declare that they have no competing interests.

Funding
L.T.S. was supported in part by The Four Year Fellowship (4YF) from the University of British Columbia. S.E.T. holds the Aubrey J. Tingle Professorship in Pediatric Immunology and is a clinical scholar of the Michael Smith Foundation for Health Research. This work was supported in part by funding from The Canadian Institutes of Health Research (CIHR) and the Allergy, Genes and Environment AllerGen) Network of Centres of Excellence (NCE).

References
1. Lyons A, O'Mahony D, O'Brien F, MacSharry J, Sheil B, Ceddia M, Russell WM, Forsythe P, Bienenstock J, Kiely B, et al. Bacterial strain-specific induction of Foxp3 + T regulatory cells is protective in murine allergy models. Clin Exp Allergy. 2010;40(5):811–9.
2. Russell SL, Gold MJ, Willing BP, Thorson L, McNagny KM, Finlay BB. Perinatal antibiotic treatment affects murine microbiota, immune responses and allergic asthma. Gut Microbes. 2013;4(2):158–64.
3. Russell SL, Gold MJ, Reynolds LA, Willing BP, Dimitriu P, Thorson L, Redpath SA, Perona-Wright G, Blanchet MR, Mohn WW, Finlay BB. Perinatal antibiotic-induced shifts in gut microbiota have differential effects on inflammatory lung diseases. J Allergy Clin Immunol. 2015;135(1):100–9.
4. Arrieta MC, Stiemsma LT, Dimitriu PA, Thorson L, Russell S, Yurist-Doutsch S, Kuzeljevic B, Gold MJ, Britton HM, Lefebvre DL, et al. Early infancy microbial and metabolic alterations affect risk of childhood asthma. Sci Transl Med. 2015;7(307):307ra152.

5. Stiemsma L, Arrieta MC, Dimitriu P, Cheng J, Thorson L, Lefebvre D, Azad MB, Subbarao P, Mandhane P, Becker A, et al. Shifts in Lachnospira and Clostridium sp. in the 3-month stool microbiome are associated with preschool-age asthma. Clin Sci (Lond). 2016;130(23):2199–207.

6. Fujimura KE, Sitarik AR, Havstad S, Lin DL, Levan S, Fadrosh D, Panzer AR, LaMere B, Rackaityte E, Lukacs NW, et al. Neonatal gut microbiota associates with childhood multisensitized atopy and T cell differentiation. Nat Med. 2016;22(10):1187–91.

7. Holgate ST. Innate and adaptive immune responses in asthma. Nat Med. 2012;18(5):673–83.

8. Mallol J, Crane J, von Mutius E, Odhiambo J, Keil U, Stewart A, Group IPTS. The International study of asthma and allergies in childhood (ISAAC) phase three: a global synthesis. Allergol Immunopathol (Madr). 2013;41(2):73–85.

9. World Health Organization: Asthma [http://www.who.int/mediacentre/factsheets/fs307/en/]. Accessed 10 Sept 2016.

10. Fact sheet: asthma's impact on the nation. In.: CDC: Centres for Disease Control and Prevention; 2015.

11. To T, Dell S, Dick P, Cicutto L. The burden of illness experienced by young children associated with asthma: a population-based cohort study. J Asthma. 2008;45(1):45–9.

12. Beasley R. ISAAC Steering Committee. Worldwide variation in prevalence of symptoms of asthma, allergic rhinoconjunctivitis, and atopic eczema: ISAAC. The international study of asthma and allergies in childhood (ISAAC) Steering committee. Lancet. 1998;351(9111):1225–32.

13. Anandan C, Nurmatov U, van Schayck OC, Sheikh A. Is the prevalence of asthma declining? Systematic review of epidemiological studies. Allergy. 2010;65(2):152–67.

14. Paaso EM, Jaakkola MS, Lajunen TK, Hugg TT, Jaakkola JJ. The importance of family history in asthma during the first 27 years of life. Am J Respir Crit Care Med. 2013;188(5):624–6.

15. Burke W, Fesinmeyer M, Reed K, Hampson L, Carlsten C. Family history as a predictor of asthma risk. Am J Prev Med. 2003;24(2):160–9.

16. Subbarao P, Mandhane PJ, Sears MR. Asthma: epidemiology, etiology and risk factors. Cent Med Assoc J. 2009;181(9):E181–90.

17. de Marco R, Locatelli F, Sunyer J, Burney P. Differences in incidence of reported asthma related to age in men and women. A retrospective analysis of the data of the European Respiratory Health Survey. Am J Respir Crit Care Med. 2000;162(1):68–74.

18. Sears MR. Growing up with asthma. Br Med J. 1994;309(6947):72–3.

19. Slager RE, Hawkins GA, Li X, Postma DS, Meyers DA, Bleecker ER. Genetics of asthma susceptibility and severity. Clin Chest Med. 2012;33(3):431–43.

20. Stiemsma L, Reynolds L, Turvey S, Finlay B. The hygiene hypothesis: current perspectives and future therapies. Immunotargets Ther. 2015;4:143–57.

21. Bach JF. The effect of infections on susceptibility to autoimmune and allergic diseases. N Engl J Med. 2002;347(12):911–20.

22. Graham-Rowe D. Lifestyle: when allergies go west. Nature. 2011;479(7374):S2–4.

23. Rodriguez A, Vaca M, Oviedo G, Erazo S, Chico ME, Teles C, Barreto ML, Rodrigues LC, Cooper PJ. Urbanisation is associated with prevalence of childhood asthma in diverse, small rural communities in Ecuador. Thorax. 2011;66(12):1043–50.

24. Malik HU, Kumar K, Frieri M. Minimal difference in the prevalence of asthma in the urban and rural environment. Clin Med Insights Pediatr. 2012;6:33–9.

25. Rodriguez A, Vaca MG, Chico ME, Rodrigues LC, Barreto ML, Cooper PJ. Migration and allergic diseases in a rural area of a developing country. J Allergy Clin Immunol. 2016;138(3):901–3.

26. Ruiz-Calderon JF, Cavallin H, Song SJ, Novoselac A, Pericchi LR, Hernandez JN, Rios R, Branch OH, Pereira H, Paulino LC, et al. Walls talk: microbial biogeography of homes spanning urbanization. Sci Adv. 2016;2(2):e1501061.

27. Almqvist C, Cnattingius S, Lichtenstein P, Lundholm C. The impact of birth mode of delivery on childhood asthma and allergic diseases—a sibling study. Clin Exp Allergy. 2012;42(9):1369–76.

28. Negele K, Heinrich J, Borte M, Berg A, Schaaf B, Lehmann I, Wichmann H, Bolte G. Mode of delivery and development of atopic disease during the first 2 years of life. Pediatr Allergy Immunol. 2004;15(1):48–54.

29. Hoskin-Parr L, Teyhan A, Blocker A, Henderson AJ. Antibiotic exposure in the first two years of life and development of asthma and other allergic diseases by 7.5 year: a dose-dependent relationship. Pediatr Allergy Immunol. 2013;24(8):762–71.

30. Kummeling I, Stelma FF, Dagnelie PC, Snijders BE, Penders J, Huber M, van Ree R, van den Brandt PA, Thijs C. Early life exposure to antibiotics and the subsequent development of eczema, wheeze, and allergic sensitization in the first 2 years of life: the KOALA Birth Cohort Study. Pediatrics. 2007;119(1):e225–31.

31. Devereux G. The increase in the prevalence of asthma and allergy: food for thought. Nat Rev Immunol. 2006;6(11):869–74.

32. Sevelsted A, Stokholm J, Bonnelykke K, Bisgaard H. Cesarean section and chronic immune disorders. Pediatrics. 2015;135(1):e92–8.

33. Azad MB, Konya T, Maughan H, Guttman DS, Field CJ, Chari RS, Sears MR, Becker AB, Scott JA, Kozyrskyj AL, et al. Gut microbiota of healthy Canadian infants: profiles by mode of delivery and infant diet at 4 months. Can Med Assoc J. 2013;185(5):385–94.

34. Azad MB, Konya T, Maughan H, Guttman DS, Field CJ, Sears MR, Becker AB, Scott JA, Kozyrskyj AL. Infant gut microbiota and the hygiene hypothesis of allergic disease: impact of household pets and siblings on microbiota composition and diversity. Allergy Asthma Clin Immunol. 2013;9(1):15.

35. Kozyrskyj AL, Ernst P, Becker AB. Increased risk of childhood asthma from antibiotic use in early life. Chest. 2007;131(6):1753–9.

36. Strachan DP. Hay fever, hygiene, and household size. Br Med J. 1989;299(6710):1259–60.

37. Strachan DP, Taylor EM, Carpenter RG. Family structure, neonatal infection, and hay fever in adolescence. Arch Dis Child. 1996;74(5):422–6.

38. Shreiner A, Huffnagle GB, Noverr MC. The "Microflora Hypothesis" of allergic disease. Adv Exp Med Biol. 2008;635:113–34.

39. Gollwitzer ES, Marsland BJ. Impact of early-life exposures on immune maturation and susceptibility to disease. Trends Immunol. 2015;36(11):684–96.

40. Pollard M, Sharon N. Responses of the Peyer's patches in germ-free mice to antigenic stimulation. Infect Immun. 1970;2(1):96–100.

41. Olszak T, An D, Zeissig S, Vera MP, Richter J, Franke A, Glickman JN, Siebert R, Baron RM, Kasper DL, et al. Microbial exposure during early life has persistent effects on natural killer T cell function. Science. 2012;336(6080):489–93.

42. Lathrop SK, Bloom SM, Rao SM, Nutsch K, Lio CW, Santacruz N, Peterson DA, Stappenbeck TS, Hsieh CS. Peripheral education of the immune system by colonic commensal microbiota. Nature. 2011;478(7368):250–4.

43. O'Hara AM, Shanahan F. The gut flora as a forgotten organ. EMBO Rep. 2006;7(7):688–93.

44. Clemente JC, Pehrsson EC, Blaser MJ, Sandhu K, Gao Z, Wang B, Magris M, Hidalgo G, Contreras M, Noya-Alarcón Ó, Lander O. The microbiome of uncontacted Amerindians. Sci Adv. 2015;1(3):e1500183.

45. Marsland BJ, Trompette A, Gollwitzer ES. The gut-lung axis in respiratory disease. Ann Am Thorac Soc. 2015;12(Suppl 2):S150–6.

46. Chieppa M, Rescigno M, Huang AY, Germain RN. Dynamic imaging of dendritic cell extension into the small bowel lumen in response to epithelial cell TLR engagement. J Exp Med. 2006;203(13):2841–52.

47. Samuelson DR, Welsh DA, Shellito JE. Regulation of lung immunity and host defense by the intestinal microbiota. Front Microbiol. 2015;6:1085.

48. Ignacio A, Morales CI, Camara NO, Almeida RR. Innate sensing of the gut microbiota: modulation of inflammatory and autoimmune diseases. Front Immunol. 2016;7:54.

49. Mikhak Z, Strassner JP, Luster AD. Lung dendritic cells imprint T cell lung homing and promote lung immunity through the chemokine receptor CCR4. J Exp Med. 2013;210(9):1855–69.

50. Schuijs MJ, Willart MA, Vergote K, Gras D, Deswarte K, Ege MJ, Madeira FB, Beyaert R, van Loo G, Bracher F, et al. Farm dust and endotoxin protect against allergy through A20 induction in lung epithelial cells. Science. 2015;349(6252):1106–10.

51. Wong JM, de Souza R, Kendall CW, Emam A, Jenkins DJ. Colonic health: fermentation and short chain fatty acids. J Clin Gastroenterol. 2006;40(3):235–43.

52. Correa-Oliveira R, Fachi JL, Vieira A, Sato FT, Vinolo MA. Regulation of immune cell function by short-chain fatty acids. Clin Transl Immunol. 2016;5(4):e73.

53. Arpaia N, Campbell C, Fan X, Dikiy S, van der Veeken J, deRoos P, Liu H, Cross JR, Pfeffer K, Coffer PJ, et al. Metabolites produced by commensal bacteria promote peripheral regulatory T-cell generation. Nature. 2013;504(7480):451–5.

54. Furusawa Y, Obata Y, Fukuda S, Endo TA, Nakato G, Takahashi D, Nakanishi Y, Uetake C, Kato K, Kato T, et al. Commensal microbe-derived butyrate induces the differentiation of colonic regulatory T cells. Nature. 2013;504(7480):446–50.

55. Trompette A, Gollwitzer ES, Yadava K, Sichelstiel AK, Sprenger N, Ngom-Bru C, Blanchard C, Junt T, Nicod LP, Harris NL, et al. Gut microbiota metabolism of dietary fiber influences allergic airway disease and hematopoiesis. Nat Med. 2014;20(2):159–66.

56. Thorburn AN, McKenzie CI, Shen S, Stanley D, Macia L, Mason LJ, Roberts LK, Wong CHY, Shim R, Robert R, et al. Evidence that asthma is a developmental origin disease influenced by maternal diet and bacterial metabolites. Nat Commun. 2015; 6.

57. Kumar H, Lund R, Laiho A, Lundelin K, Ley RE, Isolauri E, Salminen S. Gut microbiota as an epigenetic regulator: pilot study based on whole-genome methylation analysis. MBio. 2014;5(6):e02113–4.

58. Gonda TA, Kim YI, Salas MC, Gamble MV, Shibata W, Muthupalani S, Sohn KJ, Abrams JA, Fox JG, Wang TC, Tycko B. Folic acid increases global DNA methylation and reduces inflammation to prevent Helicobacter-associated gastric cancer in mice. Gastroenterology. 2012;142(4):824–33.

59. Xia M, Liu J, Wu X, Liu S, Li G, Han C, Song L, Li Z, Wang Q, Wang J, et al. Histone methyltransferase Ash1 l suppresses interleukin-6 production and inflammatory autoimmune diseases by inducing the ubiquitin-editing enzyme A20. Immunity. 2013;39(3):470–81.

60. Michel S, Busato F, Genuneit J, Pekkanen J, Dalphin JC, Riedler J, Mazaleyrat N, Weber J, Karvonen AM, Hirvonen MR, et al. Farm exposure and time trends in early childhood may influence DNA methylation in genes related to asthma and allergy. Allergy. 2013;68(3):355–64.

61. Lluis A, Depner M, Gaugler B, Saas P, Casaca VI, Raedler D, Michel S, Tost J, Liu J, Genuneit J, et al. Increased regulatory T-cell numbers are associated with farm milk exposure and lower atopic sensitization and asthma in childhood. J Allergy Clin Immunol. 2014;133(2):551–9.

62. Herbst T, Sichelstiel A, Schar C, Yadava K, Burki K, Cahenzli J, McCoy K, Marsland BJ, Harris NL. Dysregulation of allergic airway inflammation in the absence of microbial colonization. Am J Respir Crit Care Med. 2011;184(2):198–205.

63. Forsythe P, Inman MD, Bienenstock J. Oral treatment with live *Lactobacillus reuteri* inhibits the allergic airway response in mice. Am J Respir Crit Care Med. 2007;175(6):561–9.

64. Russell SL, Gold MJ, Hartmann M, Willing BP, Thorson L, Wlodarska M, Gill N, Blanchet MR, Mohn WW, McNagny KM, et al. Early life antibiotic-driven changes in microbiota enhance susceptibility to allergic asthma. EMBO Rep. 2012;13(5):440–7.

65. Hill DA, Siracusa MC, Abt MC, Kim BS, Kobuley D, Kubo M, Kambayashi T, Larosa DF, Renner ED, Orange JS, et al. Commensal bacteria-derived signals regulate basophil hematopoiesis and allergic inflammation. Nat Med. 2012;18(4):538–46.

66. Lozupone CA, Stombaugh J, Gonzalez A, Ackermann G, Wendel D, Vazquez-Baeza Y, Jansson JK, Gordon JI, Knight R. Meta-analyses of studies of the human microbiota. Genome Res. 2013;23(10):1704–14.

67. Cahenzli J, Koller Y, Wyss M, Geuking MB, McCoy KD. Intestinal microbial diversity during early-life colonization shapes long-term IgE levels. Cell Host Microbe. 2013;14(5):559–70.

68. Arnold IC, Dehzad N, Reuter S, Martin H, Becher B, Taube C, Muller A. *Helicobacter pylori* infection prevents allergic asthma in mouse models through the induction of regulatory T cells. J Clin Invest. 2011;121(8):3088–93.

69. Abrahamsson TR, Jakobsson HE, Andersson AF, Bjorksten B, Engstrand L, Jenmalm MC. Low gut microbiota diversity in early infancy precedes asthma at school age. Clin Exp Allergy. 2014;44(6):842–50.

70. Hollander WJ, Sonnenschein-van der Voort AM, Holster IL, Jongste JC, Jaddoe VW, Hofman A, Perez-Perez GI, Moll HA, Blaser MJ, Duijts L, Kuipers EJ. Helicobacter pylori in children with asthmatic conditions at school age, and their mothers. Aliment Pharmacol Ther. 2016;43(8):933–43.

71. Nembrini C, Sichelstiel A, Kisielow J, Kurrer M, Kopf M, Marsland BJ. Bacterial-induced protection against allergic inflammation through a multicomponent immunoregulatory mechanism. Thorax. 2011;66(9):755–63.

72. Huang YJ, Nariya S, Harris JM, Lynch SV, Choy DF, Arron JR, Boushey H. The airway microbiome in patients with severe asthma: associations with disease features and severity. J Allergy Clin Immunol. 2015;136(4):874–84.

73. Marri PR, Stern DA, Wright AL, Billheimer D, Martinez FD. Asthma-associated differences in microbial composition of induced sputum. J Allergy Clin Immunol. 2013;131(2):346–52.

74. Gollwitzer ES, Saglani S, Trompette A, Yadava K, Sherburn R, McCoy KD, Nicod LP, Lloyd CM, Marsland BJ. Lung microbiota promotes tolerance to allergens in neonates via PD-L1. Nat Med. 2014;20(6):642–7.

75. Teo SM, Mok D, Pham K, Kusel M, Serralha M, Troy N, Holt BJ, Hales BJ, Walker ML, Hollams E, et al. The infant nasopharyngeal microbiome impacts severity of lower respiratory infection and risk of asthma development. Cell Host Microbe. 2015;17(5):704–15.

76. Carpagnano GE, Malerba M, Lacedonia D, Susca A, Logrieco A, Carone M, Cotugno G, Palmiotti GA, Foschino-Barbaro MP. Analysis of the fungal microbiome in exhaled breath condensate of patients with asthma. Allergy Asthma Proc. 2016;37(3):41–6.

77. Huffnagle GB, Noverr MC. The emerging world of the fungal microbiome. Trends Microbiol. 2013;21(7):334–41.

78. Virgin HW. The virome in mammalian physiology and disease. Cell. 2014;157(1):142–50.

79. Marsland BJ, Gollwitzer ES. Host-microorganism interactions in lung diseases. Nat Rev Immunol. 2014;14(12):827–35.

2

Association between fractional exhaled nitric oxide, sputum induction and peripheral blood eosinophil in uncontrolled asthma

Jie Gao*[iD] and Feng Wu

Abstract

Background: The fractional exhaled nitric oxide (FeNO) and blood eosinophils are biomarkers of eosinophilic airway inflammation used in the diagnosis and management of asthma, although induced sputum is the gold standard test for phenotypic asthma. Nevertheless, the clinical application of the correlation between sputum eosinophils, FeNO and blood eosinophils is controversial.

Objective: To investigate the clinical application of the correlation between sputum eosinophils, FeNO and blood eosinophils with uncontrolled asthmatic patients. It also examined the relationships between these biomarkers in bronchial reversibility and bronchial hyper-responsiveness (BHR).

Methods: This study evaluated 75 uncontrolled asthmatic patients (symptom control and future risk of adverse outcomes). All patients underwent the following on the same day: FeNO, spirometry, BHR or bronchodilator reversibility, sputum induction and blood collection. Eosinophilic airway inflammation was defined as sputum eosinophils $\geq 2.5\%$ or FeNO levels ≥ 32 parts per billion (ppb).

Results: A significant positive relationship was between percentage of sputum eosinophils and FeNO ($r = 0.4556$; $p < 0.0001$) and percentage of blood eosinophils ($r = 0.3647$; $p = 0.0013$), and a significant negative correlation was between percentage of sputum neutrophils and FeNO ($r = -0.3653$; $p = 0.0013$). No relationship between FeNO and percentage of blood eosinophils ($p = 0.5801$). ROC curve analysis identified FeNO was predictive of sputum eosinophilia [area under the curve (AUC) 0.707, $p = 0.004$] at a cutoff point of 35.5 ppb (sensitivity $= 67.3\%$, specificity $= 73.9\%$). Percentage of blood eosinophils was also highly predictive with an AUC of 0.73 ($p = 0.002$) at a cut-off point of 1.5%, sensitivity and specificity were 61.5 and 78.3%, respectively. Although the sputum neutrophil percentage was correlated with FeNO, ROC curve of these parameters did not show useful values (AUC $= 0.297$, $p = 0.003$; AUC $= 0.295$, $p = 0.021$).

Conclusions and clinical relevance: Blood eosinophils and FeNO can accurately predict eosinophilic airway inflammation in uncontrolled asthmatic patients. FeNO is poor surrogates for sputum neutrophils and blood eosinophils. The FeNO level and blood eosinophils, which determine an optimal cutoff for sputum eosinophilia, need more studies.

Keywords: Asthma, Sputum, FeNO, Blood, Eosinophil, Neutrophil, BHR, Bronchial reversibility

*Correspondence: xiekewei-568@126.com
Department of Respiratory Medicine, The Third People's Hospital, Guangzhou Medical College, 1# Xuebei Ave., Huizhou 516002, Guangdong, China

Background

Asthma is a heterogeneous disease, characterized by the history of variable respiratory symptoms such as wheeze, shortness of breath, chest tightness and cough, usually together with variable expiratory airflow limitation. This was reached by consensus, recommended by the 2017 Global Initiative for Asthma (GINA) [1]. It has been recognized that among asthmatic patients there are clusters of demographic, clinical and/or pathophysiological characteristics, which has been called "asthma phenotypes" [1, 2]. However, to date, no strong relationship has been found between specific pathological features and particular clinical or treatment responses [3]. When examining the airway inflammation using sputum analysis, patients with asthma can be classified in four different inflammatory phenotypes. Based on the percentage of eosinophils and neutrophils in sputum, it was to define four airway inflammatory subgroups: eosinophilic asthma, neutrophilic asthma, mixed granulocytic asthma and paucigranulocytic asthma [4]. There is recent evidence from prospective clinical studies that airway inflammatory phenotype can help to optimise therapy and disease outcome. Eosinophilic asthma responds well to anti-inflammatory treatment with steroids, non-eosinophilic asthma shows little or no response [5]. This suggests that biomarkers of inflammation could be considered in identifying and monitoring of asthmatic patients in clinical practice, such as the titration of steroid treatment.

Airway inflammatory phenotype can be measured through the airway noninvasively by induced sputum analysis [2, 4] and fractional exhaled nitric oxide (FeNO) [6]. Both are considered as a direct, reliable, sensitive, simple, and repeatable method of assessing inflammatory phenotypes, widely used in clinical practice. Peripheral blood eosinophils has also been studied as another potentially biomarker; it is associated with the patient's future risk for exacerbations [7, 8], the risk factor for developing fixed airflow limitation [9], the diagnosis of eosinophilic asthma [10]. In 2016, the normal reference values of induced sputum cytology in China, defined as sputum eosinophils $\geq 2.5\%$, and increases in FeNO level ≥ 32 ppb, were identified as airway eosinophilia [11]. Nevertheless, the clinical application of the correlation between FeNO levels, sputum eosinophils and peripheral blood eosinophils is controversial.

We conducted a retrospective study to (1) evaluate the correlation between sputum eosinophils, FeNO level and peripheral blood eosinophils in patients with asthma (2) to determine the accuracy of these biomarkers as indicators of airway inflammatory phenotypes in these patients (3) assess the relationship between these biomarkers, bronchial hyper-responsiveness (BHR) and bronchodilator reversibility in asthma.

Methods

Study design and participants

We conducted a retrospective study on a series of 65 patients with asthma visiting in The Third People's Hospital of Guangzhou Medical College in Huizhou from April 2016 to June 2017. Asthma patients were diagnosed according to a clinical history of wheezing, cough, chest tightness or shortness of breath, as well as the presence of bronchial hyper-responsiveness or bronchodilator reversibility, based on the 2016 of the Chinese national Guidelines on Diagnosis and Management of Asthma [12]. Included asthma patients received initial diagnosis and were uncontrolled stage. The level of asthma control was defined by asthma symptoms control (in the past 4 weeks, has the patient had daytime asthma symptoms more than twice/week and/or any night waking due to asthma and/or any activity limitation due to asthma and/or reliever needed for symptoms' more than twice/week) and future risk of adverse outcomes (in the past 4 weeks, has the patient had $FEV_1\%$ less than normal predicated value and/or any severe exacerbation due to asthma). Uncontrolled asthmatic patient had equal to or greater than 3 features as the above.

Inclusion criteria were any patients with asthma aged ≥ 18 years who agreed to undergo detailed investigation. All the patients who had successful FeNO, lung function and sputum induction were included in the study. Data were collected during regular clinical practice and medical procedures. Their demographic and functional characteristics are summarized in Tables 1, 2 and 3.

Exclusion criteria were any patients had a history with chronic obstructive pulmonary disease (COPD), or previous doctor-diagnosed asthma-COPD overlap [(ACO),

Table 1 Patient demographics and baseline characteristics

Demographic parameter	All participants (N = 75)
Age, years, median	61 (53, 71)
Range	18–85
Males, n (%)	42 (56)
Race, n (%)	
Chinese	75 (100%)
Mean height, cm (SD)	160 (8.78)
Range	136–174
Mean weight, kg (SD)	59 (9.29)
Range	44.5–84
Mean body mass index, kg/m^2 (SD)	23.2 (3.61)
Range	16.71–34.22
Smokers, n (%)	32 (42.7)

N, total population; n, sub-group population; SD, standard deviation

Table 2 Spirometry results for the patients

Variable	All participants (N = 75)
FVC (L), mean (SD)	2.94 (0.86)
FVC% predicted, mean (SD)	97.03 (13.96)
FEV1 (L), mean (SD)	1.99 (0.57)
FEV1% predicted, mean (SD)	81.77 (11.86)
FEV1/FVC (%), mean (SD)	68.33 (8.54)
PEF (L/min), mean (SD)	5.33 (1.76)
PEF% predicted, mean (SD)	78.45 (17.64)
MMEF, mean (SD)	1.36 (0.5)
MMEF% predicted, mean (SD)	40.46 (18.25)
MEF50% (L/s), mean (SD)	1.76 (0.76)
MEF50% predicted, mean (SD)	47.55 (20.86)
MEF25% (L/s), mean (SD)	0.59 (0.26)
MEF25% predicted, mean (SD)	45.34 (19.62)

FVC, forced vital capacity; FEV1, forced expiratory volume in 1 s; PEF, peak expiratory flow; MMEF, maximum mid-expiratory flow; MEF, maximal expiratory flow

Table 3 FeNO level, induced sputum and peripheral blood result for the patients

Variable	All participants (N = 75)
FeNO level, ppb	38 (20, 72)
Eosinophil (%) in sputum	4.2 (1.1, 15.7)
Neutrophil (%) in sputum, mean (SD)	78.51 (17.3)
White blood cell (× 10^9/L)	7.6 (6.4, 9.9)
Eosinophil (%) in peripheral blood	0.1 (0, 0.3)
Eosinophil count in peripheral blood (× 10^9/L)	1.4 (0.4, 3.2)

Values are expressed as median (inter quartile range) or mean (SD)

COPD/ACO was distinguished according to the 2017 recommendation of GINA, on the basis of chronic respiratory symptoms and post-bronchodilator $FEV_1/FVC < 0.7$ or $FEV_1/FVC < 0.7$ after treatment]. Patients have used any oral or/and inhaled corticosteroid in the previous 12 weeks. Patients had a confounding pulmonary comorbidity such as a pulmonary tuberculosis, an interstitial lung disease, a lung cancer or a pulmonary infection. Patients had a cognitive impairment that may affect the collaboration or comprehension of the study.

Ethics statement

The Institutional Review Board of the Third People's Hospital of Guangzhou Medical College in Huizhou approved the study protocol and absolved the need for written informed consent from patients as the study was a retrospective study, personal identification data were anonymized.

Assessments and study procedures

On the same day the following tests or determinations were performed: FeNO test, pulmonary function test (PFT), BHR test or bronchodilator reversibility test, induced sputum and routine blood test. Clinical variables were recorded for the participants.

FeNO: FeNO level was measured before PFT according to the guidelines in the user manual training on the NO electrochemical equipment (NIOX VERO; Aerocrine AB, Solna, Sweden). Patients were required to refrain from eating, drinking, and smoking for at least 1 h prior to the FeNO measurement. Patients were instructed to inhale NO-free air to total lung capacity and immediately exhale fully into the device at a sustained flow rate of 50 mL/s for 6 or 10 s, which resulted in display of FeNO value 6. A significant increase in FeNO was considered if the FeNO value was equal to or higher than 32 parts per billion (ppb) [6].

PFT: Airway limitation was identified using lung function machine (MS-pneumo + aps; Jaeger, Friedberg, German) by an experienced technician according to the 2014 recommendations of the Chinese National Guidelines of Pulmonary Function Test. Percentage predicted values (%pred) were calculated based on reference values for healthy Chinese adults. All patients were required to undergo PFT in a reproducible way, and the best values were retained [13].

BHR test: PFT values were assessed prior to the methacholine challenge. Patients with a FEV1%pred < 60% were excluded from the BHR test (at baseline). The breath dosimeter method was used according to published guidelines from Chinese National Guidelines of Pulmonary Function Test. The test sequence included five steps: 0.9% NaCl only, 0.078, 0.312, 1.125 and 2.504 mg. Measure the FEV_1 at about 60 s from the start of one to the start on the next inhalation from the nebulizer. Obtain an acceptable-quality FEV1 at each time point. Airway responsiveness was required to induce a 20% decrease in FEV1 (PD_{20}), and the positive response was defined as $PD_{20} \leq 2.504$ mg (between NS and 2.504 mg) [13].

Bronchodilator reversibility test: Patients were asked to inhale 400 μg salbutamol via a metered-dose inhaler after baseline evaluation, and PFT was repeated not less than 20 min. Three forced expiratory maneuvers were recorded. The positive response, which was defined as $FEV_1 > 12\%$ and 200 mL after salbutamol inhalation, were obtained [13].

Sputum induction: Sputum was induced with hypertonic saline inhalation through ultrasonic atomizer. A single hypertonic saline (3%NaCl) was used. Patients were asked to inhale 400 μg salbutamol via a metered-dose inhaler 20 min before induction. Collected lower respiratory sputum portions of induced sputum were dispersed using 0.1% dithiothreitol in a water bath (37 °C) and oscillator 15 min before the 300 mesh nylon mesh filter. Subsequently, total cell count was centrifuged, smeared and stained (hematoxylin–eosin). A differential cell count was obtained from 400 cells under 400× microscope to identify the type of airway inflammation in patients with asthma. We defined percentage of sputum eosinophils ≥ 2.5% as abnormal [11].

Blood collection and analysis: Peripheral venous blood was measured using Automated Hematology Blood Analyzer (ABX Pentra DF120–1; ABX, France). The results of peripheral blood eosinophil percentage and absolute eosinophil count were obtained.

Statistical analysis

Analysis of the data was performed using SPSS 19 (IBM Corporation, Armonk, NY, USA). Continuous variables are expressed as mean ± SD or median (interquartile range) for non-normal variables when appropriate, and categorical variables with the Chi square test. Non-normally distributed variables used the Mann–Whitney test. The relationship between FeNO, sputum eosinophils, blood eosinophils, BHR and bronchodilator reversibility was assessed using the Spearman's rank correlation coefficient. Correlation between tests was performed by constructing receiver operating characteristic (ROC) curve. The optimal cutoff value was determined from the highest sum of sensitivity and specificity. Statistical significance was defined as $p < 0.05$.

Results

Characteristics of the patients

Patient demographic information is presented in Table 1. A total of 75 patients with uncontrolled asthma participated [42 (56%) males] in the study. The median age was 61 years with a range between 18 and 85 years. Smokers accounted for 42.7% of patients. All participants were Chinese. PFT results are reported in Table 2. Patients with uncontrolled asthma had a mean FEV1/FVC% of 68.33% and a mean FEV1%pred of 81.77%. The result of FeNO level, induced sputum and peripheral blood are reported in Table 3.

Sputum induction

Eosinophilic airway inflammation (sputum eosinophilia ≥ 2.5%) was present in 52 participants. The characteristics of patients are shown in Table 4. Patients in sputum eosinophilia group compared with patients in sputum noneosinophilia group showed a significantly higher FeNO level ($p = 0.011$), in peripheral blood eosinophil percentage ($p = 0.003$) and absolute eosinophil count ($p = 0.016$).

FeNO

FeNO level equal to or higher than 32 ppb was present in 45 participants. The characteristics of patients are shown in Table 5. Patients in the two groups showed a meaningless result in eosinophilic cell in peripheral blood percentage and absolute count, but a significantly increased in the percentage of sputum eosinophils ($p < 0.001$).

Peripheral blood eosinophils

Eosinophilic percentage in peripheral blood ≥ 2% was present in 28 participants. The characteristics of patients are shown in Table 6. The percentage of sputum eosinophils ($p = 0.001$) and blood absolute eosinophil count ($p < 0.001$) were significantly higher in blood eosinophilia

Table 4 FeNO levels and peripheral blood result for the patients

Variables	Sputum eosinophilia (n = 52)	Sputum noneosinophilia (n = 23)	p-value
Age, years	58 (50, 66)	64 (59, 76)	0.224
Males, n (%)	30 (57.7)	12 (52.2)	0.657
Mean body mass index, kg/m²	23.3 (3.86)	22.98 (3.03)	0.476
Smokers, n (%)	23 (44.2)	9 (39.1)	0.68
Postbronchodilator FEV1% predicted	80.48 (8.57)	84.7 (17.02)	0.07
Postbronchodilator FEV$_1$ (L)	2.06 (0.58)	1.81 (0.51)	0.548
Postbronchodilator FEV$_1$/FVC (%)	68.12 (8.95)	68.82 (7.7)	0.297
FeNO level (ppb)	48 (25, 92)	24 (19, 47)	*0.011*
Neutrophil (%) in sputum	74.36 (18.11)	87.7 (10.55)	0.062
White blood cell (×10⁹/L)	7.3 (6.2, 9.6)	8.5 (6.5, 10.3)	0.192
Eosinophil (%) in peripheral blood	1.8 (0.6, 4.8)	0.5 (0.2, 1.8)	*0.003*
Eosinophil count in peripheral blood (×10⁹/L)	0.1 (0.1, 0.3)	0 (0, 0.2)	*0.016*

Sputum eosinophilia refers to sputum eosinophils ≥ 2.5%; sputum noneosinophilia refers to sputum eosinophils < 2.5%. Significant p value < 0.05

Table 5 Sputum induction and peripheral blood result for the patients

Variables	FeNO ≥ 32 ppb (n = 45)	FeNO < 32 ppb (n = 30)	p-value
Age, years	58 (49, 65.5)	63.5 (58.5, 75.3)	0.386
Males, n (%)	26 (57.8)	16 (53.3)	0.704
Mean body mass index, kg/m²	22.62 (3.35)	24.07 (3.86)	0.396
Smokers, n (%)	21 (46.7)	11 (36.7)	0.391
Postbronchodilator FEV1% predicted	82.38 (12.68)	80.86 (10.64)	0.71
Postbronchodilator FEV1 (L)	2.12 (0.56)	1.78 (0.52)	0.875
Postbronchodilator FEV1/FVC (%)	68.22 (8.7)	68.5 (8.44)	0.953
Eosinophil (%) in sputum	9.89 (3.65, 20.53)	2.44 (0.59, 4.05)	< 0.001
Neutrophil (%) in sputum, mean (SD)	74.15 (18.56)	84.9 (12.83)	0.076
White blood cell (×109/L)	7.6 (6.3, 10.3)	7.5 (6.4, 9.6)	0.841
Eosinophil (%) in peripheral blood	1.8 (0.3, 4.8)	1.3 (0.5, 2.93)	0.97
Eosinophil count in peripheral blood (×109/L)	0.1 (0, 0.3)	0.1 (0.08, 0.23)	0.889

Significant p value < 0.05

Table 6 FeNO level and sputum induction result for the patients

Variables	Blood eosinophilia (n = 28)	Blood noneosinophilia (n = 47)	p-value
Mean age, years	58 (52.3, 71.3)	62 (53, 71)	0.496
Males, n (%)	16 (57.1)	26 (55.3)	0.878
Mean body mass index, kg/m²	22.64 (3.15)	23.54 (3.85)	0.509
Smokers, n (%)	11 (39.3)	21 (44.7)	0.648
Postbronchodilator FEV1% predicted	83.29 (7.33)	80.87 (13.87)	0.23
Postbronchodilator FEV1 (L)	2.13 (0.59)	1.9 (0.54)	0.696
Postbronchodilator FEV1/FVC (%)	68.32 (8.02)	68.34 (8.92)	0.505
FeNO level, (ppb)	48 (25, 95)	35 (19, 65)	0.103
Eosinophil (%) in sputum	9.85 (3.52, 24.83)	3.6 (0.5, 10.3)	0.001
Neutrophil (%) in sputum, mean (SD)	71.37 (19.34)	82.66 (14.51)	0.151
White blood cell (×10⁹/L)	6.9 (6, 9.2)	7.9 (6.8, 10.3)	0.069
Eosinophil count in peripheral blood (×10⁹/L)	0.3 (0.2, 0.7)	0.1 (0, 0.1)	<0.001

Blood eosinophilia refers to peripheral blood eosinophils ≥ 2%; blood noneosinophilia refers to peripheral blood eosinophils < 2%. Significant p value < 0.05

group. Nonetheless, FeNO level was not different between groups.

Associations between FeNO level, sputum induction, peripheral blood eosinophils, BHR and bronchodilator reversibility

A significant positive relationship was observed between percentage of sputum eosinophils and FeNO level (r = 0.4556; p < 0.0001) (Fig. 1a) and percentage of blood eosinophils (r = 0.3647; p = 0.0013) (Fig. 1b), and a significant negative correlation between percentage of sputum neutrophils and FeNO level (r = −0.3653; p = 0.0013) (Fig. 1c). We also found weaker but significant correlations between percentage of sputum neutrophils and percentage of blood eosinophils (r = −0.2294; p = 0.0477)

(Fig. 1d). No relationship between FeNO level and percentage of blood eosinophils (p = 0.5801).

Evidence of variable airflow obstruction was observed in 75 participants, 44 of whom had airway hyper-responsiveness based on the methacholine challenge results, and 31 had bronchodilator reversibility. There were no significant relationship between PD20 and percentage of sputum eosinophils (p = 0.2505), PD20 and FeNO level (p = 0.0955), PD20 and blood eosinophil percentage/count (p = 0.4517; p = 0.4933; respectively). There were also no significant relationship between ΔFEV1 (Δ, improvement in FEV1 after 400 μg of salbutamol) and percentage of sputum eosinophils (p = 0.3645). Neither FeNO level (p = 0.281) nor blood eosinophil percentage/

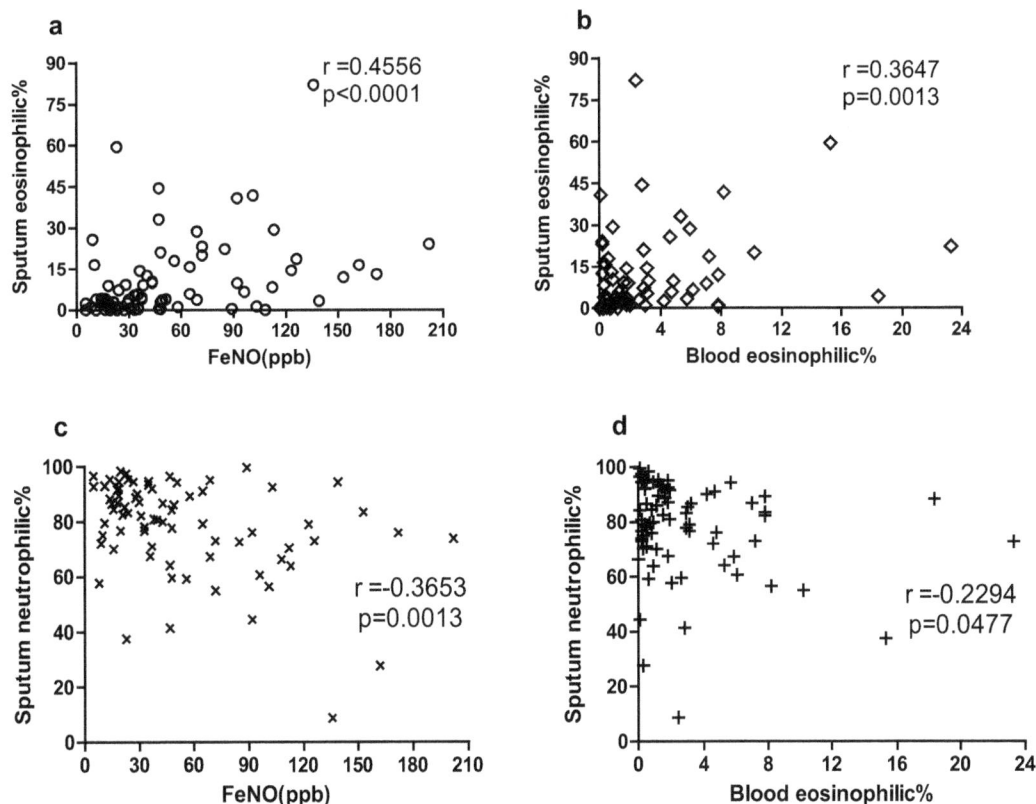

Fig. 1 Scatter plots of correlation between sputum eosinophil/neutrophil percentage, FeNO level and peripheral blood eosinophil percentage. **a** Correlation between sputum eosinophil percentage and FeNO level. **b** Correlation between sputum eosinophil percentage and blood eosinophil percentage. **c** Correlation between sputum neutrophil percentage and FeNO level. **d** Correlation between sputum neutrophil percentage and blood eosinophil percentage

count (p = 0.6027; p = 0.1236; respectively) did not correlate with bronchodilator reversibility.

The ROC curve analysis identified FeNO level as the best predictor for sputum eosinophilia with an area under the curve (AUC) of 0.707 (p = 0.004). The optimum cut-point for FeNO level was 35.5 ppb, and this yielded a sensitivity of 67.3%, a specificity of 73.9%. The percentage of blood eosinophils was also highly predictive with an area under the curve of 0.73 (p = 0.002) at a blood eosinophils cut-off of 1.5%, sensitivity and specificity were 61.5 and 78.3%, respectively (Fig. 2a). In addition, 4.36% was the best diagnostic cut-off value of percentage of sputum eosinophils for 32 ppb of FeNO level, with an ROC AUC of 0.755 (p < 0.001), sensitivity and specificity were 68.9 and 80%, respectively (Fig. 2b). Although the sputum neutrophil percentage was correlated with FeNO level, a ROC curve of these parameters did not show useful values (AUC = 0.297, p = 0.003, Fig. 2b; AUC = 0.295, p = 0.021, Fig. 2c). Percentage of blood eosinophils (p = 0.97) failed in the correlation of FeNO level.

There was no difference between blood eosinophil percentage (p = 0.089) and absolute blood eosinophil count (p = 0.14) in the prediction of sputum neutrophilia.

Discussion

This study assessed the correlation of FeNO level, sputum eosinophils and blood eosinophils in initial diagnosis and uncontrolled asthma. All the people in the study were Chinese. FeNO level and percentage of blood eosinophils can accurately predict sputum eosinophilia. Percentage of sputum neutrophils was correlated with FeNO level and percentage of blood eosinophils, but not enough to be clinically useful. We also identified some additional findings, namely $PD_{20}/\Delta FEV_1$ association with FeNO level and percentage of sputum/blood eosinophils, which may reflect nothing.

There is a need to include simple and accessible biomarkers in the management of asthmatic airway inflammatory subtype, FeNO and blood eosinophils are markers of local and systemic eosinophilic inflammation, respectively. According to the literature, biomarkers of airway eosinophilic inflammation (FeNO, blood

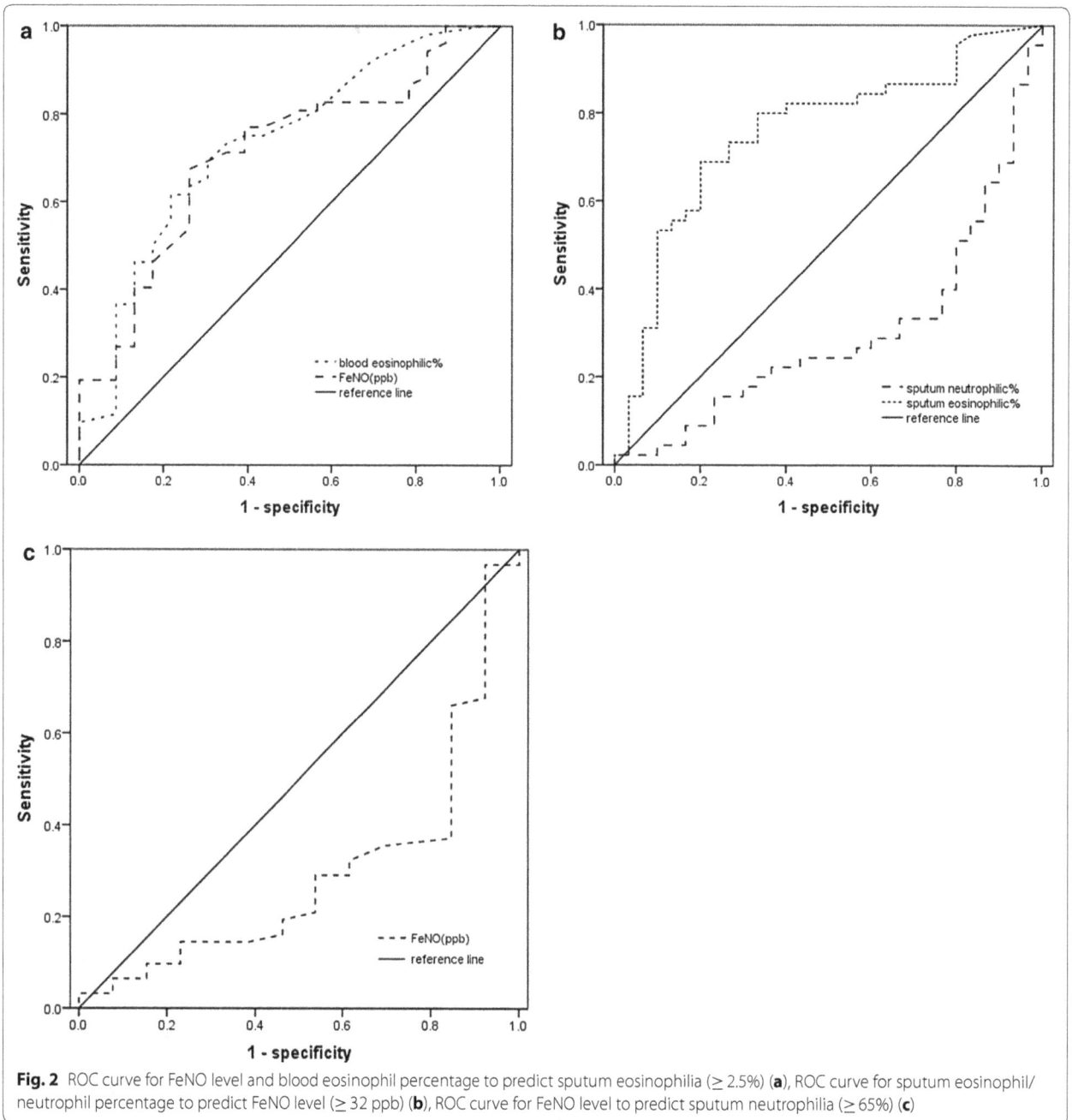

Fig. 2 ROC curve for FeNO level and blood eosinophil percentage to predict sputum eosinophilia (≥ 2.5%) (**a**), ROC curve for sputum eosinophil/neutrophil percentage to predict FeNO level (≥ 32 ppb) (**b**), ROC curve for FeNO level to predict sputum neutrophilia (≥ 65%) (**c**)

eosinophils and others, such as the sputum eosinophils) are well correlated with each other [14–16]. However, there is disagreement in the literature as to the value of FeNO level and sputum/blood eosinophils and there is no study following the diagnostic criteria of China [17, 18]. Few studies have used ROC to assess the ability of FeNO and peripheral blood eosinophils to detect airway eosinophilic phenotypes. Our results resolve these issues by showing that FeNO level and peripheral blood eosinophils were an excellent predictor of sputum eosinophilia

in the clinically important subgroup of patients who received initial diagnosis and were uncontrolled asthma.

Following the 2016 recommendations of the Chinese National Guidelines on Diagnosis and Management of Cough, eosinophilic airway inflammation was defined as percentage of eosinophils ≥ 2.5% in induced sputum [11]. As shown in Table 4, FeNO level and peripheral blood eosinophils percentage/count were different. Although induced sputum has been considered the "gold standard" for airway inflammatory phenotypes, measurement of

FeNO has achieved wide acceptance in routine clinical practice because it is easy to perform and readily available readout. The 2016 recommendation also suggested that a significant increase in sputum eosinophils ≥ 2.5% was considered if the FeNO level was ≥ 32 ppb [11]. As shown in Table 5, the percentage of sputum eosinophils was significantly different; however, the difference in peripheral blood eosinophil percentage and absolute count were not significant. According to the 2017 recommendation of GINA, which recently published an evidence-based clinical research guideline, eosinophil, such as in induced sputum or peripheral venous blood, can predict the risk of exacerbations [1]. We predicted that sputum eosinophilia was considered if the peripheral blood eosinophil percentage was ≥ 2%. As shown in Table 6, percentage of sputum eosinophils was different; however, the difference between FeNO in the two groups was not significant.

In clinical practice, there is a tendency to generalize the correlation between FeNO and percentage of sputum eosinophils, although the two methods are useful to assess the eosinophilic airway inflammation [19–21]. Our present optimal cutoff point (35.5 ppb) is similar to this optimal cut-off point (32 ppb) in the 2015 recommendation of China. These results showed that FeNO was to distinguish the patients with uncontrolled asthma with sputum eosinophilia from those without, thereby indicating its potential use as a diagnostic biomarker for eosinophilic asthma. However, there are confounding factors that may affect FeNO values in many cases. As a nitrate-rich diet or the contamination of nasal NO increase, and smoking or spirometry decrease FeNO, these factors should be avoided or taken into account when measuring FeNO [6]. The cutoff value has been a question in dispute because normal or low FeNO levels do not exclude the presence of disease. Optimal cutoff points by calculating sensitivity and specificity on an ROC curve to assess diagnostic biomarkers of eosinophilic airway inflammation may not be clinically applicable, given that their sensitivity and/or specificity is often suboptimal compared to that of reference standard tests [22]. Furthermore, FeNO has a limited value to assess the sputum neutrophilia, our study provided that sputum neutrophil percentage was correlated with FeNO level, a ROC curve of these parameters did not show useful values (AUC = 0.297, p = 0.003; AUC = 0.295, p = 0.021). Bronchial induced sputum cytology provides a more accurate approximation of airway inflammation phenotypes in asthma patients than FeNO.

The 2017 GINA recently published an evidence-based clinical research guideline that blood eosinophils may be a biomarker of exacerbation risk in patients with a history of exacerbation and can predict the effects of ICS on exacerbation prevention [1]. Because of their accuracy and convenience, blood eosinophils can be used in the clinic for detecting airway eosinophilia in uncontrolled asthma. One study in uncontrolled asthma has shown that peripheral blood eosinophil percentage (2.7%) and absolute count (0.26×10^9/L) can serve as a diagnostic biomarker of sputum eosinophilia (≥ 3%) (AUC 0.907, sensitivity = 92.2%, specificity = 75.8%; AUC 0.898, sensitivity = 83.1%, specificity = 82.8%, respectively) [10]. These finding also indicates that percentage of blood eosinophils has a higher relevance than FeNO with eosinophil sputum in patients with asthma. These results suggest that blood eosinophils can be useful in assessing eosinophilic asthma and may have a role in selecting add-on therapy. However, there was no correlation between FeNO level and blood eosinophil percentage/count (p = 0.5801) in our study.

Limitations and future research
One limitation of the study was that the p-value (p = 0.0477) changed slightly under 0.05, and the correlation coefficients (r = − 0.2294) were very low, as shown in Fig. 1d. The given number of data points may not be taken as strong evidence for such a relationship. It is possible that no relevant correlation between sputum neutrophil percentage and blood eosinophil percentage exists in the clinical practice.

The other was smoking cigarette factor. It is well known that smoking decreases FENO level [23]. Furthermore, some studies of the general population have reported that smoking increase blood eosinophils [24–26]. Other studies have reported blood eosinophils seems to be lower in asthmatic smokers than in asthmatic non-smokers [20, 27–29], and one study indicated that FeNO and blood eosinophils were significantly correlated in patients who have never smoked and former smokers but not in current smokers. There is disagreement in the literature as to the value of blood eosinophils [30]. Further investigation of smoking or no smoking factor in asthma would also benefit from bigger sample sizes.

Conclusion
This study provides that inflammatory biomarkers, including sputum eosinophils, FeNO level and blood eosinophils, can accurately predict sputum eosinophilia in patients with uncontrolled asthma. It suggests that peripheral blood eosinophil is a useful tool better than FeNO level for monitoring sputum eosinophilia in uncontrolled asthma. FeNO level is poor surrogates for sputum neutrophils and blood eosinophils. These data may be useful for identifying patients with eosinophilic airway inflammation who will have a beneficial response to treatment with an ICS, and it is important to help guide treatment and management of asthmatic patients.

Abbreviations

FeNO: fractional exhaled nitric oxide; BHR: bronchial hyper-responsiveness; GINA: the Global Initiative for Asthma; FVC: forced vital capacity; FEV1: forced expiratory volume in 1 s; PEF: peak expiratory flow; MMEF: maximum mid-expiratory flow; MEF: maximal expiratory flow.

Authors' contributions

GJ performed data collection and analysis, and was a major contributor in writing the manuscript. WF analyzed and interpreted the patient data with asthma. Both authors read and approved the final manuscript.

Acknowledgements

The study was supported by Health and Family Planning Commission of Guangdong, People's Republic of China (grant ID: A2017535).

Competing interests

The authors declare that they have no competing interests.

Funding

Not applicable.

References

1. Global Initiative for Asthma. Global strategy for asthma management and prevention. http://ginasthma.org/2017-pocket-guide-for-asthma-management-andprevention/. Accessed 19 Jan 2017.
2. Bel EH. Clinical phenotypes of asthma. Curr Opin Pulm Med. 2004;10:44–50.
3. Anderson GP. Endotyping asthma: new insights into key pathogenic mechanisms in a complex, heterogeneous disease. Lancet. 2008;372:1107–19.
4. Simpson JL, Scott R, Boyle MJ, Gibson PG. Inflammatory subtypes in asthma: assessment and identification using induced sputum. Respirology. 2006;11:54–61.
5. Petsky HL, Cates CJ, Lasserson TJ, et al. A systematic review and meta-analysis: tailoring asthma treatment on eosinophilic markers (exhaled nitric oxide or sputum eosinophils). Thorax. 2012;67:199–208.
6. Dweik RA, Boggs PB, Erzurum SC, et al. An official ATS clinical practice guideline: interpretation of exhaled nitric oxide levels (FENO) for clinical applications. Am J Respir Crit Care Med. 2011;184:602–15.
7. Belda J, Giner J, Casan P, Sanchis J. Mild exacerbations and eosinophilic inflammation in patients with stable, well-controlled asthma after 1 year of follow-up. Chest. 2001;119(4):1011–7.
8. Ulrik CS. Peripheral eosinophil counts as a marker of disease activity in intrinsic and extrinsic asthma. Clin Exp Allergy. 1995;25(9):820–7.
9. Ulrik CS. Outcome of asthma: longitudinal changes in lung function. Eur Respir J. 1999;13:904–18.
10. Zhang XY, Simpson JL, Powell H, et al. Full blood count parameters for the detection of asthma inflammatory phenotypes. Clin Exp Allergy. 2014;44:1137–45.
11. Asthma Workgroup of Chinese Society of Respiratory Diseases (CSRD), Chinese Medical Association. The Chinese national guidelines on diagnosis and management of cough (2015). Chin J Tuberc Respir Dis. 2016;39:321–39.
12. Asthma Workgroup of Chinese Society of Respiratory Diseases (CSRD), Chinese Medical Association. The Chinese national guidelines on diagnosis and management of asthma (2016). Chin J Tuberc Respir Dis. 2016;39:675–97.
13. Pulmonary Function Workgroup of Chinese Society of Respiratory Diseases (CSRD), Chinese Medical Association. The Chinese national guidelines of pulmonary function test (2014). Chin J Tuberc Respir Dis. 2014;37(8):566–71.
14. Payne DN, Adcock IM, Wilson NM, Oates T, Scallan M, Bush A. Relationship between exhaled nitric oxide and mucosal eosinophilic inflammation in children with difficult asthma, after treatment with oral prednisolone. Am J Respir Crit Care Med. 2001;164:1376–81.
15. Jatakanon A, Lim S, Kharitonov SA, Chung KF, Barnes PJ. Correlation between exhaled nitric oxide, sputum eosinophils, and methacholine responsiveness in patients with mild asthma. Thorax. 1998;53:91–5.
16. Silvestri M, Spallarossa D, Frangova Yourukova V, Battistini E, Fregonese B, Rossi GA. Orally exhaled nitric oxide levels are related to the degree of blood eosinophilia in atopic children with mild-intermittent asthma. Eur Respir J. 1999;13:321–6.
17. Ullmann N, Bossley CJ, Fleming L, Silvestri M, Bush A, Saglani S. Blood eosinophil counts rarely reflect airway eosinophilia in children with severe asthma. Allergy. 2013;68:402–6.
18. Gutierrez V, Prieto L, Torres V, et al. Relationship between induced sputum cell counts and fluid-phase eosinophil cationic protein and clinical or physiologic profiles in mild asthma. Ann Allergy Asthma Immunol. 1999;82:559–65.
19. Berry MA, Shaw DE, Green RH, Brightling CE, Wardlaw AJ, Pavord ID. The use of exhaled nitric oxide concentration to identify eosinophilic airway inflammation: an observational study in adults with asthma. Clin Exp Allergy. 2005;35:1175–9.
20. Lex C, Ferreira F, Zacharasiewicz A, et al. Airway eosinophilia in children with severe asthma: predictive values of noninvasive tests. Am Respir Crit Care Med. 2006;174:1286–91.
21. Schleich FN, Seidel L, Sele J, et al. Exhaled nitric oxide thresholds associated with a sputum eosinophil count 3% in a cohort of unselected patients with asthma. Thorax. 2010;65:1039–44.
22. Korevaar DA, Westerhof GA, Wang J, et al. Diagnostic accuracy of minimally invasive markers for detection of airway eosinophilia in asthma: a systematic review and meta-analysis. Lancet Respir Med. 2015;3:290–300.
23. Bjermer L, Alving K, Diamant Z, et al. Current evidence and future research needs for FeNO measurement in respiratory diseases. Respir Med. 2014;108:830–41.
24. Sørensen LT, Toft BG, Rygaard J, et al. Effect of smoking, smoking cessation, and nicotine patch on wound dimension, vitamin C, and systemic markers of collagen metabolism. Surgery. 2010;148:982–90.
25. Freedman DS, Flanders WD, Barboriak JJ, Malarcher AM, Gates L. Cigarette smoking and leukocyte subpopulations in men. Ann Epidemiol. 1996;6:299–306.
26. Hou L, Lloyd-Jones DM, Ning H, et al. White blood cell count in young adulthood and coronary artery calcification in early middle age: coronary artery risk development in young adults (CARDIA) study. Eur J Epidemiol. 2013;28:735–42.
27. Sunyer J, Springer G, Jamieson B, et al. Effects of asthma on cell components in peripheral blood among smokers and non-smokers. Clin Exp Allergy. 2003;33:1500–5.
28. Telenga ED, Kerstjens HAM, Ten Hacken NHT, Postma DS, van den Berge M. Inflammation and corticosteroid responsiveness in ex-, current and never-smoking asthmatics. BMC Pulm Med. 2013;13:58.
29. Thomson NC, Chaudhuri R, Heaney LG, et al. Clinical outcomes and inflammatory biomarkers in current smokers and exsmokers with severe asthma. J Allergy Clin Immunol. 2013;131:1008–16.
30. Giovannelli J, Chérot-Kornobis N, Hulo S, et al. Both exhaled nitric oxide and blood eosinophil count were associated with mild allergic asthma only in non-smokers. Clin Exp Allergy. 2016;46:543–54.

3

Asthma pressurised metered dose inhaler performance: propellant effect studies in delivery systems

William F. S. Sellers[*]

Abstract

Background: Current pressurised metered dose asthma inhaler (pMDI) propellants are not inert pharmacologically as were previous chlorofluorocarbons, have smooth muscle relaxant, partial pressure effects in the lungs and inhaled hydrofluoroalkane 134a (norflurane) has anaesthetic effects. Volumes of propellant gas per actuation have never been measured.

Methods: In-vitro studies measured gas volumes produced by pMDIs on air oxygen (O_2) levels in valved holding chambers (VHC) and the falls in O_2% following actuation into lung ventilator delivery devices.

Results: Volumes of propellant gas hydrofluoroalkane (HFA) 134a and 227ea and redundant chlorofluorocarbons (CFC) varied from 7 ml per actuation from a small salbutamol HFA inhaler to 16 ml from the larger. Similar-sized CFC pMDI volumes were 15.6 and 20.4 ml. Each HFA salbutamol inhaler has 220 full volume discharges; total volume of gas from a small 134a pMDI was 1640 ml, and large 3885 ml. Sensing the presence of liquid propellant by shaking was felt at the 220th discharge in both large and small inhalers. Because of a partial pressure effect, VHC O_2% in air was reduced to 11% in the smallest 127 ml volume VHC following 10 actuations of a large 134a salbutamol inhaler. The four ventilator delivery devices studied lowered 100% oxygen levels to a range of 93 to 81% after five actuations, depending on the device and type of pMDI used.

Conclusion: Pressurised inhaler propellants require further study to assess smooth muscle relaxing properties.

Keywords: Metered dose inhalers, Propellants, Valved holding chambers (spacers), Ventilator inhaler devices, Toxicology

Background

Inhaled therapy delivery devices for asthma and chronic lung disease such as oxygen driven jet nebulisers, pressurised metered dose inhalers (pMDI), and valved holding chambers (VHC) have little evidence or research to support their efficacy [1, 2]; historical use determines current practice. The amounts of drugs deposited, and in which part of the respiratory tract absorption occurs, is based on intuition rather than research. Inhaled asthma drugs are erroneously considered to act directly through local absorption into receptors, and not systemically. The physical and pharmacological properties of the propellant and drugs in pMDIs gives a scientific explanation and reason for the increasing use of pMDIs and VHCs to manage acute severe asthma in place of evidence-baseless jet nebulisation of beta2-agonists in saline. Inhaled anaesthetic agents and stupefants (glue, butane) descend deep into the lung architecture where bronchial and alveolar absorption into blood is followed by vascular delivery to the whole body. Beta2-agonists in respiratory disease arrive at bronchial smooth muscle receptors from bronchial arteries, and one cardiac cycle later by pulmonary arteries. Inhaled terbutaline has been studied for uterine tocolysis. Upper respiratory tract and oral absorption also play an unknown-percentage part in the delivery of inhaled drugs to target organs. There are corticosteroid receptors in the bronchial epithelial lining

*Correspondence: wfssellers@hotmail.com
Broadgate House, 22 Broadgate, Great Easton, Leicestershire LE16 8SH, UK

cells, which may account for the thought that inhaled drugs act locally and remain in the lungs. The propellants of pMDIs have had little scrutiny, either of previous chlorofluorocarbon (CFC) di-chlorodi-fluoro and tri-chlorofluoro methanes, current hydrofluoroalkanes (HFA) 134a and 227ea. HFA (hydrofluorocarbon) inhaler propellants replaced chlorofluorocarbons in the late 1990s, but propellant toxicological research was incomplete and an anaesthetic effect of HFA134a was missed. Asthma inhaler actuation produces a measurable volume of propellant gases, CFCs, HFA134a, HFA227ea, and as per John Dalton's Law of partial pressures, oxygen and nitrogen in air are reduced in the lungs during inhalation. Inhaler abuse for recreational purposes occurs and Olympic endurance athletes with asthma have outperformed their healthy rivals since the year 2000 [3, 4], interestingly mirroring replacement of inert CFCs by the improved delivery effects of pharmacologically active HFA propellants.

Volumes of propellant produced by metered dose inhalers have not before been measured, nor the volumes of valved holding chambers (VHC) or the gas (percentage) changes inside them after actuations of pMDIs. Devices specifically made to be inserted into ventilated patient circuits for actuation of aluminium pMDI cartridges have received little scientific appraisal. Toxicology studies on safety for human use of HFA134a and 227ea neither appreciated nor studied the physical and pharmacological properties of the propellant at higher doses than 0.8% in humans [5, 6]. HFA134a and 227ea are gases at room temperature. All fluorinated hydrocarbon inhalational anaesthetic agents have smooth muscle relaxing properties in the gut, vasculature, uterus, and lungs (bronchial smooth muscle) via a calcium channel blocking effect, which is the mechanism of action of magnesium sulphate and beta2-agonists. Both HFA propellants interfered with infra-red anaesthetic agent operating theatre monitors [7]. In a review it was noted that up to twelve actuations of metered dose inhalers into valved holding chambers before a single inhalation were being used to treat acute severe asthma in children's hospitals in Melbourne and Sydney, Australia and there was a similar use by United Kingdom paediatricians [2]. A closer examination of metered dose inhaler publications revealed a lack of information of the pharmacological and physical effects of current propellants. This review looks at the performance of pressurised metered dose inhalers in vitro and discusses toxicology studies performed to assess propellant safety and publications comparing CFC and HFA inhalers. Some of the results presented have been published as abstracts [8, 9]. Simple measurements in vitro were made of CFC and HFA pMDIs, valved holding chambers, and tracheal delivery pMDI apparatus [10].

Methods

In vitro experiments were performed using anaesthetic equipment and oxygen monitors; pMDIs were well shaken prior to actuation.

Actuation volumes of inhalers

HFA134a propelled salbutamol small aluminium canister (Salamol^R, IVAX Pharmaceuticals, Waterford, Ireland), salbutamol large aluminium canister (Ventolin™, Allen & Hanburys, Uxbridge, UK) inhalers and a large Clenil^{R}Modulite^R (Chiesi, Cheadle, UK) beclometasone corticosteroid steroid inhaler containing 13% ethanol (which aids corticosteroid solubility); HFA227ea propelled sodium cromogliate (Intal™, SanofiAventis, Guildford, Surrey, UK) and budesonide/eformoterol (Vannair™ 100/6, AstraZeneca, Auckland, NZ), CFC (trichlorofluoromethane and dichlorodi-fluoromethane) propelled small canister salmeterol (Serevent™), expiration date 2005, and large salbutamol (Ventolin™), expiration 1995 (both Allen & Hanburys), were placed inside 500 ml green reservoir bags of an anaesthetic circuit (Intersurgical, Wokingham, UK). The bags were sealed and evacuated to empty, and shaken inhaler actuations by hand, from outside the reservoir bag, were counted until the bag was deemed full (Fig. 1). This was repeated three times for each inhaler, the bag was evacuated using a 60 ml syringe until empty. The volume in the bag was divided by the number of actuations to give a volume in millilitre (ml) per actuation or "puff".

Weights, total volumes and volumes toward exhaustion of pMDI propellant

Small and large salbutamol pMDI full and empty aluminium cannisters were weighed on hospital biochemistry

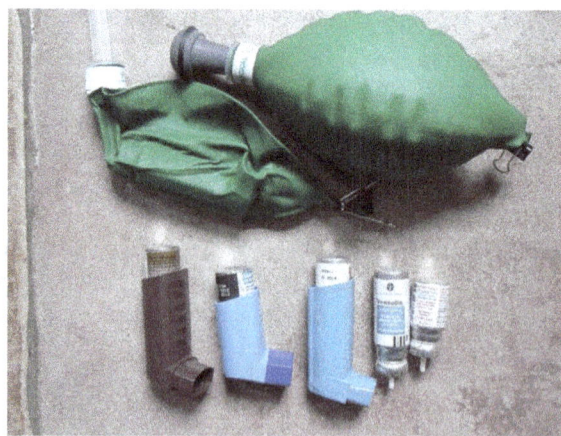

Fig. 1 Full and evacuated 500 ml anaesthetic reservoir bags. The evacuated contains an inhaler and other inhalers and cartridges are shown

laboratory scales. Total volumes were measured until exhaustion of the inhaler by reservoir bag insertion, as above. Volumes were measured after every 50 actuations. At 150 and up to 200, 210, 220 and 230 discharges, the pMDI was removed from the reservoir bag and propellant liquid movement was "sensed" by both shaking and listening within close earshot. After 200 discharges, each 10 actuations were measured until exhaustion. Using Avogadro's Hypothesis or Law (Gram molecular weight = 22.4 l) but without subtracting salbutamol powder weight (>20mg) and the 1% weight by volume of ethanol, theoretical volumes of each net weight of propellant were found.

Actuations into valved holding chambers (spacers)

Four types of VHCs, recommended in order to reduce the velocity of the expelled propellant, to improve timing of inhalation and to warm the propellant and drug [11] were studied. A valve at the inspiratory end retains gas and drug in the chamber reducing leakage to atmosphere before inhalation. A large salbutamol Ventolin[R] pMDI was activated into an Ablespacer[TM] (Clement Clarke International, Essex, UK), Vortex[R] (Pari, VA, USA), BabyHaler[R] (GlaxoSmithKline, Evreux, France) and Volumatic[TM] (Allen and Hanbury, Middlesex, UK). The volumes of the spacers (which were unknown), were determined by filling them with water, emptying and collecting the water, weighing the water and assuming 1 g of water represents 1 ml volume. Oxygen falls were measured after one, two and ten actuations of a large salbutamol pMDI into the four spacers using oxygen and CO_2 tubing inserted into the spacers, which delivered the gases to a Datex paramagnetic oxygen analyser (measuring gas as a percentage) sampling at 150 ml/min. Spacers have inspiratory valves which help reduce leak of propellant and drug from the device; on a deep inhalation air will be entrained though the pMDI. VHCs are "leaky" and addition of pressurised gas from pMDIs displaces existing air and pressure remains atmospheric. The Vortex VHC has an aluminium interior sleeve which is said to reduce a static effect which can cause adherence of drug to the walls of pure plastic spacers.

Oxygen falls in a ventilator circuit reservoir bag using four pMDI delivery devices

An anaesthetic ventilator and circle absorber tubing delivered 100% oxygen with a tidal volume of 500 ml at a rate of 12 breaths per minute in turn through each pMDI delivery device attached to a size 7 mm id 28 cm length cuffed tracheal tube inserted and sealed by tracheal cuff inflation in the opening of a 1 l anaesthetic reservoir bag. From the distal end of the bag gas contents were sampled by a Philips MP70 G5-O_2 analyser. When 100% oxygen content of the reservoir bag was seen, shaken inhalers of norflurane propelled ipratropium and levalbuterol (Duolin[TM], Rex Medical Ltd, Auckland, NZ), salbutamol (Respigen[TM], Mylan, Auckland, NZ) and apaflurane propelled sodium cromoglycate (Intal[TM], SanofiAventis, Surrey, UK) and budesonide and eformoterol (Vannair[TM], AstraZeneca, Auckland, NZ) were separately actuated five times during the short period between ventilations into the devices. Puff volumes were determined as in Method 2. The DDS Spirale[R] (Armstrong Medical, Coleraine, NI, UK) system was used in "open" position when it has a volume of 133 ml. It has no leak from the inhaler port when in "closed" position. The following three devices have "caps" that seal the inhaler port when not being used; an MDI delivery connector, (1964001, Intersurgical, Berkshire, UK), a single swivel tube inhaler, L-Trace (60-60-009, Jackson Allison, Auckland, NZ) and a "Three in one respiratory care system" RT 200 (Fisher & Paykel Healthcare, Auckland, NZ) which has a port as part of the distal "Y" of the tubing. The fall in oxygen percentages was recorded for each inhaler and device.

Results

Volumes after actuations of different inhalers

Table 1—A small salbutamol 134a pMDI produced 7 ml per actuation, larger 16 ml per puff. Larger corticosteroid produced 11.75 ml and Intal[R] produced 13.5 ml. A small salmeterol CFC pMDI produced 15.6 ml and large

Table 1 Propellant volumes from different pMDIs

HFA 134a norflurane	Salamol, (IVAX) small	490/70 puffs = 7 ml per puff
	Ventolin (A&H) large	480/30 puffs = 16 ml per puff
	Clenil Modulite[TM] (Chiesi) large	400/35 puffs = 11.75 ml per puff
HFA 227ea apaflurane	Intal[TM] (Sanofi-Aventis) large	465/35 puffs = 13.5 ml per puff
	Vannair[TM] (AstraZeneca) small	480/53 puffs = 9 ml per puff
CFC[a]	Serevent[TM] (A&H) small	530 ml/35 puffs = 15.6 ml per puff
	Ventolin[TM] (A&H) large	490/24 puffs = 20.4 ml per puff

[a] CFCs dichlorodifluoromethane Cl_2F_2C; trichlorofluoromethane Cl_3FC plus lecithin

salbutamol 20.4 ml per actuation. Table 1 shows volumes of propellant and drug of different pMDIs that were actuated to fill the reservoir bag. The reservoir bag cooled as the low boiling point propellant was expelled into the bag; with a large salbutamol HFA134a inhaler, the temperature fall was from 20 °C room temperature to minus 6 °C, measured with a meat thermometer, and caused little change in volume.

Total weights and volumes

Table 2—220 full volume HFA propellant doses are available, after this, no liquid is sensed on shaking small or large aluminium cartridges, when removed from their plastic surrounds.

Avogadro's hypothesis theoretical gas volumes at 20 °C were: Small pMDI 1730 ml (measured 1640 ml): Large 4075 ml (measured 3885 ml).

Falls in oxygen

Table 3—maximum fall after 10 puffs in the smallest spacer was from 21 to 11%.

Table 2 Weights and volumes of salbutamol HFA134a propellant pMDIs

	Small salbutamol Salamol^R	Large salbutamol Ventolin™
Actuations of a first full pMDI		
Cartridge weight		
Full	15.64 g	28.75 g
Empty	7.76 g	11.43 g
Total volume	1640 ml	3885 ml^a
Actuations of a second full pMDI		
151–200 (50)	350 ml	800 ml
201–210 (10)	70 ml	160 ml
211–220	70 ml (last "sensing")	160 ml (last "sensing")
221–230	65 ml	100 ml
231–240	30 ml	70 ml
241–250	5 ml	40 ml
251–260	0 ml	15 ml
Total volume	1640 ml	3745 ml^a

^{a} 140 ml less total propellant gas volume of second large pMDI

Table 3 Valved holding chamber type; their volumes; and drop in oxygen percentage from 21% air per actuation

Spacer type	Volume (ml)	1 puff (O$_2$ %)	2 puffs (O$_2$ %)	10 puffs (O$_2$ %)
Ablespacer™	126	19	17	11
Vortex™	180	19	18	13
BabyHaler™	393	20	19	16
Volumatic™	788	20	19	17

Oxygen falls in ventilated circuit reservoir bag

Table 4 shows fall in oxygen from 100% after five actuations of HFA 134a and HFA 227ea propellant pMDIs. The results of ×5 actuations of HFA 227ea gas propelled Intal™ (total of 80 ml), delivered during in vitro ventilation into a 1 l bag should decrease oxygen percentage by $80/1000 × 100\% = 8\%$, therefore 92% should be the theoretical percentage result, the range was 79–91%. Interference by HFA 227ea with the oxygen analyser, poor mixing in the reservoir bag, the research methods and execution may explain these results.

Discussion

No research has been performed to quantify the bronchodilating actions of HFA134a and 227ea. Delivery from pressurised metered dose inhalers (pMDIs) relies on these two fluorinated hydrocarbon propellants with low boiling points. The majority of pMDIs use hydrofluoroalkane (HFA) 134a, norflurane, formula CF_3CFH_2, an anaesthetic agent of intermediate potency, described in 1967. The gas was studied in dogs, cats and monkeys, and required 50% in oxygen to anaesthetise dogs: "Action was rapid and readily reversible, overdosage is difficult and vital functions appear to be protected even at very high concentrations". No human studies were performed on anaesthetic effects. This publication is not cited in any toxicology study of the propellants, possibly because the Shulman and Sadove [12] publication title used the alternative name for HFA134a of 1,1,1,2-tetrafluoroethane (TFE). This has a similar chemical structure to the inhalational anaesthetic agent halothane; a bromine and chlorine is replaced by an additional fluorine and hydrogen. Halothane and all other hydrofluorocarbon (hydrofluoroalkane) anaesthetic agents are potent smooth muscle relaxants of gut, vasculature, uterus and bronchi. HFA 227ea, apaflurane, CF_3CFHCF_3, the other pMDI propellant, is chemically similar to the inhalational anaesthetic agent isoflurane but has no anaesthetic activity. Both propellants are refrigerants, the boiling point of HFA 134a is minus 26.3 °C, and of HFA227ea is minus 17.3 °C. Corticosteroid pMDIs contain 13% ethanol to improve solubility, one salbutamol pMDI (Respigen™, Mylan, Auckland, NZ) has 7% ethanol; all other salbutamol HFA MDIs have 1% ethanol added. The high percentage of ethanol is the likely reason for cough following inhalation of corticosteroid.

For 50 years in the United States of America, an over-the-counter-purchase adrenaline (epinephrine) CFC pMDI, delivered 220 mg of adrenaline per puff, and for solubility reasons contained 34% ethanol. A proposed new HFA134a pMDI delivering 125 mg of adrenaline with 1% ethanol was not passed for public use by the Federal Drugs Administration in 2014 [13].

Table 4 Falls in percentage from 100% oxygen after five actuations of pMDIs into four ventilator delivery devices

	5× Duolin™ 45 ml (O₂ %)	5× Respigen™ 60 ml (O₂ %)	5× Vannair™ 45 ml (O₂ %)	5× Intal™ 67.5 ml (O₂ %)
L-Trace™	88	87	89	81
Spirale™	86	87	89	82
Intersurgical™	87	86	87	79
RT 200 (ventilator tubing)	90	91	93	91

The results of these simple easily repeatable experiments may have more educational and research use than clinical relevance, but demonstrate why it is correct for health carers, patients and parents to use multiple actuations of pMDIs through VHCs. Oxygen driven jet nebulisation of saline diluted bronchodilator drugs has limited pulmonary absorption, because water vapour carriage of drugs can only achieve a partial pressure of 47 mmHg (6.3 kPa) which is the pressure of saturated water vapour at 37 °C. This limits the amount of drug that can be delivered below the carina, unlike the gas HFA134a which produces a partial pressure related to the percentage in that breath, and hence carries particles of asthma drugs down to alveoli. Falls in oxygen levels because of high inhaled gas percentage displacing oxygen may have implications of hypoxia for recreational users of asthma inhalers, who are known as "huffers". Purloined asthma inhalers, when actuated into balloons, empty plastic drink bottles, or other vessels, give a "high" to the person inhaling, and the inhaled gas will have a low oxygen content [14, 15]. In CFC propellant metered dose inhalers it was thought that salbutamol rather than the propellant caused a "high", because there were no cases of cortico steroid inhaler abuse [16, 17]; an additional anaesthetic or stupifiant effect is likely with current HFA134a pMDIs.

Patients or doctors who use multiple actuations of pMDIs at one time into VHCs, spacers, and ventilator delivery devices in acute severe and life-threatening asthma, or for reversal of bronchospasm in anaphylaxis, may be affected by a reduction of oxygen and a slight sedative effect of HFA134a. HFA 134a (also known as R134a) is used as an automobile air conditioner refrigerant, but because it has a global warming potential (GWP) of 1410, is likely to be withdrawn from use, as only compounds with a GWP of less than 150 will be allowed. GWP is a 100 year warming potential of 1 kg of a gas relative to 1 kg of carbon dioxide, which has a GWP of 1. In pharmaceutical factories, HFA134a and HFA227ea, and asthma medication with added ethanol to aid solubility, are introduced into different sized drawn aluminium bottles by a "cold transfer method" at minus 55 °C (Information from

manufacturers of Airomir^R, 3 M Health Care Ltd), the propellant is a liquid with a saturated vapour above.

A toxicology study looked at eight volunteers, four male, four female, who inspired pure HFA 134a, HFA 227ea and CFC in air when inside a whole body exposure chamber, up to a maximum of 8000 parts per million (0.8%) for HFAs, and 4000 ppm CFC for 1 h on eight separate occasions. Why an 8000 ppm concentration was chosen is not explained. EKG (ECG), blood pressure, pulse, and lung function by peak expiratory flow rate (PEFR), measured 75 min after cessation of exposure, and serial blood samples were taken. There were no statistical changes in clinical evaluation parameters [6]. However, after 75 min, a bronchodilating effect of HFA 134a on normal tone bronchial muscle which may change PEFR, would be long-gone.

In the introduction the authors of this study mention unpublished data suggesting that; "The threshold for cardiac sensitisation in dogs was 75,000 ppm (7.5%) for HFA 134a and 100,000 ppm (10%) for HFA 227ea", but do not explain what they mean by cardiac sensitisation or describe the delivery gas which may have been air. They do not reference Shulman and Sadove's publication which stated that at 50–80% of TFE inhalational agent (HFA 134a) delivered in oxygen to dogs; "The electrocardiograph is usually quite stable, with either a sinus or a nodal rhythm". Exposure of rats up to 50,000 ppm (5%) HFA 134a 6 h per day, 5 days a week for 2 years produced an increase in Leydig cell tumours, common in rats, but not humans.

Another toxicology study gave pure HFA 134a; HFA 134a with salbutamol; and pure CFC metered dose inhalers to twelve healthy male volunteers of up to 16 inhalations from pMDIs [5]. Pulmonary function, (FEV_1, $FEF_{25-75\%}$), cardiovascular performance, (heart rate and blood pressure) were measured after each incremental dose. HFA 134a-salbutamol produced statistically significant dose-related increases in heart rate, systolic blood pressure and tremor and a significant dose—related decrease in serum potassium. A spirometric respiratory function test was performed 20 min after the last of the

16 MDI doses, and although HFA 134a salbutamol statistically improved FEV_1 and $FEF_{25-75\%}$, an opportunity to see if there was a bronchodilating effect of HFA 134a alone may have been lost because of this delay and a consequent wash out of the propellant; no statistical change was seen. A further study exposed five subjects to pure HFA 134a in air via a one way face mask (the manufacturer of the mask was not described) to see what happened on exposure if HFA 134a was used as a flame suppressant. Subject #3 at 4000 ppm (0.4%) exhibited a rapid drop in pulse and blood pressure and fainted, and subject #5 exhibited an increase in blood pressure and heart rate about 10 min after initiation of the exposure. Subject #1 was exposed to HFA 227ea at 6400 ppm (0.64%) for 3 min and, quote; "pulse rose rapidly and uncontrollably to double the baseline (pre-exposure) value. The exposure was terminated after 3.5 min. The subject's pulse returned to its pre-exposure level within 30 s after exposure was terminated". A day later the breathing system without HFA227ea was used by the same subject with no untoward effect. No further exposures were attempted [18]. Malignant hyperpyrexia (MH) is triggered in a dose related fashion by inhalational anaesthetic agents in susceptible individuals; research is required to see if HFA134a and HFA227ea have this undesirable property. R134a, the refrigerant in automobile air conditioning units is available for study. The single volunteer subject #5, breathing HFA134a, as previously mentioned, who had an increase in blood pressure and a tachycardia, lead to the experiments being abandoned.

A reduction in oxygen concentration in spacers causing mixtures low in oxygen to be inhaled should have little untoward consequence. A benefit of bronchodilation and a subsequent breath of air containing 21% oxygen, should counter a breath of low inhaled oxygen. If spacer inhalation therapy interrupts continuous oxygen delivery via a face mask during a severe asthma attack, this reduces the danger of a hypoxic inhaled mixture. A child with a 1600 ml lung volume inhaling 10×16 ml from a large salbutamol inhaler will have a maximum 10% of HFA134a in that breath which is meant to be held as long as possible. After this breath hold the spacer may be empty of gas and drug, so further deep breaths from this spacer are pointless. The time for gas to escape from a VHC has not been determined.

"Asthma spacers used with MDIs remove the need for coordination between actuation and inhalation, reduce the velocity of the aerosol and allow time for evaporation (and warming) of the propellant so that a larger proportion of the particles can be inhaled and deposited in the lungs" [11]. After activation of the metered dose inhaler, the nomenclature of the product is variously described in literature as an "aerosol", "vapour", or "gas", at that particular temperature; HFA134a and HFA227ea act as gases in the lung.

A large difference in lung deposition of corticosteroid carried by HFA 134a and CFC propellant has been seen in nine healthy volunteers breathing either HFA134a or chlorofluorocarbon (CFC) propellant carrying radioactive labelled beclometasone. 53% with HFA and 4% CFC lung deposition occurred. A smaller particle size of HFA134a beclometasone of 1.1 μ to CFC beclometasone of 3.5 μ was thought to account for the difference. Particle size distribution from the pMDIs was determined by an Andersen 1 ACFM Particle Sizing Sampler (Mark 11; Andersen Samplers; Atlanta, GA) and a Quartz Crystal Microbalance Cascade Impactor System (California Measurements; Sierra Madre, CA) [19]. A corticosteroid "carrier" effect of HFA 134a as a vapour or gas, and a reduction in resting bronchial tone because of a bronchial smooth muscle relaxing effect is another reason for better lung distribution. Particle or droplet size is measured in vitro, but in the lungs, droplets must evaporate before absorption, and particles can descend further within a partial pressure generating gas.

Conclusion

A greater volume of HFA134a propellant per actuation is produced by large salbutamol metered dose inhalers, 16 ml versus 7 ml for the smaller. If this propellant on its own relaxes bronchial smooth muscle and the gas aids drug delivery (including corticosteroid), then large metered dose inhaler actuation gives maximum bronchodilation for patients and athletes (and huffers). Exhaustion of pMDIs can be sensed by shaking, inhalers are now produced using a mechanical system with a numbered dial to count down each actuation. Further research on bronchial smooth muscle effects of HFAs may be performed with available propellant—only pressurised metered dose inhalers which are used to assess efficiency of inhalation by patients.

Abbreviations

HFA: hydrofluoroalkane; CFC: chlorofluorocarbon; pMDI: pressurised metered dose inhaler; VHC: valved holding chamber; GWP: global warming potential.

Acknowledgements

None.

Competing interests

The author declare that he has no competing interests.

Funding

Self-funded.

References

1. Boe J, Dennis JH, O'Driscoll BR. European respiratory society guidelines on the use of nebulisers. Eur Respir J. 2001;18:228–42.
2. Sellers WFS. Inhaled and Intravenous treatment in acute severe and life-threatening asthma. Br J Anaesth. 2013;110:183–90.
3. McKenzie DC, Fitch KD. The asthmatic athlete: inhaled Beta-2 agonists, sport performance, and doping. Clin J Sport Med. 2011;21:46–50.
4. Arie S. Asthma in athletes. What can we learn? BMJ. 2012;344:20–2.
5. Donnell D, Ward S, Harrison LI, et al. Acute safety of the CFC-free propellant HFA 134a from a metered dose inhaler. Eur J Clin Pharmacol. 1995;48:473–7.
6. Emmen HH, Hoogendijk EMG, Klopping-Ketelaars WAA, et al. Human safety and pharmacokinetics of the CFC alternative propellants HFA 134a (1,1,1,2-tetrafluoroethane) and HFC 227 (1,1,1,2,3,3,3-heptafluoropropane) following whole-body exposure. Regul Toxicol Pharm. 2000;32:22–35.
7. Levin PD, Levin D, Avidan A. Medical aerosol propellant interference with infrared anaesthetic gas monitors. Br J Anaesth. 2004;92:865–9.
8. Sellers WFS. Jet (wet) nebuliser and metered dose inhaler (MDI) delivery of drugs [Abstract]. Br J Anaesth. 2012;109:666–7.
9. Sellers WFS. Ventilator delivery systems for asthma inhalers [Abstract]. Br J Anaesth. 2013;110:871–2.
10. Kusukar A, Macartney NJD, Hingston CD, Holmes TW, Wise MP, Walker A. Airway emergency during anaesthesia using a metered dose inhaler. I, II, III, and IV. Anaesthesia. 2011;66:519–31.
11. British National Formulary. Respiratory system; 2011.
12. Shulman M, Sadove MS. 1, 1, 1, 2-tetrafluoroethane: an inhalational agent of intermediate potency. Anesth Analg. 1967;46:629–35.
13. FDA Advisory Committee Briefing Materials. Epinephrine HFA MDI (E004)—a proposed reformulation to replace OTC Primatene® Mist CFC NDA 205920 joint meeting of the nonprescription drugs advisory committee and the pulmonary-allergy drugs advisory committee meeting. February 25, 2014.
14. Sellers WFS. Preventing out-of-hospital asthma deaths. Thorax. 2015. doi:10.1136/thoraxjnl-2015-207207.
15. Sellers WFS. Misuse of anaesthetic gases. Editorial. Anaesthesia. 2016;71:1140–3. doi:10.1111/anae.13551.
16. Pratt HF. Abuse of salbutamol inhalers in young people. Clin Allergy. 1982;12:203–9.
17. Perron BE, Howard MO. Endemic asthma inhaler abuse among antisocial adolescents. Drug Alcohol Depen. 2008;96:22–296.
18. Vinegar A, Jepson GW, Cook RS et al. Human inhalation of Halon 1301, HFA 134a and HFA 227ea for Collection of Pharmokinetic Data. Occupational Environmental Health Directorate, Toxicology Division, Armstrong Laboratory, Wright Patterson Air Force Base Report No. AL/OE-TR-1997-0116. [For copies please contact NTIS, 5285 Port Royal Road, Springfield, Virginia 22161]; 1997.
19. Leach CL, Davidson PJ, Hasselquist BE, et al. Lung deposition of hydrofluoroalkane-134a beclometasone is greater than that of chlorofluorocarbon fluticasone and chlorofluorocarbon beclometasone. Chest. 2002;122:510–6.

4

Seasonal variation in circulating group 2 innate lymphoid cells in mugwort-allergic asthmatics during and outside pollen season

Qing Miao, Yan Wang, Yong-ge Liu, Yi-xin Ren, Hui Guan, Zhen Li, Wei Xu and Li Xiang*

Abstract

Background: Group 2 innate lymphoid cells (ILC2s) are a newly identified cell population with the potent capability to produce Th2-type cytokines in a non-antigen specific manner. Previous study demonstrated that enhanced circulating ILC2s in cat-allergic patient after experimental allergen challenge, whereas the effects of natural allergen exposure on peripheral ILC2s are still unclear. We therefore examined the variations in circulating ILC2s among asthmatic patients sensitized to different allergens in- and outside- pollen season.

Methods: 10 patients sensitized to mugwort, 10 patients sensitized to house dust mites (HDM) and 12 healthy controls were recruited into this study. Blood samples were collected from the patients in- and outside- pollens season, 2–3 months apart. ILC2s (Lin-CD127+ CRTH2+) were enumerated by flow cytometry, as well as intracellular IL-5 and IL-13 expression. The levels of IL-5 and IL-13 in supernatants of Lineage- and Lineage+ cells stimulated with IL-25 and/or IL-33 in the presence of IL-2 were measured using a Milliplex human cytokine array kit.

Results: An obvious seasonal increases in percentages of total and IL-13+ ILC2s were observed in patients with mugwort sensitization during natural pollen exposure, however, the percentages of peripheral ILC2s in HDM-allergic patients were not affected significantly. A positive correlation between FeNO and IL-13$^+$ILC2s was found in patients sensitized to mugwort. A mixture of IL-33 and IL-25 induced a significant production of IL-13 and IL-5 from Lineage$^-$ cells of both mugwort-allergic and HDM-allergic asthmatics. Stimulation with IL-33 alone induced a significantly greater quantity of IL-13 by Lineage-cells from mugwort-allergic asthmatic compared with that from HDM-allergic asthmatics, whereas IL-25 induced a significantly greater amount of IL-5 by the Lineage-cells from mugwort-allergic asthmatic compared with that from HDM-allergic asthmatics.

Conclusion: Within pollen season the frequencies and function profiles of circulating ILC2s among asthmatic children are altered dynamically, which may be closely related to the sensitized type of allergens.

Keywords: Asthma, Group 2 innate lymphoid cells, Mugwort, Pollen, House dust mites

Background

Asthma is a heterogeneous inflammatory disorders characterized by reversible airway obstruction and bronchial hyper-reactivity and airway inflammation [1, 2]. A nationwide survey in China reported that the prevalence rate of asthma in urban children is 3.02% [3], however, the overall asthma control level is still unsatisfactory [4].

Group 2 innate lymphoid cells (ILC2s) are an important early source of type 2 cytokines and are activated by epithelium-derived alarmins, including interleukin-25 (IL-25), IL-33 and thymic stromal lymphopoietin (TSLP), highlighting the potential critical role of ILC2s in the development of type 2 inflammation [5, 6]. Previously, Doherty et al. have demonstrated that a significant elevation of circulating ILC2s in cat-allergic patients after experimental nasal challenge, suggesting that the effects of allergen exposure on peripheral ILC2s [7]. However, there is little information about the variations

*Correspondence: drxiangli@163.com
Department of Allergy, Beijing Children's Hospital, Capital Medical School, No. 56 Nanlishi Road, Xicheng District, Beijing 100045, China

in ILC2s during natural allergen exposure. In order to determine whether natural seasonal allergen exposure causes changes in percentage and function of ILC2s in asthma patients, we therefore chose to carry out multiply sampling to observe the changes in peripheral ILC2s at the beginning and outside the pollen season. Unlike the experimental allergen challenge model where a large dose of allergen antigen is given at a single time-point, the strength of seasonal studies design was to observe the whole inflammation process starting from cellular activation and subsequent cytokine production after a continuous allergens exposure within a limited time period. In addition, to further verify whether the role of ILC2s may vary among asthmatics sensitized to different allergens, we investigated the phenotypic and functional characteristics of ILC2s between mugwort and HDM-allergic asthmatics.

Methods

Study group

10 subjects with mugwort-allergic asthma and 10 subjects with HDM-allergic asthma were recruited for this study. The diagnosis and selection criteria were based on the global initiative for asthma (GINA). Allergy was confirmed by a positive skin prick testing (SPT) and by the presence of specific IgE. Patients with symptoms of perennial allergy or with concomitant allergy to other seasonal allergens with overlapping time of symptoms occurrence were excluded from this study. If a patient had been taking anti-histamines, steroids, or leukotriene receptor antagonists within 4 weeks, or undergoing immunotherapy for any allergen within the past 3 years prior to the study were excluded. Another 12 healthy, non-atopic children matched for age and sex and with no history of allergy, asthma and other inflammation diseases were enrolled as healthy controls. The research protocol was reviewed and approved by the Beijing Children's Hospital Human Research Ethic Committee, and informed written consent was obtained from patients' representatives before enrollment. The study protocol conforms to the ethical guidelines of the Declaration of Helsinki.

Study design

Blood samples were collected from all enrolled subjects on two occasions through whole season pollen. Test period 1 (August to September, 2016): during pollen season immediately following the appearance of symptoms. At the onset of symptoms, after blood samples collection, all patients were started on treatment with antihistamines. Test period 2 (November, 2016): outside pollen season, when the patients' symptoms subsided and anti-inflammation treatment was discontinued. At each visit,

the patients' clinical data, including blood eosinophil count, FeNO, and pulmonary function test were record.

Isolation and preparation of peripheral blood mononuclear cells (PBMCs)

Blood samples were processed within 6 h of sample collection. PBMCs were separated by using Ficoll density gradient solution (HAOYANG, Tianjin, China) at 2000 rpm for 20 min at 4 °C. The PBMCs were collected and washed twice with cold PBS containing 2% fetal calf serum (Gibco, USA) and used for flow cytometric staining (FACS staining).

ILC2s identification and intracellular staining

Peripheral ILC2s (Lin$^-$CD127$^+$ CRTH2$^+$ cells) in present study were identified as previously reported [8], which were detected by flow cytometric analysis. The PBMCs cell pellet was collected, washed, and then stained with a FITC-conjugated monoclonal antibodies (mAbs) against human Lineage cocktail (CD3, CD14, CD16, CD19, CD34, CD123, CD11c, TCRαβ, and TCRγδ expressed on T cells, monocytes, macrophages, B cells, mast cells, dendritic cells, and hematopoietic progenitor cells), PE-conjugated antibodies against human CD127 (eBioscience, CA, USA), and APC-conjugated antibodies against human CRTH2 (CD294) (Biolegend, CA, USA) at room temperature in the dark for 30 min. We gated on cells lacking Lineage markers and examined expression of CD127 and CRTH2 within lympho-mononuclear region (low side scatter/low forward scatter), and the number of ILC2s is expressed as a percentage of all Lineage negative cells (Fig. 1). For the intracellular staining of cytokines, cells were incubated in Perm/Fix buffer (eBioscience, CA, USA) and optimal concentration of intracellular stains of anti-IL-5-PerCP (BD bioscience) and anti-IL-13-PerCP antibodies (BD bioscience) were added. Gating in the lympho-mononuclear region (low side scatter/low forward scatter) and following acquisition of 100,000 events, data were analyzed using FlowJo program to enumerate intracellular IL-5 and IL-13 levels in ILC2s (Lin-CD45+ CD127+ CRTH2+) (Fig. 2).

Correlation analysis between ILC2s and asthma clinical parameters

The percentages of IL-13$^+$ILC2s were counted among asthma patients subgroups, and its correlations with clinical parameters were analyzed between patients subgroup.

FACS sorting of ILC2s and in vitro cell culture

Blood derived mononuclear cells were stained with the FITC-Lineage cocktail as described above and then separated into Lineage$^+$ and Lineage$^-$ cells by using a

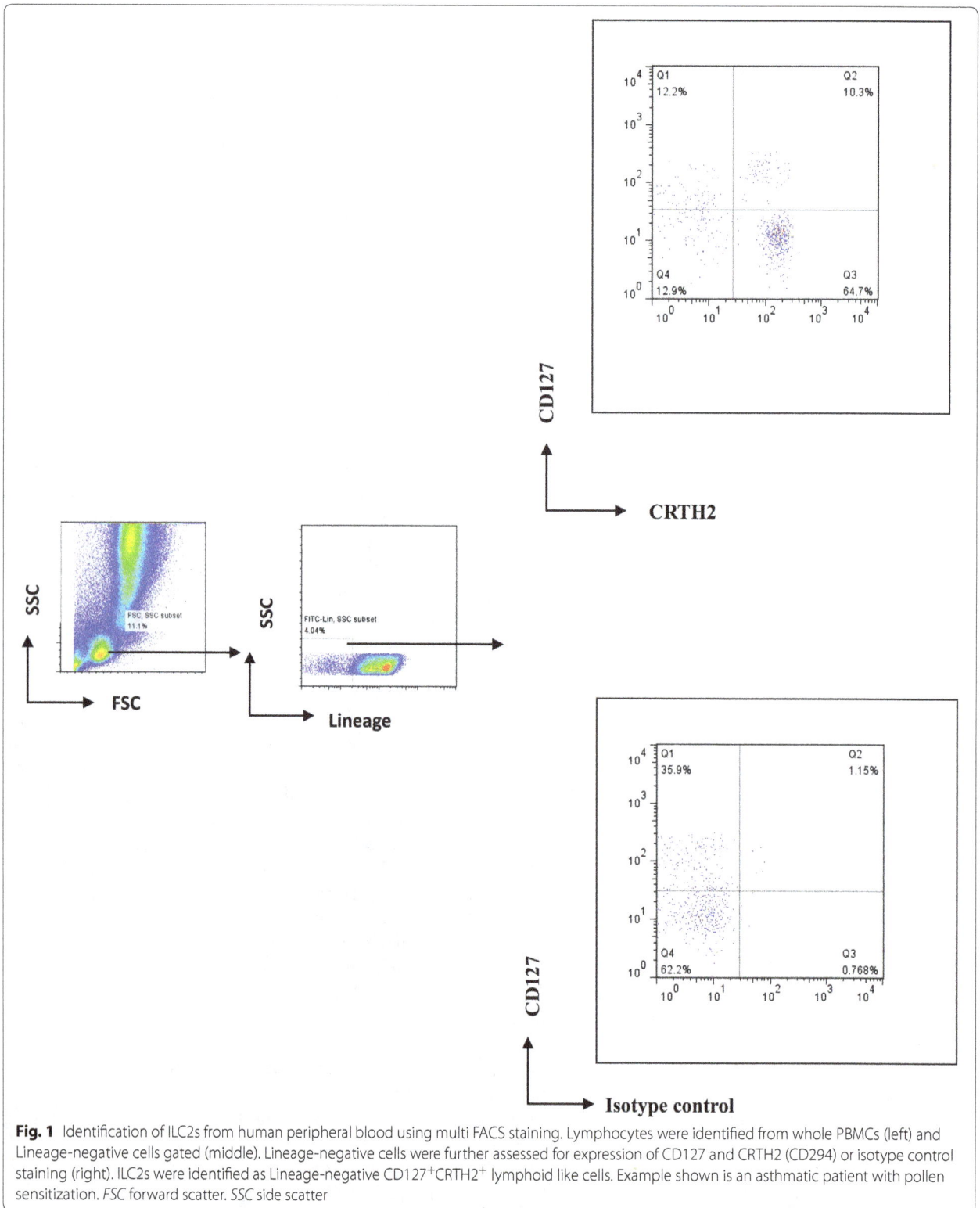

Fig. 1 Identification of ILC2s from human peripheral blood using multi FACS staining. Lymphocytes were identified from whole PBMCs (left) and Lineage-negative cells gated (middle). Lineage-negative cells were further assessed for expression of CD127 and CRTH2 (CD294) or isotype control staining (right). ILC2s were identified as Lineage-negative CD127+CRTH2+ lymphoid like cells. Example shown is an asthmatic patient with pollen sensitization. *FSC* forward scatter. *SSC* side scatter

fluorescence-activated cell sorter (BD FACSAriaII; BD Biosciences). The sorted Lineage⁻ cells were at 5×10^4 cells/mL in 96-well tissue culture plates for 7 days (37 °C,

5% CO_2) in the presence of medium alone, or IL-2 (20 U/ mL) alone, or IL-25 alone (25 ng/mL) (rhIL-25, R&D Systems Inc., Minneapolis, MN, USA, Cat. NO. 8134)

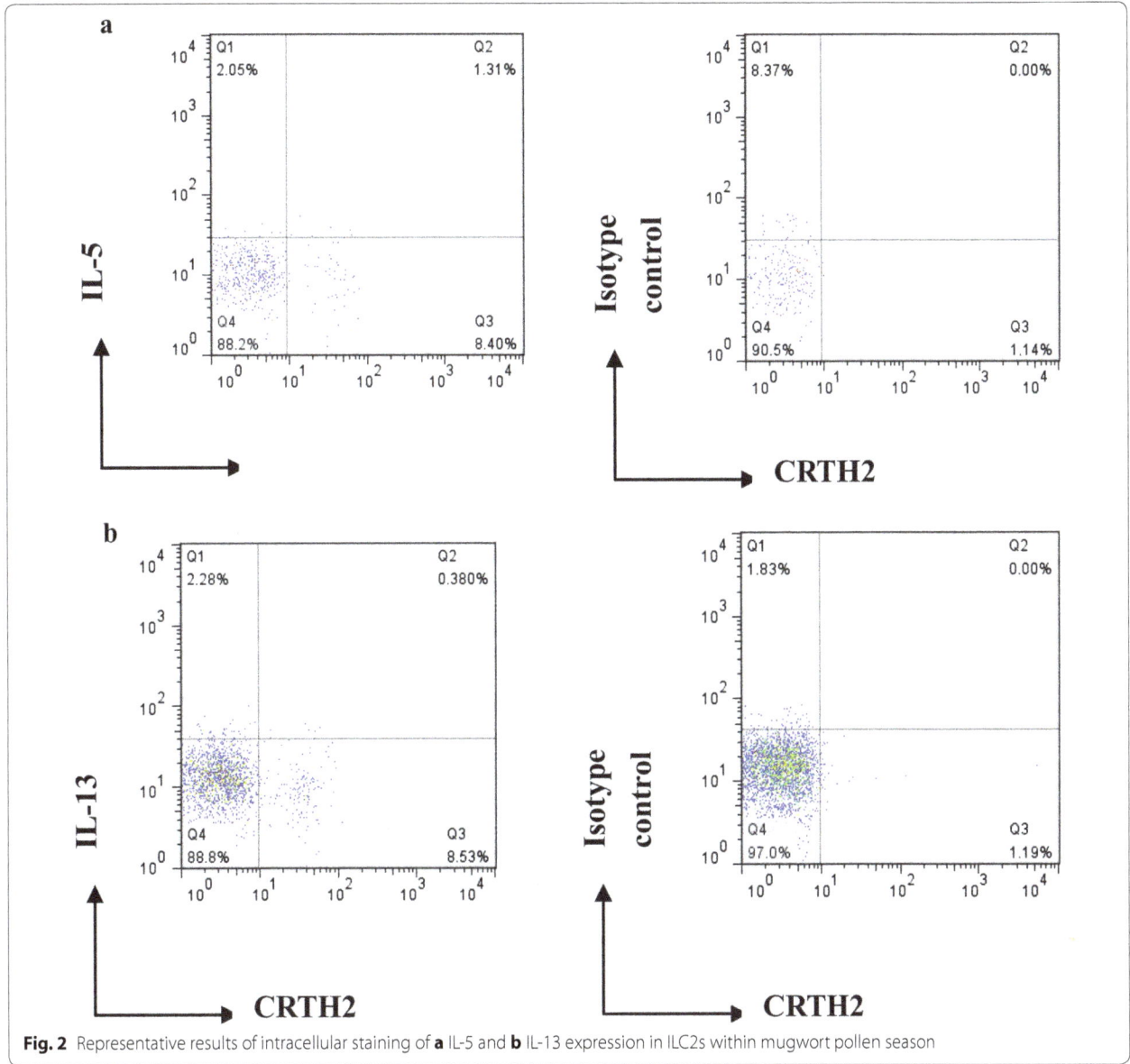

Fig. 2 Representative results of intracellular staining of **a** IL-5 and **b** IL-13 expression in ILC2s within mugwort pollen season

plus IL-2 (20 U/mL), or IL-33 alone (25 ng/mL) (rhIL-33, R&D Systems Inc., Minneapolis, MN, USA, Cat. NO. 3625) plus IL-2 (20 U/mL), or their combinations.

Multiplex analysis of cytokines production in ILC2s cell culture

The concentrations of IL-5 and IL-13 in cell culture supernatants were measured using a Milliplex human cytokine array kit (Millipore, St. Charles, MO, USA) as recommended by the manufacturer.

Statistical analysis

Statistical analysis was performed using SPSS 19.0 software (SPSS, Chicago, IL, USA) and graphs were generated using the prism software (GraphPad, LaJolla, CA, USA). All data were representative of at least three independent experiments. Results were expressed as the Mean $\pm$ SD. Comparison of ILC2% among different groups was performed using unpaired t test, and the association between ILC2% and clinical parameters was analyzed using Pearson's correlation test. All tests were 2-tailed, and P value of less than 0.05 was considered as significant.

Results

Study subjects

A total of 20 asthmatic children (including 10 patients with mugwort pollen-allergic asthma and 10 patients with HDM-allergic asthma) and 12 healthy controls were enrolled into this study. Detailed information and clinical parameters on these enrolled subjects were shown in Table 1. No significant differences were found in sex, mean age and BMI between patient groups and healthy subjects. However, the differences in FeNO, blood eosinophil counts and FEV1% predicted were statistically significant between two patients subgroups (all $P < 0.05$, respectively).

Peripheral ILC2s were significantly increased in mugwort pollen-allergic asthmatics compared to HMD-asthmatic patients during pollen season

In present study, we first compared the levels of ILC2s in peripheral blood among patients group and healthy controls group during pollen season, showing that the mean number of ILC2s in peripheral blood was significantly increased in asthmatic patients compared to healthy controls ($15.01 \pm 6.21\%$ vs. $1.69 \pm 0.87\%$, $P < 0.01$). Furthermore, a subgroup analysis indicated the level of ILC2s was higher in subjects with mugwort pollen-allergic asthma compared with those with HDM-allergic asthma ($23.09 \pm 7.86\%$ vs. $6.84 \pm 3.85\%$, $P < 0.01$). When outside pollen season, it was observed that the number of ILC2s was dramatically higher in pollen-allergic asthma group ($11.3 \pm 2.45\%$) compared to the number from health controls ($1.32 \pm 0.91\%$), moreover, the difference between mugwort pollen- and HDM-allergic asthmatics was significant ($16.9 \pm 3.12\%$ vs. $3.76 \pm 1.96\%$, $P < 0.05$) (Fig. 3).

A seasonal change in percentages of IL-13⁺ILC2, but not IL-5⁺ILC2s, was observed in pollen-allergic asthmatics

Previous studies demonstrated that ILC2s contribute to production of key cytokines IL-5 and IL-13 in response to epithelium-derived cytokines, such as IL-25 and IL-33 [9, 10]. Accordingly, we further investigated the intracellular cytokine expression of IL-5 and IL-13 in ILC2s. During pollen season, the number of IL-13⁺ILC2s was significantly higher in peripheral blood of pollen-allergic

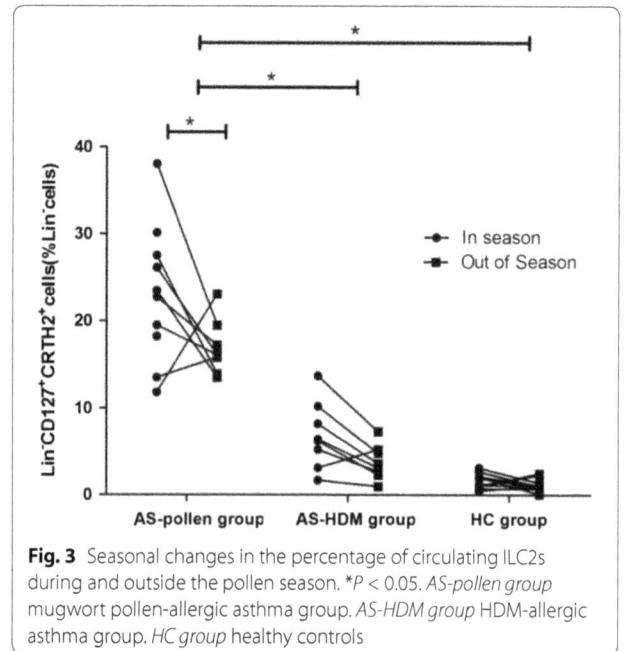

Fig. 3 Seasonal changes in the percentage of circulating ILC2s during and outside the pollen season. *$P < 0.05$. *AS-pollen group* mugwort pollen-allergic asthma group. *AS-HDM group* HDM-allergic asthma group. *HC group* healthy controls

patients ($6.94 \pm 3.16\%$) compared to HDM-allergic patients ($1.89 \pm 0.70\%$) as well as compared to HCs ($0.51 \pm 0.50\%$). When outside pollen season, an obvious decline tendency of IL-13⁺ILC2s was found in patients with pollen-allergic asthma ($6.94 \pm 3.16\%$ vs. $4.17 \pm 1.98\%$, $P < 0.05$) and in those with HDM-allergic asthma ($1.89 \pm 0.70\%$ vs. $1.44 \pm 0.55\%$, $P < 0.05$), respectively. However, the percentage of IL-13⁺ILC2s in healthy controls was not affected ($0.51 \pm 0.50\%$ vs. $0.45 \pm 0.30\%$, $P > 0.05$) (Fig. 4a). A similar analysis was performed to evaluate percentage of the IL-5⁺ILC2s percentage in each group, however, no significant changes were observed in samples from any of the study groups (Fig. 4b). Therefore, IL-13⁺ILC2s were used for the further correlation analysis.

Table 1 The clinical characteristics of enrolled subjects

	Pollen-allergic asthmatics	HDM-allergic asthmatics	Healthy controls	P value
Numbers of patients	10	10	12	–
Boys (%)	5 (50.0)	5 (50.0)	7 (58.3)	–
Age (years)	7.8 ± 3.4	10.2 ± 3.7	9.8 ± 4.0	> 0.05
BMI	15.3 ± 1.6	16.7 ± 1.9	16.0 ± 1.3	> 0.05
FEV1% predicted	77.1 ± 14.6	75.6 ± 13.4	ND	< 0.05
Blood EOS (10⁹/L)	0.51 ± 0.28	0.53 ± 0.23	ND	< 0.05
FeNO (ppb)	56.1 ± 28.1	57.1 ± 24.5	ND	< 0.05

Data expressed as Mean ± SD

ND not determined

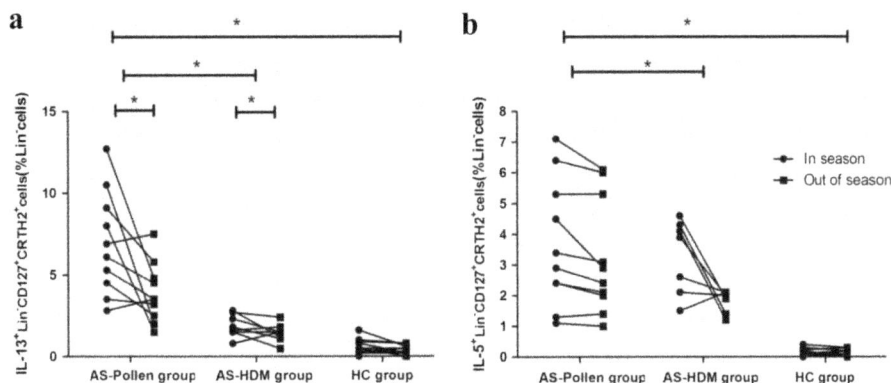

Fig. 4 Seasonal changes in **a** IL-13$^+$ILC2s **b** IL-5$^+$ILC2s during and outside the pollen season. *$P < 0.05$. *AS-pollen group*: mugwort pollen-allergic asthma group. *AS-HDM group* HDM-allergic asthma group. *HC group* healthy controls

Circulating IL-13$^+$ILC2s numbers were positively correlated with clinical parameters

A further correlation analysis between IL-13$^+$ILC2s levels and clinical parameters, including eosinophils counts, FeNO, FEV1% of predicted was performed. Within the pollen season, a positive correlation between the percentages of circulating IL-13$^+$ILC2s and FeNO levels was observed in patients with pollen-allergic asthma ($r = 0.8785, P < 0.001$). In contrast, no strong correlations were identified between circulating IL-13$^+$ILC2s numbers and blood eosinophils counts ($r = 0.3247, P > 0.05$), and FEV1% of predicted ($r = - 0.5252, P > 0.05$). Besides, no significant relationship was found between IL-13$^+$ILC2s levels and clinical parameters in HMD-allergic asthmatics (Fig. 5).

Distinct cytokines expression from IL-25 and/or IL-33-induced Lineage$^-$ cells between pollen-allergic and HDM-allergic asthmatics

We performed subsequent mechanistic studies to investigate the potential role of ILC2s as source of type 2 cytokines in the pathogenesis of allergic conditions, and to verify whether this effect was varied among patients sensitized to different types of allergens. Our data showed the Lineage-cells from both mugwort-allergic asthma group and HDM-allergic asthma group could produce significant amounts of IL-5 and IL-13 after the stimulation with IL-33 when compared to IL-2 alone (all $P < 0.05$, respectively), or medium alone (all $P < 0.05$, respectively). Similarly, higher levels of IL-5 and IL-13 were observed in IL-25-stimulated Lineage-cells from both patients subgroups (all $P < 0.05$, respectively). Furthermore, subgroup analysis showed that IL-33 stimulation had a stronger effect on the Lineage-cells from mugwort-allergic asthmatic to release IL-13, whereas a significant elevation in IL-5 release was observed in

IL-25-stimulated Lineage-cells from mugwort-allergic asthmatic compared with that of HDM-allergic asthmatics (Fig. 6).

Discussion

In present study, our date demonstrated that within mugwort pollen season a significantly higher percentage of circulating ILC2s was detected in asthma patient subgroups than healthy controls. Our results are consistent with the previous finding presented by Zhang et al. showing that an increased circulating ILC2s was observed in HDM-allergic patients, indicating the important role of ILC2s in airway allergic reactions. Moreover, a subgroup analysis of asthma patients in present study demonstrated that within pollen season the frequencies of ILC2s were significantly increased in mugwort-allergic asthmatics than that in HDM-allergic asthmatics. When outside the pollen season, an obvious decline trend of circulating ILC2s was observed in pollen-allergic patients, however, no seasonal changes in the proportions of circulating ILC2s were observed HDM-allergic asthmatics. Similarly, Fan et al. had reported that a distinct phenotypic and functional profiles in ILC2s frequencies existed between HDM-sensitized and mugwort-sensitized allergic rhinitis patients, and the main cause for this discrepancy was assumed to be related to the difference in allergenicity between HDM and mugwort [11]. Pollen of mugwort (*Artemisia vulgaris*) is one of the main causes of allergic reactions in late summer and autumn [12]. Among patients suffering from pollinosis, the incidence of allergic disease caused by mugwort pollen is 10–14% [13]. In Northern areas of China, mugwort pollination commonly occurs at the end of July, with the peak pollen period ranging from August to September [14]. Previous studies reported that the incidence of pollinosis was consistent to airborne pollen peak time, in contrast, a negative relationship was observed between airway

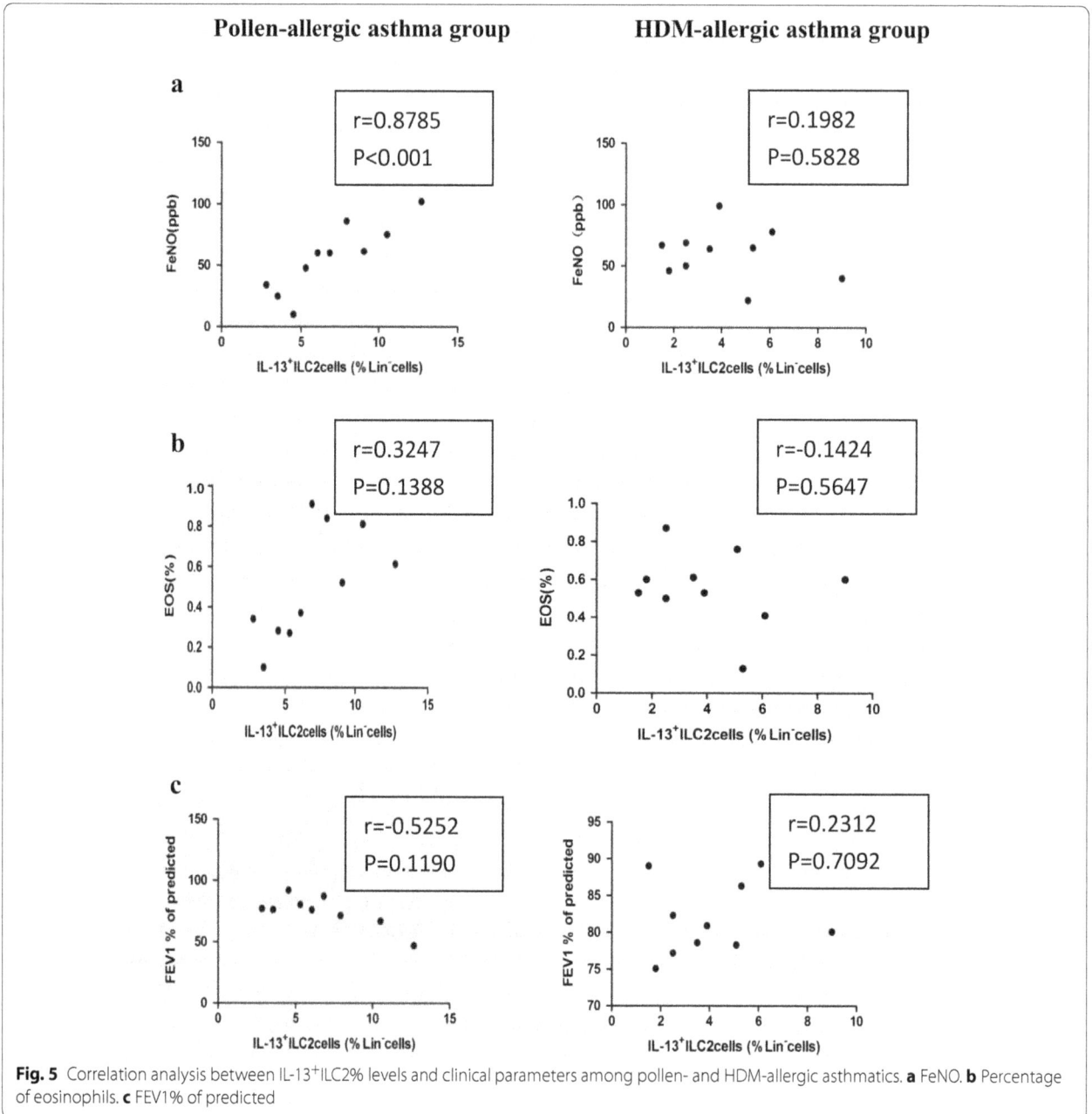

Fig. 5 Correlation analysis between IL-13⁺ILC2% levels and clinical parameters among pollen- and HDM-allergic asthmatics. **a** FeNO. **b** Percentage of eosinophils. **c** FEV1% of predicted

responsiveness and airborne pollen concentration [15, 16]. Recently, the major allergen in mugwort pollen has been determined, Art v 1, which is a highly glycosylated protein with an apparent molecule mass of 24–28 kDa react with IgE from > 95% of patients allergic to mugwort. In striking contrast to other allergens that contain multiple T cell epitopes, the T cell responses to Art v 1 is characterized by one strong immunodominant epitope [17]. Jahn-Schmid et al. had further characterized the T responses of mugwort allergic patients to natural Artv1 (nArt v 1), demonstrating that all Art v 1-specific T cell clones expressed

the CD4+ CD8-TCR α β + phenotype, and the majority exhibited a Th2 cytokine profiles [18]. In contrast, house dust mites (HDM) are a type of common, persistent, and perennial allergen that is present almost everywhere in the world. HMD and their fecal pellets contain several trypsin/chymotrypsin-like enzymes which could directly lead to tissue damage and increase the passage of allergens across the epithelial barrier, these actions might further stimulate allergic reactions through difference pathway, such as greater epithelial cell-derived IL-33 release [19, 20]. IL-33 has been shown to be a potent stimulus for ILC2s

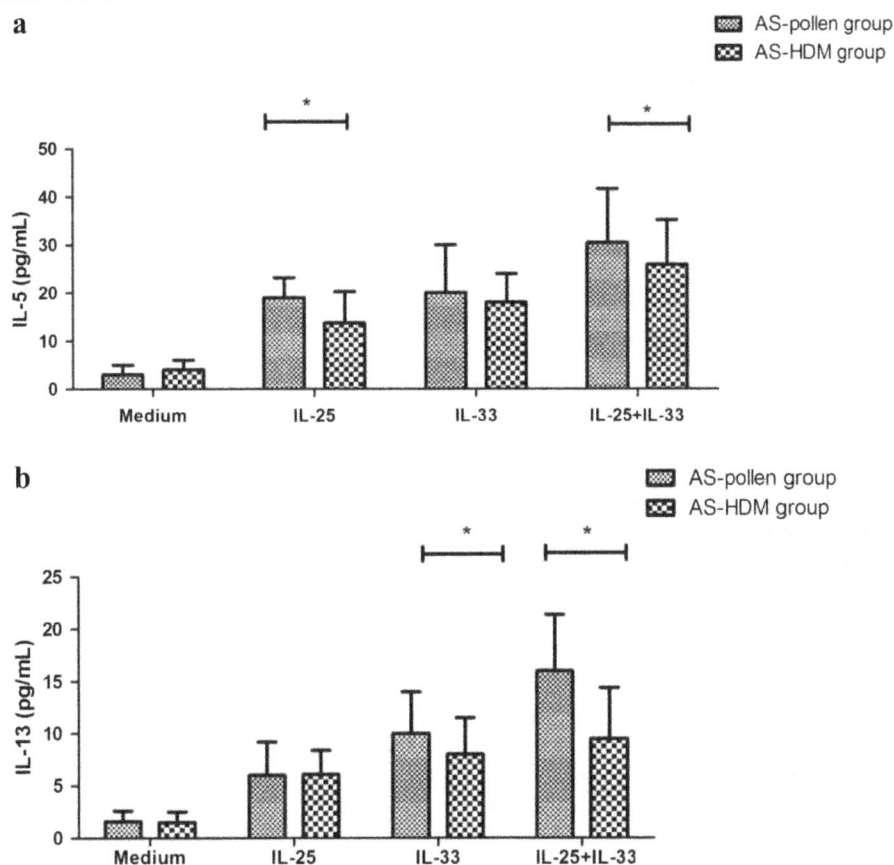

Fig. 6 Distinct cytokines expression from IL-25 and/or IL-33-induced Lineage⁻ cells between pollen-allergic and HDM-allergic asthmatics. The Lineage⁻ cell fraction was isolated from subjects with who were mono-sensitized to pollen (AS-pollen group) and with who were mono-sensitized to HDM (AS-HDM group) and then cultured for 7 days with medium, IL-2 (20 U/mL), IL-33 (25 ng/mL) alone, IL-33 (25 ng/mL) alone or a combination of IL-25 and IL-33. The levels of **a** IL-5 and **b** IL-13 in cell-free supernatants were measured by a Milliplex human cytokine array kit. The lower limit of Multiplex tested for detection was IL-5: 0.6 pg/mL, IL-13: 0.7 pg/mL, respectively). *$P < 0.05$

activation and migration in vitro, and promote the expansion of ILC2s into the airway in the initiation of HDM-induced Th2 immunity [21]. Although in present study the detail mechanism of increased peripheral blood ILC2s remains unclear, it is possible to estimate that mite allergen exposure and its direct interaction with airway epithelial cells could exert an important effect on the generation of peripheral ILC2s.

We further identified that the sorted ILC2s produced IL-5 and IL-13, and demonstrating there was a positive correlation between IL-13⁺ILC2s numbers and FeNO levels in pollen-allergic asthmatics, however, no similar results were found in HDM-allergic asthma patients. Yi et al. had demonstrated that the tendency of IL-13⁺ILC2s percentages was incrementally higher following the enhancement of asthma control levels, and a strong positive relationship was found between IL-13⁺ILC2s and GINA scores, FeNO level, respectively [22]. A recent study showed that after repeated allergen exposure, a

positive feedback between ILC2s and Th2 cell was indispensable for persistent asthma, in which IL-13 produced by ILC2s and Th2 cells further induce IL-33 production and then induce more ILC2 [23]. Therefore, the incidence of IL-13+ ILC2s may provide us with a surrogate marker of the inflammatory status of the disease, and the physiological function of IL13+ ILC2 among asthma patients with distinct clinical characteristic should be further investigated.

Next, we performed subsequent mechanistic studies to investigate whether there were differences in type 2 cytokines production from Lineage-cells among asthmatics sensitized to different allergens, showing that IL-33 can induce a significantly greater release of IL-13 by the Lineage-cells from mugwort pollen-allergic asthmatic compared to that of HDM-allergic asthmatics, whereas a significant elevation in IL-5 release was observed in IL-25-stimualted Lineage⁻cells from mugwort pollen-allergic asthmatic than that from

HDM-allergic asthmatics. Although IL-25 and IL-33 were confirmed to be potent type2-inducing cytokines, experimental mouse studies suggest that IL-33 plays a critical role in the rapid induction of airway contraction by stimulating the prompt expansion of IL-13-producing type 2 innate lymphoid cells, whereas IL-25-induced responses are slower and less potent [24]. In current study, although we did not perform an exact comparison in stimulations magnitude between mugwort pollen and HDM, our findings might raise the possibility that distinct cytokine profiles in airway microenvironment among asthma patients with different sensitized patters could exert different effects on the peripheral ILC2s generation.

In summary, we found that during pollen season there was an elevation in ILC2s in peripheral blood, and a positive relationship between ILC2s and FeNO levels among asthmatics with mugwort pollen-allergy. However, a limitation of the study is its relatively small sample size, which precludes us from performing subgroup analysis. Besides, it has not fully explored the upstream signals in driving circulating ILC2s cell generation and maturation. Clearly, clinical studies with different study designs and larger sample size are necessary to answer the above questions, which could provide insights to understand the immunopathology of asthma and to design of new therapeutic strategies.

Abbreviations
FeNO: fractional exhaled NO; ILC2s: group 2 innate lymphoid cells; EOS: eosinophils.

Authors' contributions
QM study concepts; study design; definition of intellectual content; literature research; clinical studies; statistical analysis; manuscript review. YW and YGL, performing flow cytometry measurement, interpretation of data. YXR patients recruitment and clinical assessment. LI Zhen performing lung function testing. GH acquisition of clinical data. WX study design, patients recruitment and clinical assessment, acquisition of clinical data. LX guarantor of integrity of the entire study; study concepts; study design; definition of intellectual content; manuscript editing. All authors read and approved the final manuscript.

Acknowledgements
Not applicable.
Competing interests
The authors declare that they have no competing interests.

Funding
This work was supported by a grant from Beijing natural science foundation (No. 7172074), from Beijing Municipal Administration of Hospitals Incubating Program (PX2018049), and from the special research grant for non-profit public service (No. 2015SQ00136).

References
1. Borish L. The immunology of asthma: asthma phenotypes and their implications for personalized treatment. Ann Allergy Asthma Immunol. 2016;117(2):108–14.
2. Lambrecht BN, Hammad H. The immunology of asthma. Nat Immunol. 2015;16:45–56.
3. National Cooperative Group on Childhood Asthma, Institute of Environmental Health and Related Product Safety, Chinese Center for Disease Control and Prevention, Chinese Center for Disease Control and Prevention. Third nationwide survey of childhood asthma in urban areas of China. Zhonghua Er Ke Za Zhi. 2013;51(10):729–35 **(Article in Chinese)**.
4. Xiang L, Zhao J, Zheng Y, Liu H, Hong J, Bao Y, Chen A, Deng L, Ji W, Zhong N, Shen K. Uncontrolled asthma and its risk factors in Chinese children: a cross-sectional observational study. J Asthma. 2016;53(7):699–706.
5. Artis D, Spits H. The biology of innate lymphoid cells. Nature. 2015;517:293–301.
6. Kabata H, Moro K, Koyasu S, Asano K. Group 2 innate lymphoid cells and asthma. Allergol Int. 2015;64(3):227–34.
7. Doherty TA, Scott D, Walford HH, Khorram N, Lund S, Baum R, Chang J, Rosenthal P, Beppu A, Miller M, Broide DH. Allergen challenge in allergic rhinitis rapidly induces increased peripheral blood type 2 innate lymphoid cells that express CD84. J Allergy Clin Immunol. 2014;133(4):1203–5.
8. Mjösberg JM, Trifari S, Crellin NK, Peters CP, van Drunen CM, Piet B, Fokkens WJ, Cupedo T, Spits H. Human IL-25- and IL-33-responsive type 2 innate lymphoid cells are defined by expression of CRTH2 and CD161. Nat Immunol. 2011;12(11):1055–62.
9. Spits H, Artis D, Colonna M, Diefenbach A, Di Santo JP, Eberl G, Koyasu S, Locksley RM, McKenzie AN, Mebius RE, Powrie F, Vivier E. Innate lymphoid cells–a proposal for uniform nomenclature. Nat Rev Immunol. 2013;13(2):145–9.
10. Al-Sajee D, Oliveria JP, Sehmi R, Gauvreau GM. Antialarmins for treatment of asthma: future perspectives. Curr Opin Pulm Med. 2017. https://doi.org/10.1097/mcp.0000000000000443 **(Epub ahead of print)**.
11. Dachuan Fan, Xiangdong Wang, Min Wang, Yang Wang, Liang Zhang, Ying Li, Erzhong Fan, Feifei Cao, Koen Van Crombruggen, Luo Zhang. Allergen-dependent differences in ILC2s frequencies in patients with allergic rhinitis. Allergy Asthma Immunol Res. 2016;8(3):216–22.
12. Hirschwehr R, Heppner C, Spitzauer S, Sperr WR, Valent P, Berger U, Horak F, Jäger S, Kraft D, Valenta R. Identification of common allergenic structures in mugwort and ragweed pollen. J Allergy Clin Immunol. 1998;101(2 Pt 1):196–206.
13. Oberhuber C, Ma Y, Wopfner N, Gadermaier G, Dedic A, Niggemann B, Maderegger B, Gruber P, Ferreira F, Scheiner O, Hoffmann-Sommergruber K. Prevalence of IgE-binding to Art v 1, Art v 4 and Amb a 1 in mugwort-allergic patients. Int Arch Allergy Immunol. 2008;145(2):94–101 **(Epub 2007 Sep 7)**.
14. He HJ, Zhang DS, Qiao BS. Preliminary approach of the relationship between Airborne pollen amount and meteorological factors in Beijing urban area. Chin J Microbiol Immunol. 2001;21(S2):31–3 **(Article in Chinese)**.
15. Zhu R, Li W, Wang Z, Chen H, Zhang W, Liu G. A survey of airborne pollen in Wuhan and its relationship to pollinosis. Lin Chung Er Bi Yan Hou Tou Jing Wai Ke Za Zhi. 2008;22(14):647–50 **(Article in Chinese)**.
16. Jahn-Schmid B, Sirven P, Leb V, Pickl WF, Fischer GF, Gadermaier G, Egger M, Ebner C, Ferreira F, Maillére B, Bohle B. Characterization of HLA class II/peptide-TCR interactions of the immunodominant T cell epitope in Art v 1, the major mugwort pollen allergen. J Immunol. 2008;181(5):3636–42.
17. Jahn-Schmid B, Kelemen P, Himly M, Bohle B, Fischer G, Ferreira F, Ebner C. The T cell response to Art v 1, the major mugwort pollen allergen, is dominated by one epitope. J Immunol. 2002;169(10):6005–11.
18. Chen CL, Lee CT, Liu YC, Wang JY, Lei HY, Yu CK. House dust mite Dermatophagoides farinae augments proinflammatory mediator productions and accessory function of alveolar macrophages: implications for allergic sensitization and inflammation. J Immunol. 2003;170:528–36.
19. Yu CK, Chen CL. Activation of mast cells is essential for development of house dust mite Dermatophagoides farinae-induced allergic airway inflammation in mice. J Immunol. 2003;171(7):3808–15.

20. Chu DK, Llop-Guevara A, Walker TD, Flader K, GoncharovaS Boudreau JE, et al. IL-33, but not thymic stromal lymphopoietin or IL-25, is central to mite and peanut allergic sensitization. J Allergy Clin Immunol. 2013;131:187–200.

21. Jia Y, Fang X, Zhu X, Bai C, Zhu L, Jin M, Wang X, Hu M, Tang R, Chen Z. IL-13+ type 2 innate lymphoid cells correlate with asthma control status and treatment response. Am J Respir Cell Mol Biol. 2016;55(5):675–83.

22. Christianson CA, Goplen NP, Zafar I, Irvin C, Good JT Jr, Rollins DR, Gorentla B, Liu W, Gorska MM, Chu H, Martin RJ, Alam R. Persistence of asthma requires multiple feedback circuits involving type 2 innate lymphoid cells and IL-33. J Allergy Clin Immunol. 2015;136(1):59–68.

23. Barlow JL, Peel S, Fox J, Panova V, Hardman CS, Camelo A, Bucks C, Wu X, Kane CM, Neill DR, Flynn RJ, Sayers I, Hall IP, McKenzie AN. IL-33 is more potent than IL-25 in provoking IL-13-producing nuocytes (type 2 innate lymphoid cells) and airway contraction. J Allergy Clin Immunol. 2013;132(4):933–41.

24. Ouyang YH, Zhang DS, Fan EZ, Li Y, Zhang L. Correlation between symptoms of pollen allergic rhinitis and pollen grain spreading in summer and autumn. Zhong hua Er Bi Yan Hou Tou Jing Wai Ke Za Zhi. 2012;47:623–7 **(Article in Chinese)**.

5

Evaluation of eczema, asthma, allergic rhinitis and allergies among the Grade-1 children of Iqaluit

Ahmed Ahmed[1][*] [iD], Amir Hakim[2] and Allan Becker[3]

Abstract

Background: Little is known about the prevalence of asthma, allergic rhinitis, eczema and allergies among Canadian Inuit children, especially those living in the arctic and subarctic areas.

Methods: A cross-sectional study among Grade 1 students attending schools in Iqaluit, the capital of Nunavut, was conducted during the 2015/2016 school year. We used the International Study of Allergy and Asthma in Children questionnaire with added questions relevant to the population. In addition, skin prick tests were conducted to test for sensitization to common food and environmental allergens.

Results: The prevalence of current asthma was 15.9% (> 2:1 males) with the highest prevalence among those with any non-Inuit heritage at 38.5%. The prevalence of current and past allergic rhinitis was 6.8%, also predominant among males, with the lowest prevalence among the mixed ethnicity. Home crowdedness was inversely related to past asthma. Being ever outside Nunavut was associated with higher prevalence of current and past asthma. No statistically significant relationship was found with passive smoking or exclusive breast feeding during the first 4 months of life. The current eczema prevalence was 20.5%, with the highest prevalence recorded among the Inuit at 25% compared to 15.4% among the mixed ethnicity and 14.3% among the non-Inuit. We noted a high rate of sensitization to cat at 26.7% while absent sensitization to other common inhalant allergens.

Conclusion: Variations in the prevalence and risk factors of asthma, allergic rhinitis and eczema among different ethnicities living at the same subarctic environment may be related to genetic, gene-environment interaction and/or lifestyle factors that require further investigation.

Keywords: Asthma, Allergic rhinitis, Eczema, Allergies, Inuit, Nunavut, Subarctic, Children

Background

Little is known about the prevalence of asthma, allergic rhinitis, eczema and allergies among the Canadian Inuit children, especially those living in the Canadian territory of Nunavut. This is the first study addressing that issue among Grade 1 students in Nunavut. Improving our knowledge of those conditions among the Inuit children carries the potential of improving their prevention and management.

Nunavut is a sparsely populated area of arctic and subarctic tundra located above latitude 60° with a surface area of over 2 million sq. km, (800,000 sq. miles) and a population of 36,702 as of January 1, 2015, the vast majority being of indigenous Inuit heritage. Huge areas of its surface are sheathed in ice year-round, having more than 50% of Nunavut's landmass above the Arctic Circle with not a single tree in the entire area. The City of Iqaluit is the capital of Nunavut being the largest community with a population of around 7250. Forty-one percent of the population is under the age of 16. Iqaluit is located at latitude 63°77′North and longitude 68°54′West (Fig. 1). Winters can be very harsh with average temperatures of

*Correspondence: aahm25@uottawa.ca
[1] Department of Pediatrics, University of Ottawa, Ottawa, ON, Canada
Full list of author information is available at the end of the article

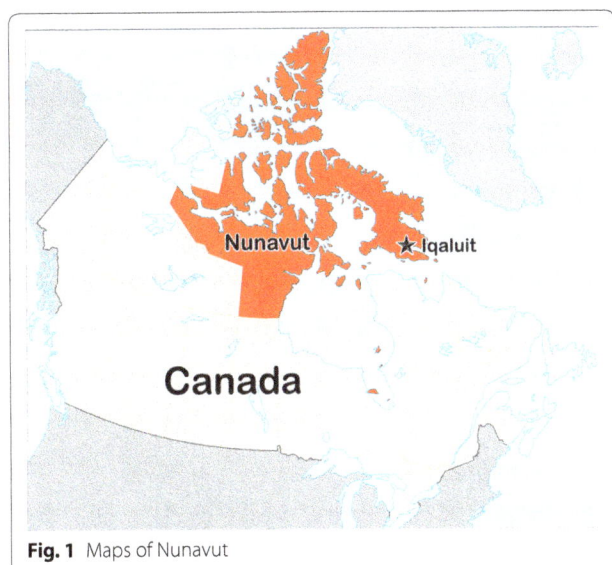

Fig. 1 Maps of Nunavut

− 27 °C in Iqaluit which limits the time of out-door activities for most of the year [1–4].

The International Study of Asthma and Allergies in Childhood (ISAAC) has shown marked variations in the prevalence of atopic diseases between countries and within countries over time [5, 6]. A number of studies have also reported a higher prevalence of allergy and eczema in colder, more northern regions [7–11].

There is a wide variation in the prevalence of asthma in Canada as found by Hong-Yu Wang et al. with the highest prevalence of asthma in Halifax at 33%, was more than double the lowest found in Vancouver at 13.7% [12]. The ISAAC study has never been conducted in Nunavut. Forsey found an eczema rate of 16.5% among Inuit children (age 2–12 years) in the Labrador area (a province south eastern to Nunavut with an Inuit minority). Two-thirds of these children presented with moderate or severe eczema, with a high female/male ratio of 2:1. Food specific IgE antibody assays showed that 32, 23, and 5% of Inuit children with eczema were sensitized to egg, milk, and wheat, respectively, while none of the controls were sensitized [13].

Asthma and allergies are among the most common chronic conditions reported by parents/guardians of indigenous children under the age of 6 years [14, 15]. Chang et al. found that children and adults with Inuit ancestry, but living outside Nunavut and off the First Nations reserves in other provinces, had a significantly lower prevalence of asthma and allergies compared to children from other indigenous groups [16].

In a study of Inuit school children in northern Quebec (a Canadian province southern to Nunavut), specific sensitization to dust mite was very unusual with almost complete absence of mite allergen in house dust (none of 50 dust samples taken from the mattress or bedroom floor contained 1 mg or more of allergen per gram of dust) [17]. Alaskan native children residing in rural Alaska have a low prevalence of allergic sensitization to inhalant allergens [18].

There is an increased burden of Tuberculosis (TB) among children in Nunavut, where over 12% of their reported cases were pediatric cases, compared to 7% for Canada [19]. All children born in Nunavut are eligible to receive the Bacille Calmette–Guérin (BCG) vaccine at birth. Many studies have tried to determine whether a relationship exists between TB infection, BCG vaccine and the prevalence of atopic diseases but reported inconsistent findings [20–23].

This study was part of a bigger research project (evaluation of eczema, asthma and allergies among the children of Iqaluit; EAACI). It also investigated if there is any discrepancy between the Inuit and non-Inuit children living in the same harsh environment as well as any possible relation to certain risk/protecting factors.

Methods

The city of Iqaluit was chosen because it is the most populated city in Nunavut so that a larger cohort can be studied. The study was approved by the Research Ethics Board at the University of Manitoba and received permission from the Nunavut Research Institute.

Study design

The study was conducted between November 2015 and February 2016 at the Qikiqtani General Hospital (Iqaluit). It is cross-sectional with the study population being all Grade 1 students attending the four elementary schools at Iqaluit during the academic year 2015/2016, a total of one hundred and thirty students, with no exclusion criteria. The families were contacted multiple times over 2 months through the schools by delivery of the study invitation and questionnaire to the students and over the phone by the study assistants. Because of major concerns expressed related to the issue of research conducted during the era of residential schools and clearly un-ethical aspects of that research, we were not allowed any other form of recruitment. The study included two components; a questionnaire and skin prick testing.

The questionnaire

A questionnaire of 30 questions (see Additional file 1: Appendix S1) adopted with modification from the ISAAC study with additional questions relevant to the Nunavut population including locally applicable risk factors (see Additional file 2: Appendix S2). The consent form and assent form were available in English and Inuktitut languages, all the parents were satisfied to use the English one. Two study coordinators were hired, one is a local

Inuit that speaks Inuktitut, to minimize the language barrier bias, and however, most of the Inuit in Iqaluit are fluent in English.

The skin prick test

The skin testing was performed to 14 common allergens (food and inhalant), see Additional file 3: Appendix S3. It was performed and interpreted by Dr. Ahmed Ahmed at the Qikiqtani General Hospital outpatient clinic over 2 days in February 2016. The skin prick epicutaneous testing was performed to a variety of common food and inhalant allergens with positive histamine and negative saline controls. The allergen extracts and the testing devices were products of Lincoln Diagnostics, New York, USA (ALK-Abello Pharmaceuticals, Inc, Mississauga, Ontario, Canada).

The food extracts included common six food allergens: cow's milk, soy, egg white, wheat, peanut and tree nut mix (equal portions of almond, Brazil nut, pecan nut and pistachio). The answered questionnaires did not have evidence for fish or shellfish allergy and these were not included in the food panel. The environmental inhalant allergens included tree mix (nine equal parts of Alder, Ash, Elm, Birch, Maple, Hickory, Oak, Poplar and Sycamore trees), Grass mix [mixture of five standardized grass pollens: Timothy (*Phleum pratense*), Orchard (*Dactylis glomerata*), June (*Poa pratensis*), Redtop (*Agrostis alba*) and Sweet Vernal (*Anthoxanthum odoratum*)], Ragweed mix (two equal parts of short and tall ragweed), Weed mix (four equal parts of Rough, Pigweed, English plantain and Lamb's quarters), Mold mix (four equal parts of Alternaria, Sphaerospermum, Mixed-Aspergillus and Mixed-Penicillium), House dust mite (HDM) (two equal parts of Dermatophagoides pteronyssinus and Dermatophagoides farinae), cat (standardized cat pelt) and dog Epithelium. Histamine (10 mg/mL) and saline solution (0.9%) were used as positive and negative controls, respectively. On the day of testing, the skin prick testing method and consent forms were reviewed with the parent and the child. In addition, an assent form was discussed with the child with either a verbal or written assent confirmed.

The skin prick test was epicutaneous and read at 15–20 min by Dr. Ahmed. A wheal with a mean diameter of at least 3 mm greater than the saline control was considered positive. There were no negative histamine control or any positive saline control.

Data analysis

The statistical analyses was performed using IBM SPSS v.22 (BM Corp. Released 2013. IBM SPSS Statistics for Windows, Version 22.0. Armonk, NY: IBM Corp.)

Data were analyzed using correlations, cross tabulations (Chi square; Fisher's exact test), and cross tabulations with risk analyses (odds ratios, 95% confidence interval).

Results

There were 130 Grade 1 students in Iqaluit at the time of the study. Forty-four families (33.8%) provided consent for the child to be enrolled in the study (all of them agreed to participate in both parts of the study; the questionnaire and the skin prick test) but only thirty children (23.1% of the total cohort) attended the skin prick testing despite a reminder call a day earlier.

Study demographics

The ethnic distribution of participants who completed the questionnaire (44 cases) was as follows: Inuit 54.5%, non-Inuit 15.9% and mixed ethnicity (one of the parents is Inuit) 29.5%. Of those who attended the skin prick test, 56.7% were Inuit, 20% non-Inuit and 23.3% of the mixed ethnicity. There were 26 males and 18 females.

Asthma prevalence

Following a standard ISAAC approach, based on the ISAAC questionnaire primary question, the prevalence of current asthma was 15.9% and the male to female ratio was 2.5:1 (Table 1). The prevalence of current asthma in this population was highest among those children of mixed ethnicity at 38.5% and lowest among the Inuit at 4.2% with prevalence amongst non-Inuit of 14.3%, this difference among ethnicities was statistically significant (Fisher's exact test 6.798 and p = 0.016)

One quarter of the 44 participants had a previous history of asthma, highest among the mixed ethnicity at 46.2% and lowest among the non-Inuit at 14.3% Inuit at 16.7% (Fig. 2).

Prevalence of allergic rhinitis

The prevalence of both past and current allergic rhinitis was 6.8% (Fig. 3).

Interestingly, only Inuit children had a current diagnosis of allergic rhinitis, whereas both Inuit and non-Inuit children only had a past history consistent with allergic rhinitis. The prevalence of current allergic rhinitis amongst Inuit children was 12.5% of the enrolled Inuit students. The male to female ratio was 2:1. The overall prevalence of past allergic rhinitis was 6.8% with two-thirds of the cases amongst Inuit children and one-third amongst non-Inuit. Prevalence of past or current allergic rhinitis amongst mixed-ethnicity children was zero. The prevalence of past allergic rhinitis among the non-Inuit was higher than the Inuit, 14.3% compared to 8.3%. The male to female ratio was 2:1 (Table 2).

Table 1 Summary of the findings in relation to current and past asthma

The questionnaire was completed by 44 subjects	Current asthma	Past asthma
Male:female	5:2	7:4
Odds ratio	1.91	1.29
95% CI	[0.33, 11.12]	[0.32, 5.28]
Ethnicity	1 (4.2)	4 (16.7)
Inuit, n (%)	5 (38.5)	6 (46.2)
Mixed, n (%)	1 (14.3)	1 (14.3)
Non-Inuit, n (%)	7 (15.9)	11 (25.0)
Total, n (%)	6.80 (0.02)	3.96 (0.15)
Chi square (p-value)		
Smoker in the home (yes:no)	3:4	4:7
Odds ratio	1.39	1.0
95% CI	[0.27, 7.15]	[0.24, 4.13]
Crowdedness correlation (p)	0.165 (0.29)	0.285 (0.06)
Cat owner (yes:no)	1:3	1:5
Odds ratio	3.0	1.60
95% CI	[0.20, 44.36]	[0.12, 21.59]
Dog owner (yes:no)	2:3	4:5
Odds ratio	1.0	1.28
95% CI	[0.15, 6.91]	[0.28, 5.93]
Exclusive breast feeding (yes:no)	4:3	5:6
Odds ratio	0.81	0.42
95% CI	[0.16, 4.18]	[0.10, 1.67]
Being ever outside Nunavut (yes:no)	7:0	11:00
Odds ratio	n/a	n/a
95% CI	n/a	n/a
Previous respiratory hospitalization (yes:no)	2:5	3:8
Odds ratio	1.71	1.69
95% CI	[0.27, 10.74]	[0.34, 8.31]
TB vaccination (yes:no)	6:0	9:1
Odds ratio	n/a	0.96
95% CI	n/a	[0.09, 10.45]
Family history of food allergy (yes:no)	1:4	2:6
Odds ratio	1.04	1.5
95% CI	[0.10, 10.77]	[0.24, 9.34]
Family history of environmental allergy (yes:no)	1:4	4:4
Odds ratio	0.63	3.57
95% CI	[0.6, 6.30]	[0.71, 18.04]
Family history of asthma (yes:no)	2:4	4:5
Odds ratio	3.1	8.0
95% CI	[0.44, 21.63]	[1.36, 47.02]
Family history of eczema (yes:no)	3:4	5:5
Odds ratio	2.25	3.71
95% CI	[0.42, 12.03]	[0.83, 16.55]

CI confidence interval

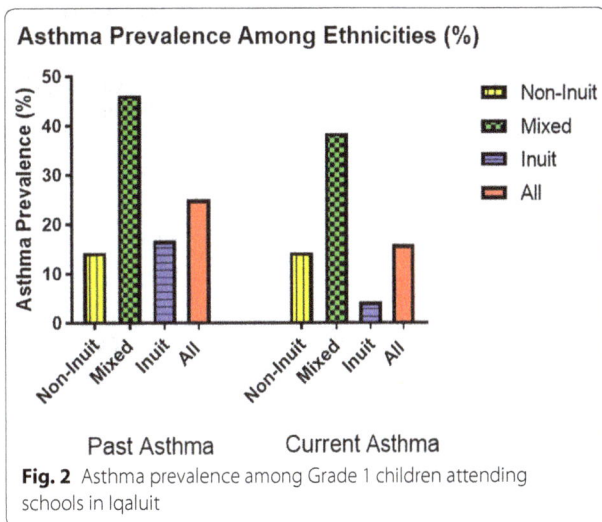

Fig. 2 Asthma prevalence among Grade 1 children attending schools in Iqaluit

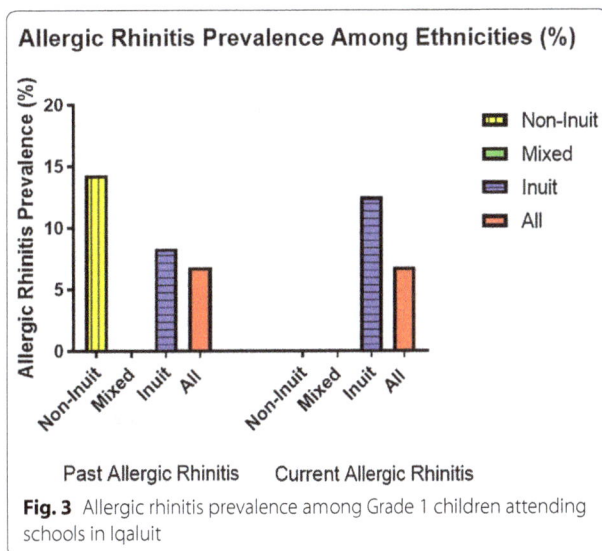

Fig. 3 Allergic rhinitis prevalence among Grade 1 children attending schools in Iqaluit

Prevalence of eczema

The prevalence of current eczema amongst the 44 Grade 1 children was 20.5%, with two-thirds of the cases amongst Inuit children (Fig. 4). Specifically, prevalence amongst Inuit, mixed ethnicity and non-Inuit was as follows 25, 15.4 and 14.3%. The male to female ratio was 1:1.25. In contrast, prevalence of past eczema amongst Inuit, mixed ethnicity and non-Inuit were as follows, 20.8, 23.1 and 28.5%, respectively. The male to female ratio was 1:1 (Table 3).

Prevalence of reported food and environmental allergy

The prevalence of a history of food allergy as reported by parents was 11.4%, with the highest prevalence among the non-Inuit at 14.3% followed by the Inuit at 8.3% (Fig. 5). Whereas, prevalence of food allergy amongst the

Table 2 Summary of the findings in relation to current and past allergic rhinitis

The questionnaire was completed by 44 subjects	Current allergic rhinitis	Past allergic rhinitis
Male:female	2:1	2:1
Odds ratio	1.42	1.42
95% CI	[0.12, 16.91]	[0.12, 16.91]
Ethnicity		
Inuit, n (%)	3 (12.5)	2 (8.3)
Mixed, n (%)	0	0
Non-Inuit, n (%)	0	1 (14.3)
Total, n (%)	3 (6.8)	3 (6.8)
Chi square (p-value)	1.69 (0.56)	1.78 (0.41)
Smoker (yes:no)	2:1	1:2
Odds ratio	3.86	0.87
95% CI	[0.32, 46.32]	[0.07, 10.38]
Crowdedness correlation (p)	− 0.225 (0.14)	− 0.176 (0.25)
Cat owner (yes:no)	0:0	1:0
Odds ratio	n/a	n/a
95% CI	n/a	n/a
Dog owner (yes:no)	2:0	1:0
Odds ratio	n/a	n/a
95% CI	n/a	n/a
Exclusive breast feeding (yes:no)	1:2	1:2
Odds ratio	0.29	0.29
95% CI	[0.02, 3.46]	[0.02, 3.46]
Being ever outside Nunavut (yes:no)	3:0	3:0
Odds ratio	n/a	n/a
95% CI	n/a	n/a
Previous respiratory hospitalization (yes:no)	1:2	1:2
Odds ratio	2.06	2.06
95% CI	[0.17, 25.68]	[0.17, 25.68]
TB vaccination (yes:no)	3:0	3:0
Odds ratio	n/a	n/a
95% CI	n/a	n/a
Family history of food allergy (yes:no)	1:1	0:2
Odds ratio	4.57	n/a
95% CI	[0.25, 82.25]	n/a
Family history of environmental allergy (yes:no)	1:1	0:2
Odds ratio	2.80	n/a
95% CI	[0.16, 49.10]	n/a
Family history of asthma (yes:no)	2:1	1:2
Odds ratio	13.6	2.75
95% CI	[1.03, 179.03]	[0.21, 35.33]
Family history of eczema (yes:no)	2:1	1:2
Odds ratio	6.0	1.32
95% CI	[0.49, 73.45]	[0.11, 16.04]

CI confidence interval

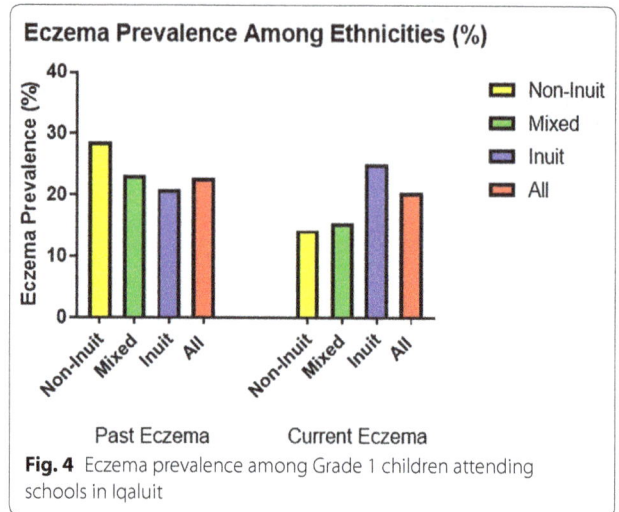

Fig. 4 Eczema prevalence among Grade 1 children attending schools in Iqaluit

mixed population was 7.7%. The male to female ratio was 1:1.5. On the contrary, the prevalence of a history of environmental allergy as reported by parents was 4.5%, none of them were non-Inuit children, while the prevalence among the mixed ethnicity was 7.7% and among the Inuit 4.2%. The male to female ratio was 1:1 (Table 4).

Prevalence of smoking and hospitalization due to a respiratory condition

Having at least one smoker living in the household was 36.4% with the highest rate among the mixed ethnicity at 53.8% while lower among the Inuit at 33.3% and the least among non-Inuit at 14.3% (Fig. 6). No statistically significant relationship was found between current or past asthma and having a smoker at home.

None of the non-Inuit students have been previously hospitalized due to bronchiolitis or respiratory infections, on the other side, one-quarter of the Inuit students had a history of at least one admission and a similar rate of 23.1% among the mixed ethnicity.

Prevalence of breast feeding

Almost two-thirds (61.4%) of the children were exclusively breastfed during the first 4 months of life, with a higher percentage among the non-Inuit children at 71.4% while 61.5% among the mixed ethnicity and a little bit lower among the Inuit students at 58.3%. No statistically significant relationship was found between exclusive breastfeeding during the first 4 months of life and asthma, allergic rhinitis or eczema.

Pet ownership

Having a dog at home was relatively common at 40.9% with the highest rate among the mixed ethnicity at 61.5% followed by the Inuit at 33.3% and lastly by the non-Inuit

Table 3 Summary of the findings in relation to current and past eczema

The questionnaire was completed by 44 subjects	Current eczema	Past eczema
Male:female	4:5	1:1
Odds ratio	0.47	0.62
95% CI	[0.11, 2.08]	[0.15, 2.56]
Ethnicity		
Inuit, n (%)	6 (25)	5 (20.8)
Mixed, n (%)	2 (15.4)	3 (23.1)
Non-Inuit, n (%)	1 (14.3)	2 (28.6)
Total, n (%)	9 (20.5)	10 (22.7)
Chi square (p-value)	0.58 (0.88)	0.45 (0.89)
Smoker (yes:no)	3:6	4:6
Odds ratio	0.85	1.22
95% CI	[0.18, 3.97]	[0.29, 5.20]
Crowdedness correlation (p)	− 0.135 (0.38)	0.047 (0.76)
Cat owner (yes:no)	0:2	1:3
Odds ratio	n/a	3.0
95% CI	n/a	[0.20, 44.36]
Dog owner (yes:no)	6:2	5:3
Odds ratio	7.13	3.33
95% CI	[1.18, 43.14]	[0.65, 17.18]
Exclusive breast feeding (yes:no)	4:5	6:4
Odds ratio	0.42	0.93
95% CI	[0.09, 1.85]	[0.22, 3.93]
Being ever outside Nunavut (yes:no)	7:2	9:1
Odds ratio	1.26	3.91
95% CI	[.22, 7.23]	[.44, 35.15]
Previous respiratory hospitalization (yes:no)	3:6	3:7
Odds ratio	2.42	2.00
95% CI	[0.47, 12.47]	[0.40, 10.05]
TB vaccination (yes:no)	8:0	9:1
Odds ratio	n/a	0.96
95% CI	n/a	[0.09, 10.45]
Family history of food allergy (yes:no)	2:5	2:6
Odds ratio	1.87	1.5
95% CI	[0.29, 12.01]	[0.24, 9.34]
Family history of environmental allergy (yes:no)	3:4	5:3
Odds ratio	2.34	7.22
95% CI	[0.43, 12.77]	[1.34, 38.92]
Family history of asthma (yes:no)	3:5	3:6
Odds ratio	4.5	3.63
95% CI	[0.77, 26.45]	[0.64, 20.57]
Family history of eczema (yes:no)	5:4	6:4
Odds ratio	4.82	6.75
95% CI	[1.02, 22.84]	[1.44, 36.60]

CI confidence interval

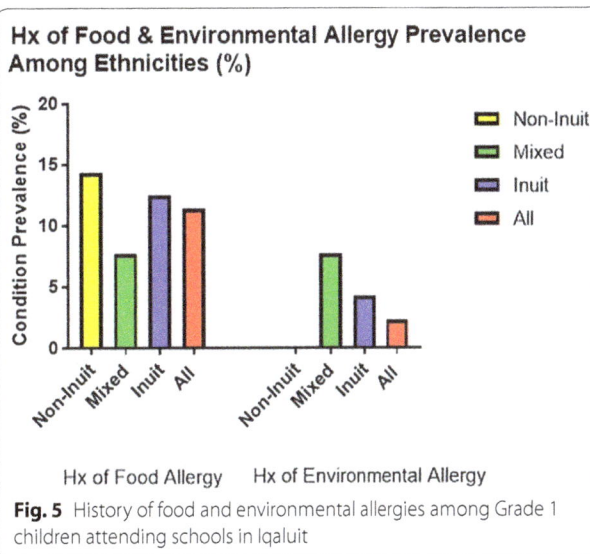

Fig. 5 History of food and environmental allergies among Grade 1 children attending schools in Iqaluit

at 28.6% (Fig. 7). A completely different picture was noticed in regard to having a cat at home with a general rate of 15.9%, with the highest among the non-Inuit at 57% compared with the Inuit at 4.2% while the mixed ethnicity at 15.4%.

No statistically significant relationship was found between pet ownership and asthma or allergic rhinitis. Three-quarters of those with current eczema had a dog at their home (OR 7.13, CI 1.18–43.14). Interestingly, none of those with current eczema have a cat at home. Almost two-thirds (62%) of those with past eczema had a dog at their home while only a quarter have a cat.

Having a family history of eczema was a risk factor to had a current eczema (OR 4.82, CI 1.02–22.84) and past eczema (OR 6.75, CI 1.44–31.60).

Family history of environmental allergy was associated with having past eczema (OR 4.39, CI 1.26–15.37).

No statistically significant relationship was found between exclusive breastfeeding during the first 4 months of life and having current or past eczema.

None of those who were not BCG vaccinated had current eczema. (OR 0.78, CI 0.66–0.93).

Prevalence of sensitization to the tested food

The prevalence of allergy to egg white as confirmed by history and skin prick testing is 3.3%, with that single case being a non-Inuit. The prevalence of allergy to peanut as confirmed by history and skin prick testing is 3.3%, with that single case being an Inuit. The prevalence of allergy to tree nuts as confirmed by history and skin prick testing is 6.7%, none of them was non-Inuit. None of those that were allergic to egg white, peanut or tree nut had current asthma or eczema. No child was sensitized to cow's milk, soy or wheat.

Table 4 Summary of the findings in relation to reported history of food and environmental allergies

The questionnaire was completed by 44 subjects	Reported food allergy	Reported environmental allergy
Male:female	2:3	1:1
Odds ratio	0.42	0.68
95% CI	[0.06, 2.79]	[0.04, 11.63]
Ethnicity		
Inuit, n (%)	3 (12.5)	1 (4.2)
Mixed, n (%)	1 (7.7)	1 (7.7)
Non-Inuit, n (%)	1 (14.3)	Zero
Total, n (%)	5 (11.4)	2 (4.5)
Chi square (p-value)	0.559 (1.0)	0.913 (1.0)
Smoker(s) at home (yes:no)	3:2	1:1
Odds ratio	3.00	1.80
95% CI	[0.45, 20.24]	[0.11, 30.90]
Crowdedness correlation (p)	− 0.172 (0.27)	− 0.128 (0.41)
Cat ownership (yes:no)	1:2	0:0
Odds ratio	4.75	n/a
95% CI	[0.29, 78.74]	n/a
Dog ownership (yes:no)	1:2	1:0
Odds ratio	0.73	n/a
95% CI	[0.06, 8.92]	n/a
Exclusive breast feeding (yes:no)	2:3	0:2
Odds ratio	0.37	n/a
95% CI	[0.06, 2.51]	n/a
Being ever outside Nunavut (yes:no)	4:1	2:0
Odds ratio	1.43	n/a
95% CI	[0.14, 14.35]	n/a
Previous respiratory hospitalization (yes:no)	1:4	2:0
Odds ratio	0.97	n/a
95% CI	[0.10, 9.91]	n/a
TB vaccination (yes:no)	5:0	2:0
Odds ratio	n/a	n/a
95% CI	n/a	n/a
Family history of food allergy (yes:no)	0:4	0:0
Odds ratio	n/a	n/a
95% CI	n/a	n/a
Family history of environmental allergy (yes:no)	0:4	0:0
Odds ratio	n/a	n/a
95% CI	n/a	n/a
Family history of asthma (yes:no)	2:3	1:0
Odds ratio	4.27	n/a
95% CI	[0.57, 32.24]	n/a
Family history of eczema (yes:no)	1:4	2:0
Odds ratio	0.61	n/a
95% CI	[0.06, 6.13]	n/a

CI confidence interval

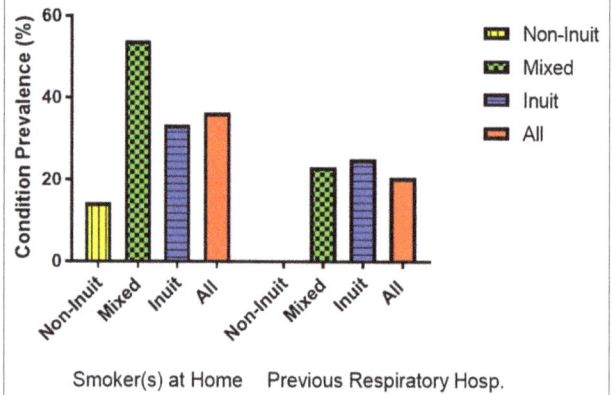

Fig. 6 The prevalence of having smoker(s) at home and history of previous respiratory hospitalization among Grade 1 children attending schools in Iqaluit

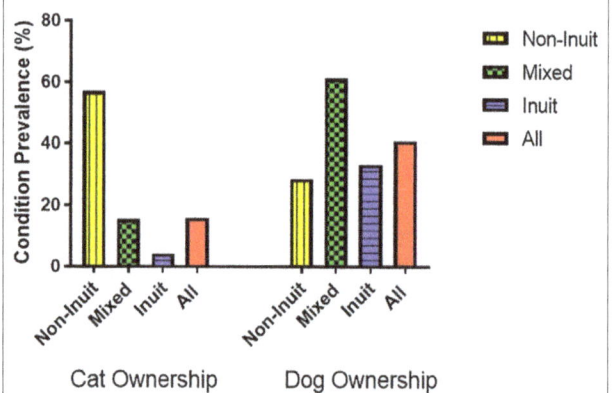

Fig. 7 The prevalence of having a pet among Grade 1 children attending schools in Iqaluit

Prevalence of sensitization to the tested environmental allergens

The prevalence of sensitization to cat was surprisingly high at 26.7% with the highest prevalence among the non-Inuit at 50% followed by the Inuit at 23.5% then the mixed ethnicity at 14.3%. The prevalence of sensitization to tree pollen was 13.3%, none of them was non-Inuit with the highest prevalence among the mixed ethnicity at 42.9% while only 5.9% among the Inuit

(Fisher's exact test 5.130, p = 0.06). On the other hand, the prevalence of sensitization to grass was low at 6.7%, with higher prevalence among the mixed ethnicity at 14.3% compared to 5.9% among the Inuit (Table 5). No child was sensitized to house dust mite, mold, weed, ragweed or dog.

Environmental exposures

Almost three-quarters of the 44 Grade 1 children (72.7%) had been at least once outside Nunavut. The rate was double amongst male students compared to females, with the highest, as expected, among the non-Inuit children at 100% with mixed ethnicity at 92.3% and Inuit lowest at 54%.

Those children with current asthma were less likely to have never been outside Nunavut [11 out of 43 were never outside Nunavut and has no current asthma, OR 0.78, CI 0.65–0.94; and the same applies to those with past asthma (OR 0.66, CI 0.51–0.84)] (Table 1).

Three-quarters of those sensitized to trees were ever outside Nunavut while none of those sensitized to grass were ever outside Nunavut. 88% of those sensitized to cat have were outside Nunavut.

Table 5 **Summary of the findings in relation to positive skin prick tests (environmental)**

	Skin prick test tree	Skin prick test grass	Skin prick test cat
Male:female	3:1	2:0	5:3
Odds ratio	2.20	n/a	1.15
95% CI	[0.20, 24.09]	n/a	[0.22, 6.10]
Ethnicity			
Inuit, n (%)	1 (5.9)	1 (5.9)	4 (23.5)
Mixed, n (%)	3 (42.9)	1 (14.3)	1 (14.3)
Non-Inuit, n (%)	0	0	3 (50.0)
Total, n (%)	4 (13.3)	2 (6.7)	8 (26.7)
Chi square (p-value)	5.13 (0.06)	1.30 (0.69)	2.15 (0.39)
Smoker(s) at home (yes:no)	1:1	1:1	3:5
Odds ratio	1.6	1.5	0.87
95% CI	[0.19, 13.24]	[0.09,27.36]	[0.16, 4.58]
Crowdedness correlation (p)	0.010 (0.95)	− 0.160 (0.40)	0.010 (0.94)
Cat ownership (yes:no)	0:0	0:1	2:1
Odds ratio	n/a	n/a	24.0
95% CI	n/a	n/a	[1.03, 560.2]
Dog ownership (yes:no)	3:0	1:1	5:1
Odds ratio	n/a	1.20	10.00
95% CI	n/a	[0.07, 21.72]	[0.94, 105.92]
Exclusive breast feeding (yes:no)	1:3	0:2	1:1
Odds ratio	0.29	n/a	1.0
95% CI	[0.03, 3.12]	n/a	[0.20, 5.05]
Being ever outside Nunavut (yes:no)	3:1	0:2	7:1
Odds ratio	1.33	n/a	4.0
95% CI	[0.12, 14.87]	n/a	[0.41, 38.65]
Previous respiratory hospitalization (yes:no)	1:1	0:2	1:7
Odds ratio	7.67	n/a	0.64
95% CI	[0.77, 76.45]	n/a	[0.06, 6.80]
TB vaccination (yes:no)	3:1	2:0	7:0
Odds ratio	0.14	n/a	n/a
95% CI	[0.01, 2.80]	n/a	n/a
Family history of food allergy (yes:no)	1:1	0:2	1:6
Odds ratio	4.20	n/a	0.53
95% CI	[0.22, 79.32]	n/a	[0.05, 5.55]
Family history of environmental allergy (yes:no)	1:1	0:2	0:7
Odds ratio	3.17	n/a	n/a
95% CI	[0.17, 58.70]	n/a	n/a
Family history of asthma (yes:no)	1:2	0:2	0:7
Odds ratio	2.10	n/a	n/a
95% CI	[0.16, 28.02]	n/a	n/a
Family history of eczema (yes:no)	1:1	0:2	0:7
Odds ratio	3.17	n/a	n/a
95% CI	[0.17, 58.70]	n/a	n/a

n/a not applicable, *CI* confidence interval

The average figure for crowdedness index at households (the number of tenants divided by the number of bedrooms) was about 1.65 for all the students enrolled in the study, with both the non-Inuit and mixed ethnicities below that average at 1.37 and 1.49 respectively while the Inuit students lived in a more crowded houses with the average index of 1.82. The crowdedness tended to be inversely related to having past asthma (Pearson correlation 0.285, p = 0.061) (Table 1).

Ninety percent of the students were vaccinated against TB, this included 100% of the Inuit children, 84.6% of the mixed ethnicity and 71.4% of the non-Inuit students. Having the BCG vaccine was associated with having current asthma, none of those who were not BCG vaccinated (4 students) had current asthma (OR 0.84, CI 0.73–0.97).

No statistically significant relationship was found between family history of asthma and having current asthma, while there was a positive relationship between having a family history of asthma and having past asthma (OR 8.0, CI 1.36–47.02).

Interestingly, none of those reported to have food allergy had a family history of food allergy (OR 1.18, CI 1.02–1.36).

No statistically significant relationship was found between exclusive breastfeeding during the first 4 months of life and the various studied allergy conditions. Though, it is worth mentioning that three-quarters of those sensitized to trees and all those sensitized to grass, peanut and tree nuts were not exclusively breastfed during the first 4 months of life.

All those sensitized to tree pollen have a dog and 83% of those sensitized to cat have a dog at home. Only a quarter of those sensitized to cat have a cat at home while two-thirds of those having a cat at home are sensitized to cats (OR 24, CI 1.03–560.18).

One-third of those sensitized to trees had a family history of asthma while none of those sensitized to grass had a family history of asthma. None of those sensitized to cat had a family history of asthma (OR 1.44, CI 1.10–1.88).

Sensitization to trees was highly associated with having current asthma, eczema, and allergic rhinitis, while sensitization to grass was only associated with having current eczema. The sensitization to cats was associated more with current eczema followed by asthma and lastly allergic rhinitis.

All those found to be allergic to egg white, peanut and tree nut had no family history of food or environmental allergy. Similarly, none of those sensitized to grass had a family history of environmental allergy and none of those sensitized to cat had a family history of environmental allergy (OR 1.54, CI 1.12–2.12).

Discussion

For the first time, our study shows that the prevalence of asthma and allergic rhinitis among children, aged 6–7 years, in Iqaluit is 15.9 and 6.8%, respectively. Interestingly, this is not substantively different from the prevalence of these conditions in the rest of Canada (18.2 and 10.8%, respectively) [24]. The ethnic distribution of the participants in this study was representative of the actual ethnic distribution in the city of Iqaluit. Of those who completed the questionnaire 54.5% were Inuit, 29.5% were of mixed ethnicity and 15.9% were non-Inuit. Statistics Canada [25] considers any individual who has at least one parent with Inuit ancestry as an Inuit. If the above classification was adopted in our study this would suggest that 84% among the participants were Inuit, which goes with their percentage in the city of Iqaluit [2]. The findings in this study do show a much higher prevalence of asthma and special characteristics that define this mixed ethnicity group in relation to lifestyle (crowdedness, passive smoking, ever being outside Nunavut and dog ownership). However, it must be noted that the non-Inuit ethnicity does not actually represent a single ethnicity, it is mainly comprised of White Canadians (most originate from western Europe) in addition to a few other ethnicities (personal observation).

In this study, the prevalence of current asthma was statistically significantly different among the three ethnic groups, Inuit, mixed ethnicity and non-Inuit with the highest among the mixed ethnicity group at 38.5% while the least among the Inuit group at 4.2%. Asthma was reported at a similar low rate of 4% among the Inuit children as documented by the 2007–2008 health survey which also relied on parental reporting [26]. Furthermore, Chang et al. found that children with Inuit ancestry living outside Nunavut had a significantly lower prevalence of asthma than those with North American Indian and Métis ancestries [16]. The prevalence of current and ever asthma among all Aboriginal children combined was 5.7 and 14.3%, respectively. Also, similar to our study findings, the prevalence of ever asthma was greater in boys than in girls [16]. The findings of this study are in agreement with previously reported studies, where Aboriginal children (5.7%) had significantly lower levels of asthma prevalence than non-Aboriginal children (10.0%) in northern Canada [27].

The reported prevalence of lifetime wheeze among children in the southern warmer Canadian city of Toronto was 29.2%, while 14.2% reported wheeze in the past 12 months [28]. Habbik et al. has shown wide variation in asthma prevalence among Grade 1 children in different Canadian cities. Lifetime prevalence of asthma was documented as 17.2% in Hamilton and 11.2% in Saskatoon. The prevalence of wheezing in the 12 months before the survey among the children aged 6–7 years was 20.1% in Hamilton and 14.1% in Saskatoon, with the male to female ratio of 1.5:1 [29].

Interestingly, self-reported asthma among school children living in another arctic region, Norway, was similar to the prevalence observed among the non-Inuit population in Nunavut in our study [8]. A similar (to the Inuit) low rate of asthma (3.9%) was reported in Nikel, a Russian arctic city [30].

The prevalence of current allergic rhinitis is low at 6.8%, all of the reported cases were Inuit and constituting 12.5% of the enrolled Inuit students with male predominance, which is less than the reported 14.6–22.6% found in five other southern Canadian cities [12]. This difference is most likely due to less allergen exposure in Nunavut and that the above study was conducted among older children (13–14 year-old). Again, our findings were similar to the low rate of allergic rhinitis (13.9%) that was reported in Nikel, a Russian arctic city [30]. This disparity in regional variations in the prevalence rates suggests dissimilar risk factors for the development or expression of wheezing (asthma), allergic rhinitis and atopic eczema [12].

The prevalence of past allergic rhinitis was also 6.8% but being higher among the non-Inuit compared to the Inuit, 14.3 and 8.3% respectively with male predominance as well. This higher prevalence of previous allergic rhinitis among the non-Inuit could be attributed to transient symptoms when travelling outside Nunavut or being living outside Nunavut earlier in life because of an exposure to a triggering allergen that is absent or less abundant in Nunavut. It may also be due to a different mechanism behind the development of those symptoms, knowing that the non-Inuit showed less sensitization to most of the major environmental allergens that exist in the south.

Repeated cross-sectional surveys in a subarctic population in northern Norway between 1985 and 2008 demonstrated an increase in the prevalence of asthma and allergic rhinoconjunctivitis ever among school children (7–14 years) [11], this emphasizes the need for follow-up studies.

Our study findings go with the Kovesi et al. finding that the Inuit infants have extremely high rates of lower respiratory tract infections with 25% of the children had, at some time, been hospitalized for chest illness [31], interestingly, this was not associated with higher prevalence of subsequent asthma.

The finding that the Inuit are living in more crowded houses was not a surprise, a previous study of the indoor quality of Inuit houses in Nunavut have found that the mean number of occupants per house in Nunavut was 6.1 people [32]. The higher crowdedness being associated with not having previous asthma, see Fig. 8. While the hygiene hypothesis can be used to explain this; having a crowded household increases the respiratory infections and decreases asthma, on the other hand, such a higher rate of respiratory infections is expected to lead to more wheezes earlier in life which may lead to either a higher prevalence of atopy if infections were mainly RSV

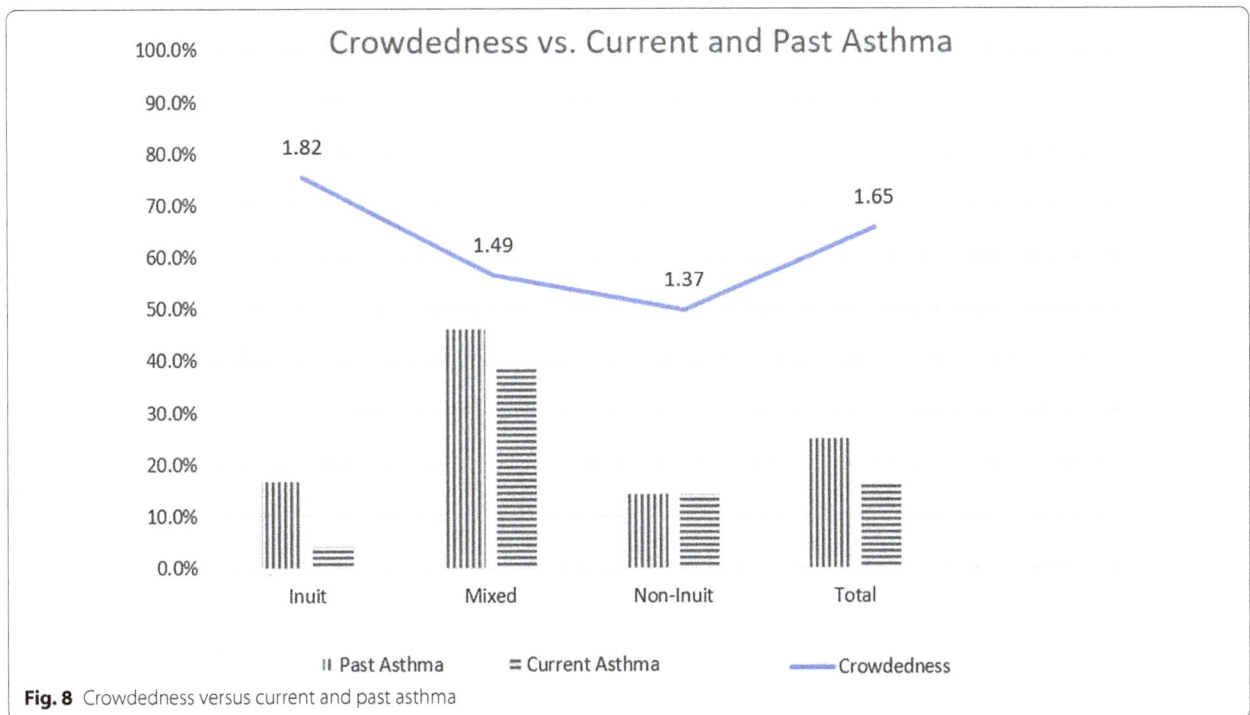

Fig. 8 Crowdedness versus current and past asthma

and HRV (especially HRV C as suggested in the COAST study) [33] or may have led to lower rates if the crowding in the home created an environment of increased endotoxin/LPS with extensive dog exposure as in the Bavarian farm families with their bovine exposure [34].

All the non-Inuit children and the vast majority of the mixed ethnicity students were ever outside Nunavut, compared to half of the Inuit. This might have a role in the degree of exposure to a higher concentration of environmental allergens in the South which might explain the significant relation between having current asthma, past asthma and being ever outside Nunavut (OR 0.78, CI 0.65–0.94) and (OR 0.66, CI 0.51–0.84) respectively. The questionnaire did not explore the timing, duration, purpose or frequency of being ever outside Nunavut. So there is not enough information to determine a causality relationship versus being a confounding factor.

A possible explanation for the relationship between the family history of asthma and past asthma but not with the current asthma is having a sibling with recurrent wheezes related to respiratory illnesses or having passive smoking with the development of wheezes among siblings, so it might be a confounding factor rather than a genetic predisposition.

The current eczema prevalence amongst the three ethnic groups was 20.5%, with the highest prevalence recorded among the Inuit at 25% compared to 15.4% among the mixed ethnicity. While 14.3% of non-Inuit recorded a current history of eczema, with more cases among the females. Interestingly, the Mushuau Inuit of Natuashish (a minority of Inuit people living in Labrador, Canada) recorded a prevalence of 16.5%, with female predominance as well (female to male ratio 2:1) [13]. In agreement with our study findings, Weiland et al. have previously reported that the prevalence of eczema symptoms correlated positively with latitude and negatively with the mean annual outdoor temperature [10], thus, making it an expected finding to get a higher eczema rate in Nunavut compared to that in southern Canada. Similarly, a high prevalence of eczema (23.6%) was reported in Arctic Norway [8] compared to a lower prevalence of 12.7% in the southern part of the same country [35, 36]. Also, in Sweden, the prevalence of atopic eczema among 7–8-year old children was reported to be higher in Kiruna in the North than in Gothenburg in the South (23% vs 18.7%) with a similar higher female to male ratio [37].

The higher prevalence of past eczema among the non-Inuit compared to the current one being highest among the Inuit might indicate that eczema is more transient among the non-Inuit while persists for a longer time in Inuit children. According to unpublished clinical experience in Nunavut, the Inuit children tend to have more

severe eczema, whether this is related to genetic predisposition, access to medical care, treatment compliance, household conditions or a combination of these factors is worth to be explored. That was out of the scope of this current study. The estimates of the annual costs of eczema in Canada is about $1.4 billion [38] which imposes a considerable financial burden on Canadian society especially among the lower socioeconomic populations in the far North.

Having a dog at home in Iqaluit is relatively common, especially among the mixed ethnicity while having a cat was the highest among the non-Inuit. There are likely a number of reasons for this; but for centuries, dogs have been used by the Inuit for work and transportation. While cats are generally not perceived to be of substantive value to the inhabitants in the Nunavut environment. In Nunavut dogs tend to be outside of the home. Owning a dog was strongly associated with the presence of current eczema (OR 7.13, CI 1.18–43.14) There was no relationship with cat ownership. These data are contrary to previous reports indicating that dog ownership significantly reduced the risk of eczema at the age of 4 years among dog-sensitized children while cat ownership combined with cat sensitization significantly increased the risk [39], though in that same article it was mentioned that children exposed to the highest dog allergen concentrations had a significantly lower risk of eczema. This is not the case in our study population, since most of the dogs are held outside the houses in Nunavut while the cats are indoors most of the time.

As expected, the study found a high correlation between having a family history of eczema and current eczema as well as past eczema. Whether this is related to atopy inheritance, household environment, exposure to the same risk factors or a familial skin barrier issue like the filaggrin mutation could not be determined in this study.

No significant relationship was found between eczema and having a family history of food allergy, which is reasonable taking into consideration the various mechanisms (intrinsic vs extrinsic) of developing those atopic diseases, especially when studied among different ethnicities.

A significant relationship was found between family history of environmental allergies and having past eczema but not with the current eczema, an explanation could be related to the fact that the current eczema was profoundly prominent among the Inuit children with less expected family history of environmental allergies because of low allergen exposure while the past eczema was more among the non-Inuit students whom their parents most probably were born and raised outside Nunavut with more allergen exposure. The study questionnaire did not address neither the place of birth of the child nor the parents.

A previous study by McIsaac [40] found that only 24.8% of the Inuit were exclusively breastfed to 6 months which is much lower than our finding, possibly because our study asked only about the first 4 months of life. There have been many studies with conflicting results in regard to a possible atopy protective effect of exclusive breastfeeding for the first 4–6 months, neither the study design nor the sample size can allow taking a side on this continued debate.

Our study shows a surprisingly high prevalence of sensitization among children, aged 6–7 years, in Iqaluit to cats, at 26.7%, which is much higher that the 8.6% prevalence among Grade 1–8 children in the province of Saskatchewan [41].

Equally surprising was the prevalence of sensitization with suggestive history of allergy to peanut and tree nut among children aged 6–7 years in Iqaluit at 3.3 and 6.7%. Especially given a prevalence of peanut allergy as tested in Montreal among children aged 4–9 years was 1.62% [42]. However, this is a small sample and food challenges were not performed.

All the non-Inuit children and the vast majority of the mixed ethnicity students were ever outside Nunavut, compared to half of the Inuit. This might have a role in the degree of exposure to a higher concentration of environmental allergens in the South which might explain the significant relation between having current asthma, past asthma and being ever outside Nunavut (OR 0.78, CI 0.65–0.94) and (OR 0.66, CI 0.51–0.84) respectively. The questionnaire did not explore the timing, duration, purpose or frequency of being ever outside Nunavut. Many of the Inuit children get outside Nunavut for the first time because of being urgently transferred to a tertiary hospital in Ontario or Manitoba (no tertiary hospital or pediatric intensive care unit in all the territory), one of the common conditions for such an urgent transfer is having a severe lower respiratory tract infection (personal observation as a pediatrician locum). So there is no enough information to determine a causality relationship versus being a confounding factor.

The prevalence of sensitization to grass being highest among the mixed ethnicity might have a similar explanation though it is worth mentioning that two of the grasses used in the skin test [June (*P. pratensis*) and Redtop (*A. alba*)] can be found in Nunavut [43, 44] which might explain the sensitization among children that have never been outside Nunavut, when compared to Greenland Inuit, the Inuit children in Greenland were more likely to be sensitized to inhaled allergens compared to the non-Inuit, with grass being the major inhaled allergen [44].

The absence of sensitization to house dust mite, mold, weed, ragweed and dog in our study is consistent with the findings in Greenland where the prevalence of sensitization to house dust mite is four times lower than that in Denmark, probably because of lower indoors house dust mite count similar to northern Norway and Iceland [45]. The overall prevalence of at least one positive skin prick test was 22.8% in Denmark compared to only 6.4% in Uummannaq (a northern community in Greenland with similarities to Iqaluit). In Denmark, the total birch pollen counts were 40–1000 times higher compared to Nuuk (Greenland), whereas the grass pollen count was 13–30 times higher in Denmark compared to Nuuk. In Denmark, house dust mites were found in 72% of households (> 10/0.1 g dust) while less than 15% of households in Greenland had measurable levels of house dust mites. Similar to my personal observation in Iqaluit, that study reported that dogs were held indoor much less frequently in Uummannaq [46], making the expected dog allergen load low inside the houses.

A study in northern Norway had similar findings with low house dust mite and mold sensitization [47], another one in northern Sweden showed that sensitization to cats was the most common at 19% while sensitization to mites and mold was uncommon [48].

A previous house survey in Nunavut have shown that although building's fungal concentrations were low, the mattress fungal levels were markedly increased, and the dust mites were virtually non-existent [31].

The strength of this study includes using a validated ISAAC questionnaire with the added relevant questions to this population and geographical area.

Limitations of this study were related mainly to the small sample size which constituted one-third of the targeted cohort. This may relate to suspicion among the families about clinical research environment which has not been conducted in this part of Canada for decades. Hopefully, this study will be a breakthrough in regard to building a positive relationship and trust with the local community in Nunavut and encourage further acceptance of research.

Given the small sample size, a post hoc power analysis revealed low power in relation to most associations, we acknowledge this limitation (Table 6, Additional file 4: Appendix S4). There is a possibility that atopy-positive families were more willing to participate. Thus, selection bias could have been possible. As well, recall bias remains a possibility as with every retrospective questionnaire-based study. Also, the study has its limits in regard to determining associations but not causality relationships. A larger scale longitudinal study is highly recommended to avoid such limitations.

Despite those limitations, we think that our study contributes to the existing literature because of the scarcity of data about allergies and allergic conditions among the Inuit population and other ethnicities living in this part of the World. Add to this, such unique baseline data serve as a benchmark for future prevalence studies.

Conclusion

Variations in the prevalence and risk factors of asthma, allergic rhinitis, eczema and sensitization among different ethnicities living at the same subarctic environment may be related to genetic, gene-environment interaction and/or lifestyle factors that require further investigation.

Abbreviations

ISAAC: International Study of Allergy and Asthma in Children; SPT: skin prick test; sq. km: square kilometer; TB: tuberculosis; BCG: Bacille Calmette–Guérin; HDM: house dust mite; OR: odds ratio; CI-95: confidence interval of 95%; AR: allergic rhinitis; L/s: liter per second; RSV: respiratory syncytial virus; HRV: human rhinovirus; LPS: lipopolysaccharide.

Authors' contributions

All the authors participated in the preparation of the study, protocol review, data analysis and script writing. Dr. Ahmed, in addition to the previous roles, did the data collection and skin prick testing. All authors read and approved the final manuscript.

Author details

[1] Department of Pediatrics, University of Ottawa, Ottawa, ON, Canada.
[2] National Heart and Lung Institute, Imperial College, London, UK. [3] Section of Allergy and Clinical Immunology, Department of Pediatrics and Child Health, University of Manitoba, Winnipeg, MB, Canada.

Acknowledgements

We are thankful to the students, their parents, principals and teachers who took part in this study. Special thanks to Dr. Jill Warner and Dr. Marta Vazquez-Ortiz for their encouragement and feedback during the initial preparation for this study.

Competing interests

The authors declare that they have no competing interests.

Funding

No external funding was received, all the expenses were paid by Dr. Ahmed Ahmed.

References

1. https://en.wikipedia.org/wiki/Portal:Nunavut. Accessed 1 Feb 2018.
2. http://www.city.iqaluit.nu.ca/i18n/english/demo.html. Accessed 20 Apr 2016.
3. http://www.gov.nu.ca/eia/information/nunavut-faqs. Accessed 7 Apr 2015.
4. http://www.stats.gov.nu.ca/en/home.aspx. Accessed 20 Apr 2016.
5. The International Study of Asthma and Allergies in, Children (ISAAC) Steering Committee. Worldwide variation in prevalence of symptoms of asthma, allergic rhinoconjunctivitis, and atopic eczema: ISAAC. Lancet. 1998;351:1225–32.
6. Odhiambo JA, Williams HC, Clayton TO, et al. The ISAAC Phase Three Study Group. Global variations in prevalence of eczema symptoms in children from ISAAC Phase Three. J Allergy Clin Immunol. 2009;124:1251–8.
7. Åberg N, Hesselmar B, Åberg B, et al. Increase of asthma, allergic rhinitis and eczema in Swedish schoolchildren between 1979 and 1991. Clin Exp Allergy. 1995;25:815–9.
8. Dotterud LK, Odland JØ, Falk ES. Atopic dermatitis and respiratory symptoms in Russian and northern Norwegian school children: a comparison study in two arctic areas and the impact of environmental factors. J Eur Acad Dermatol Venereol. 2004;18:131–6.
9. Byremo G, Rød G, Carlsen KH. Effect of climatic change in children with atopic eczema. Allergy. 2006;61:1403–10.
10. Weiland SK, Husing A, Strachan DP, et al. Climate and the prevalence of symptoms of asthma, allergic rhinitis, and atopic eczema in children. Occup Environ Med. 2004;61:609–15.
11. Hansen TE, Evjenth B, Holt J. Increasing prevalence of asthma, allergic rhinoconjunctivitis and eczema among schoolchildren: three surveys during the period 1985–2008. Acta Paediatr. 2013;102:47–52.
12. Wang H-Y, Pizzichini MM, Becker AB, et al. Disparate geographic prevalences of asthma, allergic rhinoconjunctivitis and atopic eczema among adolescents in five Canadian cities. Pediatr Allergy Immunol. 2010;21:867–77.
13. Forsey R. Prevalence of childhood eczema and food sensitization in the First Nations reserve of Natuashish, Labrador, Canada. BMC Pediatr. 2014;14:76.
14. MacMillan HL, Jamieson E, Walsh C, et al and members of the First Nations and Inuit Regional Health Survey-National Steering Committee (at the time of the 1997 data collection) and Principal Investigator Committees from the Offord Centre for Child Studies affiliated with McMaster University and Hamilton Health Sciences, Hamilton, Canada. The health of Canada's Aboriginal children: results from the First Nations and Inuit Regional Health Survey. Int J Circumpolar Health. 2010;69(2):158–67.
15. Findlay LC, Janz TA. The health of Inuit children under age 6 in Canada. Int J Circumpolar Health. 2012;71:18580.
16. Chang H-J, Beach J, Senthilselvan A. Prevalence of and risk factors for asthma in off-reserve Aboriginal children and adults in Canada. Can Respir J. 2012;19(6):e68–74.
17. Hemmelgarn B, Ernst P. Airway function among Inuit primary school children in far northern Quebec. Am J Respir Crit Care Med. 1997;156:1870–5.
18. Redding GJ, Singleton RJ, DeMain J, et al. Relationship between IgE and specific aeroallergen sensitivity in Alaskan native children. Ann Allergy Asthma Immunol. 2006;97:209–15.
19. Tuberculosis in Canada 2012 report. http://www.phac-aspc.gc.ca/tbpc-latb/pubs/tbcan12pre/index-eng.php. Accessed 17 Apr 2015.
20. Marks GB, Ng K, Zhou J, et al. The effect of neonatal BCG vaccination on atopy and asthma at age 7 to 14 years: an historical cohort study in a community with a very low prevalence of tuberculosis infection and a high prevalence of atopic disease. J Allergy Clin Immunol. 2003;111:541–9.
21. Flohr C, Nagel G, Weinmayr G, et al. the ISAAC Phase Two Study Group. Tuberculosis, bacillus Calmette–Guerin vaccination, and allergic disease: findings from the International Study of Asthma and Allergies in Childhood Phase Two. Pediatr Allergy Immunol. 2012;23:324–31.
22. Arnoldussen DL, Linehan M, Sheikh A. BCG vaccination and allergy: a systematic review and meta-analysis. J Allergy Clin Immunol. 2011;127:246–53.
23. Kiraly N, Benn CS, Biering-Sørensen S, et al. Vitamin A supplementation and BCG vaccination at birth may affect atopy in childhood: long-term follow-up of a randomized controlled trial. Allergy. 2013;68:1168–76.
24. Asher MI, Montefort S, Bjorksten B, et al. Worldwide time trends in the prevalence of symptoms of asthma, allergic rhinoconjunctivitis, and eczema in childhood: ISAAC Phases One and Three repeat multicountry cross-sectional surveys. Lancet. 2006;368(9537):733–43.

25. https://www12.statcan.gc.ca/census-recensement/2006/as-sa/97-558/note-eng.cfm. Accessed 20 Apr 2016.

26. Egeland GM, Faraj N, Osborne G. Cultural, socioeconomic, and health indicators among Inuit preschoolers: Nunavut Inuit Child Health Survey 2007_2008. Rural Remote Health. 2010;10:1365.

27. Gao Z, Rowe BH, Majaesic C, O'Hara C, et al. Prevalence of asthma and risk factors for asthma-like symptoms in Aboriginal and non-Aboriginal children in the northern territories of Canada. Can Respir J. 2008;15(3):139–45.

28. Dell SD, Foty RG, Gilbert NL, et al. Asthma and allergic disease prevalence in a diverse sample of Toronto school children: results from the Toronto Child Health Evaluation Questionnaire (T-CHEQ) Study. Can Respir J. 2010;17(1):e1–6.

29. Habbick BF, Pizzichini MM, Taylor B, et al. Prevalence of asthma, rhinitis and eczema among children in 2 Canadian cities: the International Study of Asthma and Allergies in Childhood. Can Med Assoc J. 1999;160:1824–8.

30. Dotterud LK, Odland JØ, Falk ES. Atopic diseases among schoolchildren in Nikel, Russia, an Arctic area with heavy air pollution. Acta Derm Venereol. 2001;81:198–201.

31. Kovesi T, Creery D, Gilbert NL, et al. Indoor air quality risk factors for severe lower respiratory tract infections in Inuit infants in Baffin Region, Nunavut: a pilot study. Indoor Air. 2006;16(4):266–75.

32. Kovesi T, Gilbert N, Stocco C, et al. Indoor air quality and the risk of lower respiratory tract infections in young Canadian Inuit children. Can Med Assoc J. 2007;177(2):155–60.

33. Lemanske RF Jr, Jackson DJ, Gangnon RE, et al. Rhinovirus illnesses during infancy predict subsequent childhood wheezing. J Allergy Clin Immunol. 2005;116:571–7.

34. Braun-Fahrlander C, Riedler J, Herz U, et al. for the Allergy and Endotoxin Study Team. Environmental exposure to endotoxin and its relation to asthma in school-age children. N Engl J Med. 2002;347:869–77.

35. Steen-Johnsen J, Bolle R, Holt J, et al. Impact of pollution and place of residence on atopic diseases among schoolchildren in Telemark County, Norway. Pediatr Allergy Immunol. 1995;6:192–9.

36. Dotterud LK, Kvammen B, Bolle R, et al. A survey of atopic diseases among school children in Sor-Varanger community. Possible effects of subarctic climate and industrial pollution from Russia. Acta Derm Venereol. 1994;74:124–8.

37. Hesselmar B, Aberg B, Eriksson B, et al. Allergic rhinoconjunctivitis, eczema, and sensitization in two areas with differing climates. Pediatr Allergy Immunol. 2001;12:208–15.

38. Barbeau M, Lalonde H. Burden of Atopic dermatitis in Canada. Int J Dermatol. 2006;45:31–6.

39. Epstein T, Bernstein D, Levin L, et al. Opposing effects of cat and dog ownership and allergic sensitization on eczema in an atopic birth cohort. Pediatrics. 2011;158(2):265–71.

40. McIsaac K. Factors associated with exclusive breastfeeding to 6 months among Canadian Inuit: results from the Inuit health survey for children. J Epidemiol Community Health. 2011;65(Suppl 1):A197.

41. Chu LM, Rennie DC, Cockcroft DW, et al. Prevalence and determinants of atopy and allergic diseases among school-age children in rural Saskatchewan, Canada. Ann Allergy Asthma Immunol. 2014;113(4):430–9.

42. Ben-Shoshan M, Kagan R, Alizadehfar R, et al. Is the prevalence of peanut allergy increasing? A 5-year follow-up study in children in Montreal. J Allergy Clin Immunol. 2009;123(4):783–8.

43. Aiken, SG, Dallwitz, MJ, Consaul, LL et al. 2007. Flora of the Canadian Arctic Archipelago: descriptions, illustrations, identification, and information retrieval. Ottawa: NRC Research Press, National Research Council of Canada. http://nature.ca/aaflora/data. Accessed 19 Apr 2016.

44. Adkindon Jr NF, Bochner BS, Burks AW, Busse WW, Holgate ST, Lemanske Jr RF, O'Hehir RE. Middleton's allergy: principles and practice. 8th ed, chapter 27, page 433, table 27-2. London: Elsevier Health Sciences; 2013.

45. Krause TG, Koch A, Poulsen K, et al. Atopic sensitization among children in an arctic environment. Clin Exp All. 2002;32:367–72.

46. Porsbjerg C, Linstow ML, Nepper-christensen SC, et al. Greenlandic Population Study Group. Allergen sensitization and allergen exposure in Greenlander Inuit residing in Denmark and Greenland. Respir Med. 2002;96:736–44.

47. Bakken HN, Nafstad P, Bolle R, et al. Skin sensitization in school children in northern and southern Norway. J Asthma. 2007;44(1):23–7.

48. Ronmark E, Bjerg A, Perzanowski M, et al. Major increase in allergic sensitization in schoolchildren from 1996 to 2006 in northern Sweden. J Allergy Clin Immunol. 2009;124(2):357–63.

6

Sputum cell counts to manage prednisone-dependent asthma: effects on FEV₁ and eosinophilic exacerbations

Afia Aziz-Ur-Rehman[1†], Angira Dasgupta[1†], Melanie Kjarsgaard[1], Frederick E. Hargreave[1^] and Parameswaran Nair[1,2*] (iD)

Abstract

Background: Prednisone dependence in asthma is usually described based on clinical and spirometric characteristics. It is generally believed that these patients have frequent exacerbations and lose lung function rapidly because of uncontrolled airway eosinophilia.

Objectives: The objectives of this study are to report the effect on asthma exacerbations and the change in lung function over time in prednisone-dependent asthma when severe asthma is managed using a protocol that aims to maintain normal sputum cell counts.

Methods: A retrospective survey of patients prospectively assessed in a university tertiary care asthma clinic.

Results: 52 patients (30 males, mean age 51 years, 64% non-atopic) were followed for a median period of 5.4 years (min–max: 0.2–35.2). Monitoring with the aim of keeping sputum eosinophils below 3% resulted in higher doses of corticosteroids (median daily dose of prednisone was 10 mg and for inhaled corticosteroids was 1500 μg of fluticasone equivalent) than at baseline and this was associated with predictable adverse effects. Despite the disease severity, 10 patients (19%) did not require LABA for symptom control. Most importantly, over the period of follow-up, there were only 0.3 eosinophilic exacerbations/patient/year. Overall, there was an increase in FEV1 over the period of follow-up (mean +84.6 ml/year) rather than an expected decline.

Conclusions: Monitoring of eosinophils in sputum enables to maintain symptom control and preserve FEV1 in patients with severe prednisone-dependent asthma.

Keywords: Severe asthma, Prednisone, Sputum cell counts, Eosinophils, FEV1, Exacerbations

Background

Asthma management guided by sputum cell counts has been shown to reduce eosinophilic exacerbations [1, 2] and is cost-effective [3]. This is particularly true for patients with moderate to severe asthma as most patients with mild asthma may not require a biomarker-guided treatment strategy [4]. However, it is not known if patients with the severest forms of asthma i.e. those that require daily prednisone would also benefit from a sputum-based management strategy. It is generally believed that these patients have frequent exacerbations, particularly those with persistent sputum eosinophilia [5] and that they lose lung function over time with each exacerbation [6]. These patients, although fortunately infrequent, consume the largest health care resources for asthma care [7]. They often have significant adverse effects from their doses of corticosteroids [8] and these are the patients who may benefit most with the advent of biologics that target the Th2 cytokine pathways [9].

The recent experience from the British Thoracic Society Severe Asthma program suggest that the clinical

*Correspondence: parames@mcmaster.ca
†Afia Aziz-Ur-Rehman and Angira Dasgupta contributed equally to this work
^ Deceased
2 Firestone Institute for Respiratory Health, St. Joseph's Healthcare, 50 Charlton Avenue East, Hamilton, ON L8N 4A6, Canada
Full list of author information is available at the end of the article

outcomes of patients with severe asthma are better if they are managed in specialized asthma centres than in general clinics [10]. A severe asthma clinic was set up at the Firestone clinic at St Joseph's Healthcare in Hamilton, ON in the early 1970s where patients were looked after by a respiratory physician (FEH) who was supported by a research staff of two technologists and one clinical trainee who was often a respiratory physician. The two unique features of this clinic were the introduction of quantitative cell counts in sputum to adjust initial treatment requirements and secondly (and more importantly) accessibility to these measurements within 72 h of any worsening of asthma symptoms. The main objectives of this manuscript are to describe the effects of this strategy on FEV_1 and on exacerbations in patients with prednisone-dependent asthma who were referred to this clinic.

Study design and methods

This was a retrospective descriptive chart review of patients with a physician-confirmed diagnosis of asthma (defined as episodic wheeze, chest tightness or shortness of breath and confirmed variable airflow obstruction of at least 12% and 200 ml improvement in FEV1 after inhaling 200 mcg of salbutamol or a PC20 methacholine of <8 mg/ml), and who were on a maintenance dose of at least 5 mg of prednisone daily for at least 6 months prior to the initial consultation, who were referred to a severe asthma clinic at the Firestone Institute in Hamilton, Ontario, between 1973 and 2008. Basic clinical and demographic data were documented. Pre-and post-bronchodilator reversibility were recorded according to the American Thoracic Society standards [11]. Airway responsiveness to methacholine was assessed by the tidal breathing method of Cockcroft et al. [12] if the FEV_1 was >65% of predicted. Symptoms of cough, wheeze, chest tightness, dyspnea and sputum production were documented on a 7-point Likert scale (1 being worst and 7 being best). Tools to assess "asthma control" and "asthma-specific quality of life" were not available when the first patients were recruited into this program. Sputum was induced and processed according to the methods described by Pizzichini et al. [13].

Asthma was managed according to the protocol described by Jayaram et al. [1]. Briefly, the dose of inhaled corticosteroids or prednisone was increased to maintain sputum eosinophils less than 3% (or until free eosinophil granules were no longer present). If sputum total cell count was greater than 15×10^6/g and neutrophils greater than 65%, the patients were treated with a broad spectrum antibiotic (zithromycin or amoxicillin + clavulanic acid for 5–7 days). Most importantly, the dose of steroid was not increased. Long-acting bronchodilators

(salmeterol or formoterol) were added to the inhaled steroids only after the bronchitic component was controlled and the patient continued to have shortness of breath or wheezing that required more than 2–4 puffs of short-acting bronchodilators daily. They were not added if spirometry did not show any worsening of airflow obstruction or if PC20 methacholine was greater than 8 mg/ml or had not worsened by more than one doubling dose. If the sputum eosinophil % was less than 1%, the dose of corticosteroids was reduced. Sputum was always rechecked with 6–8 weeks of any treatment change. Once the maintenance dose of steroid was identified, patients were left on this dose indefinitely and seen in follow-up on average twice a year at which time spirometry, sputum and blood counts, clinical asthma control and adverse effects of therapy were assessed by self-reported history. Methacholine airway responsiveness was also reassessed if patients reported an increase need for short-acting bronchodilators and the sputum cell counts were normal and if it was felt safe to perform the test (usually FEV_1 > 65% predicted). Adherence to prescribed medications was continuously assessed by checking the pharmacy records every year.

If patients experienced any worsening of symptoms (increase in chest tightness or wheezing requiring at least four puffs of salbutamol daily or at night, increase in sputum production or change in colour to dark yellow or green) they were instructed to call our research office. Patients were brought to the clinic within 72 h for a clinical assessment, spirometry, and collection of either spontaneously expectorated or induced sputum. They were phoned back the same evening or the next morning with instructions to change their medication dosages. If patients had seen their family doctor and had received either antibiotics or prednisone without being seen at our clinic, this information was documented in the clinic chart. All the demographic and clinical information was meticulously extracted by a research assistant (AAR) and verified by a research technologist (MK) after obtaining approval from the Hospital Research Ethics Board.

Statistical analysis

Baseline demographic and clinical data were summarized using descriptive statistics. The rates of change of FEV_1 (ml/year) were analyzed by multilevel linear regression using three time points (at baseline, time when sputum quantitative assay became normal and at the most recent assessment) for each gender and smoking status separately. As a first step, individual FEV_1s were regressed against time to find rates of change (ml/year) for each patient. In the second step of multilevel linear regression, the rates of change (ml/year) for each patient (dependent variable) were regressed with age and height as the independent variables. The final rate of change of FEV_1 in a specific group e.g. males, females, smokers and non-smokers was computed using the mean age and height of the respective groups. The analyses were carried out using SPSS (version 16). Since we did not have a comparison group of patients with milder asthma or patients with severe asthma who were not monitored using sputum cell counts, we plotted the rates of decline of our cohort against the data published by Ulrik et al. [14] for patients with mild asthma. Paired data were compared by Student's t test. P-value was considered significant if <0.05.

Results

The study included 52 (30 males and 22 females) patients. The baseline characteristics of all patients are tabulated in Table 1. The median time of follow up of all patients was 5.42 years (minimum 0.15, maximum 35.26).

Effect on sputum cell counts

Sputum eosinophil counts were normalized in all patients within a median period of 5 months (Table 2). This was associated with a trivial (but statistically significant) increase in sputum neutrophil % (Table 2; Fig. 1). The cell counts remained stable for the rest of the follow-up period.

Effect on FEV_1

The rate of change of FEV_1 from baseline value to the time point when sputum quantitative assay became normal was 1201.24 ml/year (95% CI 199.31 to 2202.7 ml/year) while the rate of change (decline) from the time sputum was normal to the time when the patient was last

Table 1 Baseline characteristics (n = 52)

Age, years (mean, SD)	51 (11)
Male (n)	30
Smoker (n)	28
Atopy (n, %)	19 (36%)
Chronic rhinosinusitis (n, %)	23 (45%)
Aspirin sensitivity (n, %)	9 (18%)
Age of onset of symptoms, years (median, min–max)	20 (9–45)
Years on prednisone prior to initial assessment (mean, SD)	7.2 (6.6)
Number of courses of prednisone over past 2 years/patient/ year (mean, SD)	1.8 (1.2)
Height, cm (mean, SD)	168.2 (10.2)
Weight, kg (mean, SD)	80.8 (14.4)
Serum IgE, KIU/l (mean, SD)	86 (18)
Blood eosinophil, $\times 10^3$/l (mean, SD)	0.4 (0.5)
ICS, µg (median)	1500
LABA (n)	22
LTRA (n)	14

Table 2 Sputum, blood counts and spirometry (mean, SD) values

	At initial visit	When sputum was normal	Current
Sputum			
Total cell count, $\times 10^6$/g	16 (24)	9 (11)	12 (8)
Eosinophil, %	22 (18)	1 (4)	2.4 (4.2)
Neutrophil, %	60 (49)	72 (28)	64 (20)
Blood			
Eosinophil count, $\times 10^3$/l	0.4 (0.5)	0.1 (0.2)	0.2 (0.3)
Eosinophil %	6 (8)	4 (8)	4 (6)
Spirometry			
FEV_1, L	2.3 (0.8)	2.5 (0.8)	2.2 (0.8)
FEV_1, %	70.7 (20.1)	76.9 (18.2)	69.4 (18.1)
VC, L	3.6 (1.1)	3.6 (0.9)	3.4 (1.1)
VC, %	88.7 (16.9)	90.9 (12.9)	84.4 (22.4)
FEV_1/VC, %	63 (14)	65 (13)	64 (14)

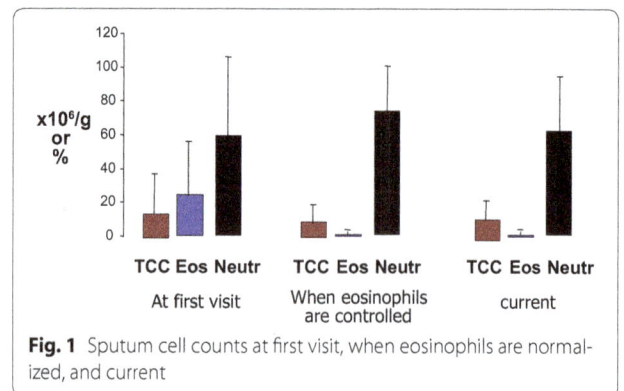

Fig. 1 Sputum cell counts at first visit, when eosinophils are normalized, and current

seen was a modest −14.9 (95% CI 53.4 to −83.2) ml/year. The overall (baseline to when last seen) rate of change of FEV_1 was 84.63 (95% CI −44.6 to 213.8) ml/year. The corresponding values in males were 970.53 (95% CI 178.5 to 1762.4) ml/year, −28.36 (95% CI −18.1 to −38.6) ml/year and the overall rate of change was 113.99 (95% CI 70.6 to 157.4) ml/year and for females were 1515.85 (95% CI −701.1 to 3732.7) ml/year, 3.44 (95% CI −115.7 to 122.6) ml/year and the overall rate of change was 44.59 (95% CI −95.6 to 184.8) ml/year. There were however no statistically significant difference between males and females in their rates of change of FEV_1. The rates of change of FEV_1 for male smokers were : from baseline to when sputum was normal 1433.13 (95% CI 199.3 to 2666.9) ml/year, from when sputum was normal to when last seen 6.09 (95% CI −113.1 to 125.3) ml/year and overall 227.31 (95% CI −91.9 to 546.5) ml/year and for females smokers were:

from baseline to when sputum was normal 663.8 (95% CI −332.4 to 1660.0) ml/year, from when sputum was normal to when last seen 21.54 (95% CI −310.1 to 353.1) ml/year and overall 82.58 (95% CI −306.6 to 471.8) ml/year. The corresponding values for male nonsmokers were: 171.48 (95% CI −78.0 to 420.9) ml/year, −87.86 (95% CI −218.7 to 43.02) ml/year and −81.73 (95% CI −190.5 to 27.1) ml/year and for female nonsmokers were: 2105.74 (95% CI −1801.4 to 6012.9) ml/year, −9.09 (95% CI −35.3 to 17.2) ml/year and 18.28 (95% CI −11.4 to 47.9) ml/year. There were no statistical differences in rates of change of FEV_1 between the genders when smokers and nonsmokers were analysed separately.

Effect on exacerbations

Over the 2 years prior to attending our clinic, the patients had reported an average of 1.9 exacerbations/patient/year that had responded to prednisone. Since sputum was not examined during these exacerbations, we cannot confirm that these were eosinophilic, but we assume they were as patients reported improvement in their asthma symptoms within 48–72 h of therapy. This was reduced to 0.3 eosinophilic exacerbations/patient/year over the course of the follow-up period. The average time of resolution of individual exacerbations was 4 days. We did not have accurate records of "non-eosinophilic" or "neutrophilic" exacerbations before their initial visit to our clinic. During the course of the follow-up, the patients had 1.2 neutrophilic exacerbations/patient/year that were treated with antibiotics.

Effects related to corticosteroids

The median duration of the steroid optimization phase was 5 months (min−max 1–7 months). During this period, the median daily dose of prednisone was 10 mg (minimum 5 mg, maximum 35 mg) and the dose of inhaled corticosteroid was 1500 mcg of fluticasone equivalent. This dose was maintained for the duration of the follow-up period. Five patients required the dose of prednisone to be increased after the maintenance dose was established. Corticosteroids caused predictable adverse effects (Table 3) that were appropriately managed.

Effects related to LABA

At initial assessment, 22 patients were on LABA (15 on salmeterol, 7 on formoterol). Over the course of the follow-up period, 20 patients were also commenced on LABA. The median period to commencement of LABA was 2 years (minimum 2 months, maximum 4 years). 10 patients have not required LABA for symptom control as their asthma severity (and airflow obstruction) was largely driven by steroid-responsive luminal eosinophilic inflammation rather than by bronchodilator-responsive smooth muscle dysfunction.

Table 3 Co-morbidities and adverse effects of prednisone

	Prevalence (%)
Co-morbidities	
GERD	70
Sinusitis	65
Recurrent bronchitis	58
Polyps	45
BMI > 30	44
NSAID sensitivity	28
Neurosis	27
Adverse effects	
Osteopenia	72
Hypertension	60
Cataract	42
Skin bruising	35
Diabetes	16
Glaucoma	14

Discussion

This retrospective study illustrates three important concepts. Firstly, when available, incorporation of timely measurements of sputum quantitative cytometry and airway hyperresponsiveness into routine clinical practice is feasible and effective in the management of severe prednisone-dependent patients with asthma. Secondly, this strategy can reduce exacerbations and preserve lung function albeit at the cost of adverse effects of glucocorticoids. Thirdly, recognition of the component of asthma that leads to severity can help to rationalize the inappropriate use of long-acting bronchodilators that are associated with asthma morbidity.

To our knowledge, this is the first study that reports the preservation of lung function in patients with severe asthma. Not only did we not observe the expected decline in FEV_1 over time that has been reported in patients with "eosinophilic severe asthma" [5, 15], but there was a modest improvement over the period of observation suggesting that the current symptom-based guideline therapies underestimate the control of airway inflammation. We analysed longitudinal data using three time points i.e. when first seen, when sputum became normal and when a patient was last seen. The rate of change of FEV_1 was positive when the rate was computed from the baseline value to the point when the airway inflammation (or the sputum quantitative assay) became normal (Fig. 2), whereas the rate of change of FEV_1 thereafter, from the time sputum was normal to the time when the patient was last seen was a modest −14 ml/year which is clearly lesser than that reported in previous longitudinal asthma studies [6, 15–18]. The overall improvement in FEV_1 in this study is possibly driven by the fact that most patients

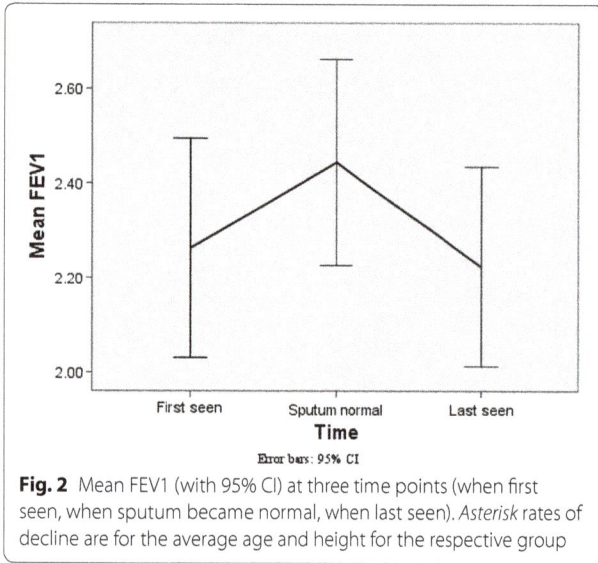

Fig. 2 Mean FEV1 (with 95% CI) at three time points (when first seen, when sputum became normal, when last seen). *Asterisk* rates of decline are for the average age and height for the respective group

had an improvement in lung function when sputum became normal after intensive anti-inflammatory therapy and that too within a short span of time resulting in high rates of improvement in FEV_1 with time. Comparison with a matched group of patients at the Firestone clinic with similar severity of asthma who were managed based on symptoms only would have certainly added strength to the study. Unfortunately, such data were not available to us. However, it is extremely unlikely that treatment based on symptoms alone would give results similar to treatment using a sputum strategy [1].

Figure 2 illustrates a comparison of rates of change of FEV_1 between this study and that by Ulrik et al. We fully realize that these two studies are not entirely comparable given the differences such as patient population, management strategies, sampling strategies etc. [14]. However, most longitudinal asthma studies are population based observational reports. We selected the Ulrick study as this is one of the larger longitudinal asthma studies and employed a similar statistical analysis method to what we performed. Various factors such as gender, smoking, age of onset, atopy, sputum eosinophilia, presence of mucous hyper secretion and use of inhaled corticosteroids have been implicated as affecting the rate of change in FEV_1 in asthmatics. However, methodological issues have led to wide variations in these observations resulting in a lot of heterogeneity in the reported rates of decline in FEV_1. Rates of decrease of FEV_1 have varied from 25.7 ml/year in severe asthma [15], 31.5 ml/year in asthmatic patients with frequent exacerbations vs 14.6 ml/year in those with infrequent exacerbations [6], 26.6 ml/year in occupational asthmatics who were exposed to low-molecular-weight sensitizers at work [16], 28.4–39.7 ml/year in adult

nonsmoker asthmatic patients in the Busselton cohort [17], to 16.1–21.5 ml/year in asthmatic patients receiving inhaled corticosteroids [18]. In the current study, the rate of decline from when sputum was normal to when last seen is similar to the decline rate reported in asthmatics with infrequent exacerbations [6]. Interestingly, in our study there were no statistical differences in rates of change of FEV_1 either between the genders (Fig. 3) or when smokers and nonsmokers were analysed (Figs. 4, 5) separately. Regardless of the fact that it may not be apt to compare studies with dissimilar populations and methodologies, we were able to demonstrate, perhaps

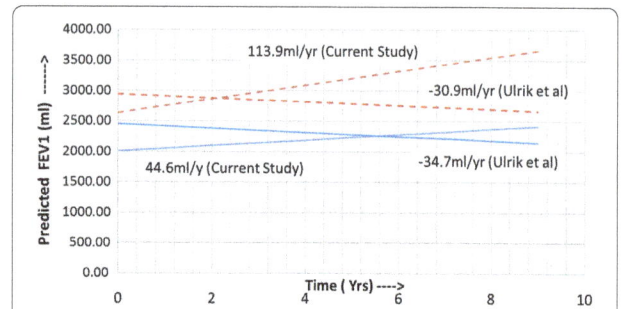

Fig. 3 Comparison of predicted (calculated) FEV1 vs time in years (Current Study vs Ulrik et al.). *Dotted lines* males, *solid line* females; predicted rates of decline and FEV1 for both studies are for the mean age (males 52.4 years, females 49.8 years) and mean height (males 173.2 cm, females 161.4 cm) of the current study population. Equations for current study: FEV1 at time t for males = (2.6795 − 0.03808*AGE +0.01124*HT) +(1.05455 − 0.00646*AGE −0.00348*HT)t; FEV1 at time t for females = (−4.27125 − 0.0253*AGE +0.04674*HT) + (−2.71234 − 0.00336*AGE +0.01812*HT)t. Equations for Ulrik et al.: FEV1 at time t for males = (−469 − 35.2*AGE +32.0*HT) − (−107 − 0.79*AGE +0.6*HT + 1.7)t; FEV1 at time t for females = (−410 − 27.6*AGE +21.2*HT) − (−107 − 0.79*AGE +0.6*HT + 3)t

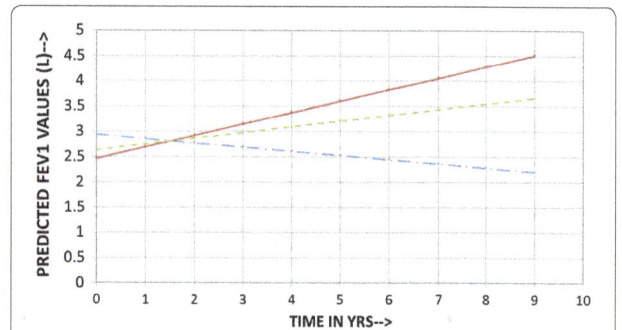

Fig. 4 Predicted (calculated) FEV1 vs time in years for males (Baseline to last seen) showing no statistical difference between smokers and nonsmokers; *dashed line* all patients, *solid line* smokers, *dash* and *dot line* nonsmokers. Predicted rates of decline and FEV1 are for the mean age and mean height for the respective group of the current study population

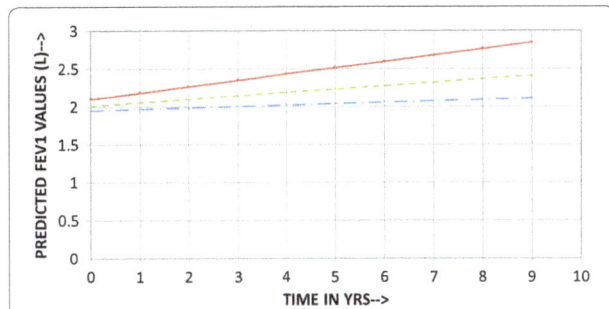

Fig. 5 Predicted (calculated) FEV1 vs time in years in females (Baseline to last seen) showing no statistical difference between smokers and nonsmokers; *dashed line* all patients, *solid line* smokers, *dash* and *dot line* nonsmokers. Predicted rates of decline and FEV1 are for the mean age and mean height for the respective group of the current study population

for the first time, a strategy that did not use biologics that could preserve lung function even when asthma is severe. Only the eosinophilic inflammatory component could be effectively targeted with corticosteroids. We did not have any effective or specific strategy (other than antibiotics) to treat neutrophilic bronchitis. We speculate that lung function could perhaps have been better preserved had broader strategies effective against non-T2 type inflammation as well been available for clinical use.

A second important point that we would like to highlight in this report is that patients could be on high doses of corticosteroids and not necessarily require long-acting beta-agonists if the severity is driven by luminal inflammation rather than by smooth muscle dysfunction. This is not often appreciated in clinical practice nor is it emphasized in the guidelines. In our cohort, the use of long-acting beta-agonist could be delayed or withheld in a small proportion of severe asthmatics in whom there is the highest concern for their adverse effects [19]. This also questions the veracity of recommendations to consider anti-eosinophil biologics (such as mepolizumab or reslizumab) as steroid-sparing therapy only after adding long-acting bronchodilators [20] when long-acting beta-agonists do not have any proven anti-eosinophil activities [21]. It is reasonable to consider biologics in patients whose disease are truly driven by eosinophils (as identified by persistent sputum eosinophils and blood eosinophils) and who have adverse effects from high doses of corticosteroids independent of their need for long-acting bronchodilators.

The major limitation of our study is the retrospective nature of data collection that spans over 25 years, the absence of a comparator group, and the lack of precision in the definition of exacerbations prior to referral to our clinic. It is also plausible that some of the exacerbations may not have been reported to us during the period

of follow up. We did not use any sophisticated method to assess compliance other than self reports and pharmacy logs.

Conclusion

In conclusion, we recommend monitoring of eosinophils in sputum in patients with severe prednisone-dependent asthma as this strategy enables to maintain symptom control, reduce exacerbations and preserve FEV_1 in these patients. The test is not intrusive and is acceptable to most patients [22]. This study was performed before anti-IL5 monoclonal antibodies were available for clinical use but the results demonstrate that most patients would not require them for improving asthma control but they would be useful to avoid the adverse effects of corticosteroids. Our experience also provides 'proof-of-principle' that 'remission' [23] can be achieved even in severe asthma by judicious use of currently available therapy, albeit at the price of adverse effects of therapy.

Abbreviations
FEV1: forced expiratory volume in the first second; PC20: provocative concentration to cause a 20% drop in FEV1; LABA: long-acting beta-agonist; ICS: inhaled corticosteroid.

Author's contributions
PN and FEH conceived the idea. MK did most of the clinical assessments. AR extracted and compiled the data. AG performed the statistical analysis. PN wrote the manuscript, All authors, except FEH, have edited the final version. All authors (except FEH) read and approved the final manuscript.

Author details
[1] Department of Medicine, McMaster University and St Joseph's Healthcare Hamilton, Hamilton, ON, Canada. [2] Firestone Institute for Respiratory Health, St. Joseph's Healthcare, 50 Charlton Avenue East, Hamilton, ON L8N 4A6, Canada.

Acknowledgements
Dr. Nair holds the Frederick E. HargreaveTeva Innovation Chair in Airway Diseases. We dedicate this manuscript to the memory of Prof. Frederick Hargreave.

Competing interests
PN is supported by the Frederick E. HargreaveTeva Innovation Chair in Airway Diseases. He has received consultancy fees from AstraZeneca, Boehringer-Ingelheim, Sanofi, Teva, Knopp, Theravance, and Roche; research support from GlaxoSmithKline, AstraZeneca, Sanofi, Roche, and Novartis; and lecture fees from Roche, AstraZeneca, and Novartis. Rest of the contributing authors do not have any competing interests to declare for this work.

Funding
The study was supported by the Canada Research Chair program.

References

1. Jayaram L, Pizzichini MM, Cook RJ, et al. Determining asthma treatment by monitoring sputum cell counts: effect on exacerbations. Eur Respir J. 2006;27:483–94.
2. Green RH, Brightling CE, McKenna S, et al. Asthma exacerbations and sputum eosinophil counts: a randomised controlled trial. Lancet. 2002;360:1715–21.
3. Dsilva L, Gafni A, Thabane L, et al. Cost analysis of monitoring asthma treatment using sputum cell counts. Can Respir J. 2008;15:370–4.
4. Nair P, Dasgupta A, Brightling CE, Chung KF. How to diagnose and phenotype asthma. Clin Chest Med. 2012;33:445–57.
5. Walsh CJ, Zaihra T, Benedetti A, et al. Exacerbation risk in severe asthma is stratified by inflammatory phenotype using longitudinal measures of sputum eosinophils. Clin Exp Allergy. 2016;46:1291–302.
6. Bai TR, Vonk JM, Postma DS, Boezen HM. Severe exacerbations predict excess lung function decline in asthma. Eur Respir J. 2007;30:452–6.
7. O'Neill S, Sweeney J, Patterson CC, et al. The cost of treating severe refractory asthma in the UK: an economic analysis from the British Thoracic Society Difficult Asthma Registry. Thorax. 2015;70:376–8.
8. Dalal AA, Duh MS, Gozalo L, et al. Dose–response relationship between long-term systemic corticosteroid use and related complications in patients with severe asthma. J Manag Care Spec Pharm. 2016;22:833–47.
9. Dasgupta A, Neighbour H, Nair P. Targeted therapy of bronchitis in obstructive airway diseases. Pharmacol Ther. 2013;140:213–22.
10. Gibeon D, Heaney LG, Brightling CE, et al. Dedicated severe asthma services improve health-care use and quality of life. Chest. 2015;148:870–6.
11. American thoracic Society. Standardization of spirometry. 1994 update. Am Rev Respir Dis. 1995;1995(152):1107–36.
12. Juniper EF, Cockcroft DW, Hargreave FE. Histamine and methacholine inhalation test: tidal breathing method, laboratory procedure and standardization. 2nd ed; 1994, p. 33–4.
13. Pizzichini E, Pizzichini MM, Efthimiadis A, Hargreave FE, Dolovich J. Measurement of inflammatory indices in induced sputum: effects of selection of sputum to minimize salivary contamination. Eur Respir J. 1996;9:1174–80.
14. Ulrik CS, Lange P. Decline of lung function in adults with bronchial asthma. Am J Respir Crit Care Med. 1994;150:629–34.
15. Newby C, AgbetileJ Hargadon B, et al. Lung function decline and variable airway inflammatory pattern: longitudinal analysis of severe asthma. J Allergy Clin Immunol. 2014;134:287–94.
16. Anees W, Moore VC, Burge PS. FEV1 decline in occupational asthma. Thorax. 2006;61:751–5.
17. James AL, Palmer LJ, Kicic E, Maxwell PS, Lagan SE, Ryan GF, et al. Decline in lung function in the Busselton Health Study: the effects of asthma and cigarette smoking. Am J Respir Crit Care Med. 2005;171:109–14.
18. Dijkstra A, Vonk JM, Jongepier H, Koppelman GH, Schouten JP, ten Hacken NH, et al. Lung function decline in asthma: association with inhaled corticosteroids, smoking and sex. Thorax. 2006;61:105–10.
19. Rodrigo GJ, Castro-Rodriguez JA. Safety of long-acting β agonists for the treatment of asthma: clearing the air. Thorax. 2012;67:342.
20. Nucala product monograph, http://ca.gsk.com/media/1209435/nucala.pdf. Accessed 25 Feb 2017.
21. Sindi A, Todd DC, Nair P. Anti-inflammatory effects of long-acting beta2-agonists in patients with asthma: a systematic review and meta-analysis. Chest. 2009;136:145–54.
22. D'silva L, Neighbour H, Gafni A, Radford K, Hargreave F, Nair P. Quantitative sputum cell counts to monitor bronchitis: a qualitative study of physician and patient perspectives. Can Respir J. 2013;20:47–51.
23. Upham JW, James AL. Remission of asthma: the next therapeutic frontier? Pharmacol Ther. 2011;130:38–45.

7

Regular follow-up visits reduce the risk for asthma exacerbation requiring admission in Korean adults with asthma

Hye Jung Park[1], Min Kwang Byun[1*] ⓘ, Hyung Jung Kim[1], Chul Min Ahn[1], Chin Kook Rhee[2], Kyungjoo Kim[2], Bo Yeon Kim[3], Hye Won Bae[4] and Kwang-Ha Yoo[5]

Abstract

Background: Asthma requires regular follow-up visits and sustained medication use. Although several studies have reported the importance of adherence to medication and compliance with the treatment, none to date have reported the importance of regular follow-up visits. We investigated the effects of regular clinical visits on asthma exacerbation.

Methods: We used claims data in the national medical insurance review system provided by the Health Insurance Review and Assessment Service of Korea. We included subjects aged ≥ 15 years with a diagnosis of asthma, and who were prescribed asthma-related medication, from July 2013 to June 2014. Regular visitors (frequent visitors) were defined as subjects who visited the hospital for follow-up of asthma three or more times per year.

Results: Among 729,343 subjects, 496,560 (68.1%) were classified as regular visitors. Old age, male sex, lack of medical aid insurance, attendance of a tertiary hospital, a high Charlson comorbidity index, and a history of admission for exacerbated asthma in the previous year were significant determining factors for regular visitor status. When we adjusted for all these factors, frequent visitors showed a lower risk of asthma exacerbation requiring general ward admission (odds ratio [OR] 0.48; 95% confidence interval [CI] 0.47–0.50; $P < 0.001$), emergency room admission (OR 0.83; 95% CI 0.79–0.86; $P < 0.001$), and intensive care unit admission (OR 0.49; 95% CI 0.44–0.54; $P < 0.001$) than infrequent visitors.

Conclusions: Regular clinical visits are significantly associated with a reduced risk of asthma exacerbation requiring hospital admission in Korean adults with asthma.

Keywords: Asthma, Compliance, Exacerbation

Background

Asthma is characterized by chronic airway inflammation that requires regular followed-up visits and continuous medication use [1, 2]. Several studies have reported that a large proportion of asthma patients (10–60%) showed poor adherence to medication [3–5]. There are numerous reasons for such poor adherence. Some patients prefer to use medication for a shorter period of time, and therefore, they do not take medication when they are asymptomatic [6–8]. Other reasons include forgetfulness, inconvenience, and unawareness of the importance of medication [9]. However, many studies have revealed that subjects with good adherence to medication use were at reduced risk for asthma exacerbation and mortality as compared with subjects with poor adherence [10–12]. Therefore, clinicians have attempted to increase adherence to obtain a better prognosis by using inhaler reminders, good partnership, and intensive patient education and training [13, 14].

Regular clinical visits may have increased the opportunity to increase adherence and compliance. When

*Correspondence: littmann@yuhs.ac
[1] Department of Internal Medicine, Gangnam Severance Hospital, Yonsei University College of Medicine, 211 Eonju-ro Gangnam-gu, Seoul 135-720, South Korea
Full list of author information is available at the end of the article

patients visit clinics frequently, clinicians can pay careful attention to the patients, educate them in detail, judge the situation more appropriately, and prescribe the proper medication. Together, this might lead to an improved prognosis; however, to date, there are no data to prove this hypothesis. We therefore investigated the hypothesis that regular visits would have a protective effect against asthma exacerbation, by using a large body of claims data from the national medical insurance review system that covers most Korean individuals.

Methods

Ethics

This study was approved by the Ethics Committee of the National Evidence-Based Healthcare Collaborating Agency. The need for informed consent was waived by the institutional review board of the Gangnam Severance Hospital, Yonsei University Health System (Approval Number: 3-2016-0332).

Data sources

Korea has adopted a single mandatory government-established health insurance system, and the Health Insurance Review and Assessment Service (HIRA) is an agency responsible for evaluating all medical claim data in Korea. As the HIRA has accumulated all medical records, most Korean citizens are thought to be covered by this system [15]. We retrospectively reviewed and analyzed the data from the HIRA database of the national medical insurance review system of Korea.

Study populations

Patients with asthma were defined as follows, based on previous articles that had used HIRA data [15, 16]; this was also concordant with the definition used by HIRA for the asthma quality evaluation program. We included all patients aged ≥ 15 years, with asthma (J45.0, J45.1, J45.8, J45.9, J46.0, J46.1, J46.8, or J46.9 from the International Classification of Diseases-10th revision) as the principal or the first additional diagnosis, from July 2013 to June 2014. The included patients were prescribed asthma-related medication (inhaled, oral, or injected) on at least two outpatient visits, or on at least one outpatient visit along with systemic corticosteroids prescribed on admission. Asthma-related medications included corticosteroids, leukotriene antagonists, long-acting β2-agonists, short-acting β2-agonists, anticholinergics, and xanthine derivatives.

Definition of terms

Regular visitors (frequent visitors) were defined as subjects who visited the hospital for clinical follow-up of asthma three or more times per year, regardless of the

visit interval and visit site; alternatively, they were classified as infrequent visitors. The Charlson comorbidity index, which is a value facilitating prediction of prognosis and mortality based on comorbidities, was calculated as previously described [17, 18]. Asthma exacerbation requiring hospital admission was defined as an admission to a general ward, emergency room (ER), or intensive care unit (ICU), with a diagnosis of asthma as the principal or the first additional diagnosis.

Statistical analysis

We used the t test and Chi square test to identify differences in continuous data and categorical variables between frequent and infrequent visitors, respectively. Univariate and multivariate analyses were used to find significant factors for regular visitor status and admission with asthma exacerbation, using logistic regression analysis. We used SPSS v18.0 (IBM Corp, Armonk, NY). A P < 0.05 was considered statistically significant.

Results

Demographics of subjects

We reviewed 729,343 subjects enrolled in National Health Insurance Database. The mean age of subjects was 57.2 years, and 40.3% were male. Most subjects (82.2%) were followed-up in a primary hospital, while others (21.7%) attended a tertiary hospital. Pulmonary function tests were performed in 21.2% of subjects. Although data was not shown, 11.1% of subjects attended more than two hospital types. Most of the subjects (66.2%) had allergic rhinitis. Hypertension, diabetes mellitus, and metabolic syndrome accompanied asthma in 15.3, 7.7, and 6.5% of patients, respectively. The mean Charlson comorbidity index was 1.3. Some subjects (2.6%) had experienced at least one additional asthma exacerbation requiring hospital admission in the previous year. A total of 68.1% of cases were regular visitors (Table 1).

Significant factors for frequent visitors

Frequent visitors were significantly older. The percentage of male patients was slightly higher in the frequent visitor group, compared with the infrequent visitor group. They had less medical aid insurance and frequently attended a tertiary hospital. They also had a high Charlson's comorbidity index, and had more frequently experienced admission with exacerbated asthma in the previous year, as compared to infrequent visitors (Table 2).

We set out to define significant factors that determine frequent visitor status. Multivariate analysis confirmed that old age (odds ratio [OR] 10.5; 95% confidence interval [CI] 1.01–1.02; P < 0.001), male sex (OR 1.05; 95% CI 1.04–1.07; P < 0.001), tertiary hospital attendance (OR 4.97; 95% CI 4.84–5.10; P < 0.001), a higher Charlson

Table 1 Demographics of subjects

Parameters	N (%)
Age (mean ± SD)	57.2 ± 17.9
Male	293,762 (40.3)
Subjects with medical aid insurance	675,479 (92.6)
Hospital type	
Primary	599,460 (82.2)
Secondary	56,484 (7.7)
Tertiary	158,043 (21.7)
Tests subjects were taken	
Chest X-rays	118,479 (16.2)
Chest CT	2291 (0.3)
Pulmonary function test	154,984 (21.2)
Co-morbidity	
Ischemic heart disease	21,191 (2.9)
Osteoporosis	16,138 (2.2)
Depressive disorder	7703 (1.1)
Arthritis	24,392 (3.3)
Diabetes mellitus	56,355 (7.7)
Pneumothorax	716 (0.1)
Congestive heart failure	10,914 (1.5)
Hypertension	111,249 (15.3)
Anemia	7412 (1.0)
Metabolic syndrome	47,605 (6.5)
Allergic rhinitis	482,540 (66.2)
Charlson's comorbidity index (mean ± SD)	1.3 ± 0.7
Subjects admitted with exacerbated asthma in previous year	18,899 (2.6)
Frequent visitor	496,560 (68.1)
Total	729,343 (100.0)

SD standard deviation, CT computed tomography

comorbidity index (OR 1.40; 95% CI 1.39–1.42; P < 0.001), and a history of admission with exacerbated asthma in the previous year (OR 1.72; 95% CI 1.64–1.80; P < 0.001)

were significant contributing factors to frequent visitor status. Subjects with medical aid insurance tended not to be frequent visitors (OR 0.69; 95% CI 0.68–0.71; P < 0.001) (Table 3).

Number of subjects with asthma exacerbation according to visit frequency

We compared unadjusted healthcare utilization with asthma exacerbation between infrequent and frequent visitors. Frequent visitors showed more frequent exacerbations requiring admission to the general ward (4.6% vs. 3.2%; P < 0.001), ER (2.8% vs. 1.2%; P < 0.00), or ICU (0.4% vs. 0.3%; P < 0.001) than did infrequent visitors (Table 4).

Regular visits are protective factors against asthma exacerbation

Concordant with the results shown in Table 3 in univariate analysis, frequent visitor status was a significant risk factor for asthma exacerbation requiring general ward admission (OR 1.44; 95% CI 1.40–1.48; P < 0.001), ER utilization (OR 2.29; 95% CI 2.20–2.39; P < 0.001), and ICU admission (OR 1.54; 95% CI 1.41–1.69; P < 0.001). However, we sought to define whether the frequent visits increased the risk for or were protective against asthma exacerbation in adjusted conditions. In multivariate analysis, in which we included all the factors significant for frequent visitor status, we found the opposite results, as follows. Old age, male sex, subjects without medical aid insurance, tertiary hospital type attendance, a higher Charlson comorbidity index, and admission with exacerbated asthma in the previous year were significant predictive factors for asthma exacerbation requiring admission. Moreover, we found that frequent hospital visits was factor protecting against asthma exacerbation requiring general ward admission (OR 0.48; 95% CI 0.47–0.50; P < 0.001), ER utilization (OR 0.83; 95% CI 0.79–0.86; P < 0.001), and ICU admission (OR 0.49; 95% CI 0.44–0.54; P < 0.001) (Table 5).

Table 2 Differences in patterns between infrequent and frequent visitors

Parameters	Infrequent visitor	Frequent visitor	P value
Age (mean ± SD)	52.9 ± 18.5	59.2 ± 17.5	< 0.001
Male	38.9%	40.9%	< 0.001
Medical aid insurance	95.1%	91.4%	< 0.001
Hospital type			< 0.001
Primary	81.3%	67.4%	
Secondary	4.6%	4.0%	
Tertiary	11.0%	13.8%	
Charlson's comorbidity index (mean ± SD)	1.2 ± 0.5	1.4 ± 0.8	< 0.001
Admission with exacerbated asthma in previous year	1.0%	3.3%	< 0.001

SD standard deviation

Table 3 Significant factors contributing to frequent visitor status

Parameters	Univariate analysis		Multivariate analysis	
	OR (95% CI)	P value	OR (95% CI)	P value
Age	1.02 (1.02–1.02)	<0.001	1.01 (1.01–1.02)	<0.001
Male	1.09 (1.08–1.10)	<0.001	1.05 (1.04–1.07)	<0.001
Medical aid insurance	0.55 (0.54–0.56)	<0.001	0.69 (0.68–0.71)	<0.001
Hospital type				
Primary	0.82 (0.81–0.83)	<0.001	3.95 (3.84–4.06)	<0.001
Secondary	1.55 (1.52–1.58)	<0.001	3.35 (3.25–3.45)	<0.001
Tertiary	2.25 (2.22–2.28)	<0.001	4.97 (4.84–5.10)	<0.001
Charlson's comorbidity index	1.71 (1.69–1.72)	<0.001	1.40 (1.39–1.42)	<0.001
Admission with exacerbated asthma in previous year	3.28 (3.14–3.42)	<0.001	1.72 (1.64–1.80)	<0.001

OR odds ratio, *CI* confidence interval

Table 4 Number of subjects with asthma exacerbations, according to visit frequency

Parameters	Number of subjects experienced asthma exacerbation in infrequent visitor (%)	Number of subjects experienced asthma exacerbation in frequent visitor (%)	P value
General ward admission	7504 (3.2)	22,697 (4.6)	<0.001
ER admission	2881 (1.2)	13,876 (2.8)	<0.001
ICU admission	596 (0.3)	1958 (0.4)	<0.001
Total	232,783 (100.0)	496,560 (100.0)	

ER emergency room, *ICU* intensive care unit

Discussion

This large retrospective population study of asthma patients defined significant decisive factors for regular hospital visitor status, and demonstrated that regular visits were significantly associated with a better asthma prognosis. Superficially, regular visits would seem to be associated with increased asthma exacerbation, as shown in the unadjusted data in Table 2. We first identified significant decisive factors for regular visitor status, although age and male sex are not clinically significant factors. Importantly, admission with exacerbated asthma in the "previous year" was a significant factor for frequent visitor status. Thus, asthma patients who suffered asthma exacerbation in the "previous year" may visit the hospital frequently. Further, we observed acute exacerbation in the "next year" in both frequent and infrequent visitors. After we controlled for the effect of asthma exacerbation in the "previous year," including the effects of other significant decisive factors on regular visitor status, we found that the risk of acute exacerbation in the "next year" was reduced in frequent visitors. Regular visits (at least three or more times per year) were significantly associated with a reduction in the risk of general ward, ER, and ICU admission for exacerbated asthma by 52, 17, and 51%, respectively, as compared to infrequent hospital visits. This study therefore revealed that regular visits

may have protective effects against asthma exacerbation. We therefore suggest that clinicians should encourage asthma patients to participate in regular and frequent follow-up visits in order to reduce the risk for asthma exacerbation requiring admission.

Asthma is a chronic airway disease that requires long-term follow-up and consistent care. It is advisable to encourage patients to attend regular follow-up visits as a first step toward achieving a good prognosis. Patients require education regarding an asthma action plan [19], inhaler technique [20], required changes of medication dose and frequency [21], and improvement of the patient-physician partnership [22], in order to improve adherence and compliance, so as to facilitate a good prognosis. Regular visits are a precondition for these factors; notably, regular visitors may receive careful attention, be educated closely, and be assured that their medication is adjusted appropriately. Thus, regular visits will lead to increased adherence and compliance, with associated improvements in prognosis.

As in many countries, the majority of asthma patients are managed at primary hospitals (82.2%) by general practitioners in Korea because the initial management of asthma can be satisfactorily carried out at a primary hospital. Moreover, the primary hospital is generally more accessible, implies lower cost, and greater convenience.

Table 5 Univariate and multivariate analyses for asthma exacerbation requiring admission

Parameters	Univariate analysis		Multivariate analysis	
	OR (95% CI)	P value	OR (95% CI)	P value
General ward admission with exacerbated asthma				
Age	1.04 (1.04–1.04)	<0.001	1.02 (1.02–1.02)	<0.001
Male	1.08 (1.06–1.11)	<0.001	0.79 (0.77–0.81)	<0.001
Medical aid insurance	0.43 (0.42–0.44)	<0.001	0.81 (0.78–0.85)	<0.001
Hospital type				
Primary	0.19 (0.19–0.20)	<0.001	1.44 (1.39–1.48)	<0.001
Secondary	7.75 (7.56–7.95)	<0.001	15.97 (15.40–16.56)	<0.001
Tertiary	12.25 (11.93–12.58)	<0.001	20.14 (19.44–20.88)	<0.001
Charlson's comorbidity index	2.11 (2.09–2.13)	<0.001	1.62 (1.60–1.64)	<0.001
Admission with exacerbated asthma in previous year	14.16 (13.70–14.63)	<0.001	4.39 (4.22–4.56)	<0.001
Frequent visitor	1.44 (1.40–1.48)	<0.001	0.48 (0.47–0.50)	<0.001
ER admission with asthma exacerbation				
Age	1.02 (1.02–1.02)	<0.001	0.99 (1.00–1.00)	0.023
Male	1.44 (1.40–1.48)	<0.001	1.10 (1.07–1.14)	<0.001
Medical aid insurance	0.48 (0.46–0.050)	<0.001	0.79 (0.75–0.83)	<0.001
Hospital type				
Primary	0.25 (0.25–0.26)	<0.001	2.03 (1.96–2.11)	<0.001
Secondary	2.93 (2.82–3.05)	<0.001	4.10 (3.91–4.30)	<0.001
Tertiary	60.61 (56.91–64.56)	<0.001	77.05 (72.11–82.33)	<0.001
Charlson's comorbidity index	1.84 (1.82–1.86)	<0.001	1.38 (1.36–1.40)	<0.001
Admission with exacerbated asthma in previous year	9.51 (9.11–9.92)	<0.001	2.55 (2.43–2.67)	<0.001
Frequent visitor	2.29 (2.20–2.39)	<0.001	0.83 (0.79–0.86)	<0.001
ICU admission with asthma exacerbation				
Age	1.08 (1.08–1.08)	<0.001	1.05 (1.05–1.06)	<0.001
Male	1.55 (1.44–1.68)	<0.001	1.16 (1.07–1.26)	<0.001
Medical aid insurance	0.39 (0.35–0.43)	<0.001	0.84 (0.75–0.94)	0.002
Hospital type				
Primary	0.19 (0.17–0.20)	<0.001	1.42 (1.30–1.54)	<0.001
Secondary	2.33 (2.10–2.59)	<0.001	2.09 (1.87–2.34)	<0.001
Tertiary	158.04 (121.81–205.04)	<0.001	122.29 (93.79–159.45)	<0.001
Charlson's comorbidity index	2.13 (2.09–2.18)	<0.001	1.51 (1.48–1.55)	<0.001
Admission with exacerbated asthma in previous year	11.68 (10.64–12.82)	<0.001	2.47 (2.23–2.72)	<0.001
Frequent visitor	1.54 (1.41–1.69)	<0.001	0.49 (0.44–0.54)	<0.001

OR odds ratio, *CI* confidence interval, *ER* emergency room, *ICU* intensive care unit

Therefore, the role of the general practitioner at primary hospitals in encouraging asthma patients to participate in regular and frequent follow-up visits is important.

In Korea, an asthma quality evaluation program was launched in 2013, to improve the quality of life of asthma patients and achieve a good prognosis. The assessment parameters included the frequency of pulmonary function tests, the frequency of prescription of mandatory asthma medications (inhaled corticosteroids and/or anti-leukotriene modifiers) [23], the frequency of prescription of non-mandatory asthma medications (beta-agonist and/or oral corticosteroids), and regular visitor status, which was defined as subjects who visited

hospitals for asthma three or more times per year. We therefore attempted to identify whether regular visits facilitated a good prognosis. We used the same definition as described in the asthma appropriateness assessment in Korea in this study.

The GINA 2016 guidelines recommend that patients should preferably be seen 1–3 months for step-up and step-down management after starting treatment, and thereafter every 3–12 months for maintenance [2]. However, there has been no clear evidence to date supporting the necessity of frequent and regular visits. The persistence rate for clinic visits is reported to be 65 and 40% after 3 and 6 months of medication initiation, respectively [24]. Our findings suggest that asthma patients should be followed-up at least every 3–4 months (at least three or more times per year), and that this may be an easy approach for achieving a favorable prognosis.

The strength of this study was that we included a large population, reflecting almost all adults with asthma in Korea. The national medical insurance review system covers nearly all Korean individuals, and therefore, the 729,343 subjects enrolled in this study might encompass all the asthma patients in Korea. This is also supported by a calculation based on an asthma prevalence of about 2% and the total population size (about 40 million) in South Korea [25]. Therefore, this indicates the trustworthiness of the data.

This study has some limitations. First, this is a cross-sectional observational study, not a cohort study. There-fore, we cannot firmly conclude that regular visits directly reduce asthma exacerbations. We cannot ascer-tain causality; instead, we suggest that regular visits are significantly associated with reduced asthma exacerba-tions. Second, we could not analyze the potential vari-ables that affect the frequency of visits and prognosis due to the retrospective nature of this study. For instance, adherence to medication, the dose of the inhaler, socio-economic status, clinical characteristics, residential dis-trict, and weather may be influential factors [26, 27]. In this retrospective study, which used claim data from a national medical insurance review system, the available variables were extremely restricted. Third, we used an operational definition for asthma diagnosis and exacerba-tion. We could not use the results of pulmonary function tests, or review the clinical charts of patients. Moreover, the operational definition of "asthma exacerbation" used in this study may contain a small number of patients who were admitted to the hospital for other reasons. This operational definition may influence the results; how-ever, the large number of subjects may overcome this bias. Fourth, we could not discriminate mild exacerba-tions that did not require admission. Outpatients with mild exacerbations may visit clinics more frequently, and this may be a confounding factor. However, a history of exacerbation in previous years, for which we adjusted in this study, will also help to overcome this bias. Fifth, we cannot ignore collider bias; medication analysis could be considered to reveal indirect effects of other variables on asthma exacerbations. Last, we did not stratify accord-ing to the number of visits. Further studies are needed to determine an optimal threshold for the number of visits.

Conclusions

This retrospective study, based on a large study popu-lation, demonstrated that regular clinic visits are sig-nificantly associated with reducing the risk of asthma exacerbation requiring hospital admission by 20–50% in Korean adults with asthma. We recommend that clini-cians encourage asthma patients to participate in regular medical visits to achieve a good prognosis.

Abbreviations
HIRA: Health Insurance Review and Assessment Service; CI: confidence inter-val; ER: emergency room; ICU: intensive care unit; OR: odds ratio.

Authors' contributions
HJP: This author contributed to the conception and design of this study. She analyzed, and interpreted the data. She drafted and revised the article and approved the final version of the article for publication. HJK, CMA, CKR, BYK, HWB, K-HY: These authors collected the data, generated and analyzed the data. They contributed to the draft, revised the article, and approved the final version of the article for publication. KK: This author, as a professional statisti-cian, possesses scientific responsibility for the analysis and interpretation of the data. MKB: This author provided critical opinion regarding the concept and design of this study, as the corresponding author. He interpreted the data and drafted and revised the articles. He approved the final version of the article for publication. All authors read and approved the final manuscript.

Author details
[1] Department of Internal Medicine, Gangnam Severance Hospital, Yonsei Uni-versity College of Medicine, 211 Eonju-ro Gangnam-gu, Seoul 135-720, South Korea. [2] Division of Pulmonary, Allergy and Critical Care Medicine, Department of Internal Medicine, Seoul St Mary's Hospital, College of Medicine, The Catho-lic University of Korea, Seoul, South Korea. [3] Healthcare Review and Assess-ment Committee, Health Insurance Review & Assessment Service, Seoul, South Korea. [4] Division of Quality Assessment Management, Health Insurance Review & Assessment Service, Seoul, South Korea. [5] Division of Pulmonary, Allergy and Critical Care Medicine, Department of Internal Medicine, Konkuk University School of Medicine, Seoul, South Korea.

Acknowledgements
HIRA (Joint Project on Quality Assessment Research) collected the raw data, provided the data to the authors, and permitted the use of data by the authors.

Competing interests
The authors declare that they have no competing interests.

Funding
Not applicable.

References
1. Kim DK, Park YB, Oh YM, Jung KS, Yoo JH, Yoo KH, et al. Korean Asthma Guideline 2014: summary of major updates to the Korean Asthma Guide-line 2014. Tuberc Respir Dis (Seoul). 2016;79(3):111–20.
2. FitzGerald JM. 2016 GINA report, global strategy for asthma management and prevention. 2016. http://ginasthma.org/2018-gina-report-global-strategy-for-asthma-management-and-prevention/.
3. Spector S. Noncompliance with asthma therapy—are there solutions? J Asthma. 2000;37(5):381–8.
4. Cerveri I, Locatelli F, Zoia MC, Corsico A, Accordini S, de Marco R. Inter-national variations in asthma treatment compliance: the results of the European Community respiratory health survey (ECRHS). Eur Respir J. 1999;14(2):288–94.
5. van der Palen J, Klein JJ, Rovers MM. Compliance with inhaled medication and self-treatment guidelines following a self-management programme in adult asthmatics. Eur Respir J. 1997;10(3):652–7.
6. Chambers CV, Markson L, Diamond JJ, Lasch L, Berger M. Health beliefs and compliance with inhaled corticosteroids by asthmatic patients in primary care practices. Respir Med. 1999;93(2):88–94.

7. Buston KM, Wood SF. Non-compliance amongst adolescents with asthma: listening to what they tell us about self-management. Fam Pract. 2000;17(2):134–8.

8. Put C, Van den Bergh O, Demedts M, Verleden G. A study of the relationship among self-reported noncompliance, symptomatology, and psychological variables in patients with asthma. J Asthma. 2000;37(6):503–10.

9. Boulet LP. Perception of the role and potential side effects of inhaled corticosteroids among asthmatic patients. Chest. 1998;113(3):587–92.

10. Otsuki M, Eakin MN, Rand CS, Butz AM, Hsu VD, Zuckerman IH, et al. Adherence feedback to improve asthma outcomes among inner-city children: a randomized trial. Pediatrics. 2009;124(6):1513–21.

11. Sturdy PM, Victor CR, Anderson HR, Bland JM, Butland BK, Harrison BD, et al. Psychological, social and health behaviour risk factors for deaths certified as asthma: a national case-control study. Thorax. 2002;57(12):1034–9.

12. Stern L, Berman J, Lumry W, Katz L, Wang L, Rosenblatt L, et al. Medication compliance and disease exacerbation in patients with asthma: a retrospective study of managed care data. Ann Allergy Asthma Immunol. 2006;97(3):402–8.

13. Foster JM, Usherwood T, Smith L, Sawyer SM, Xuan W, Rand CS, et al. Inhaler reminders improve adherence with controller treatment in primary care patients with asthma. J Allergy Clin Immunol. 2014;134(6):1260–1268.e3.

14. Clark NM, Cabana MD, Nan B, Gong ZM, Slish KK, Birk NA, et al. The clinician–patient partnership paradigm: outcomes associated with physician communication behavior. Clin Pediatr (Phila). 2008;47(1):49–57.

15. Yang MS, Lee JY, Kim J, Kim GW, Kim BK, Kim JY, et al. Incidence of Stevens–Johnson syndrome and toxic epidermal necrolysis: a nationwide population-based study using National Health Insurance Database in Korea. PLoS ONE. 2016;11(11):e0165933.

16. Lee J, Lee JH, Kim JA, Rhee CK. Trend of cost and utilization of COPD medication in Korea. Int J Chronic Obstr Pulm Dis. 2017;12:27–33.

17. Charlson ME, Pompei P, Ales KL, MacKenzie CR. A new method of classifying prognostic comorbidity in longitudinal studies: development and validation. J Chronic Dis. 1987;40(5):373–83.

18. Song SE, Lee SH, Jo EJ, Eom JS, Mok JH, Kim MH, et al. The prognostic value of the Charlson's comorbidity index in patients with prolonged acute mechanical ventilation: a single center experience. Tuberc Respir Dis (Seoul). 2016;79(4):289–94.

19. Larson A, Ward J, Ross L, Whyatt D, Weatherston M, Landau L. Impact of structured education and self management on rural asthma outcomes. Aust Fam Physician. 2010;39(3):141–4.

20. Prabhakaran L, Lim G, Abisheganaden J, Chee CB, Choo YM. Impact of an asthma education programme on patients' knowledge, inhaler technique and compliance to treatment. Singapore Med J. 2006;47(3):225–31.

21. Aftab RA, Khan AH, Sulaiman SAS, Ali I, Hassali A, Saleem F. An assessment of adherence to asthma medication guidelines: findings from a tertiary care center in the state of Penang, Malaysia. Turk J Med Sci. 2016;46(5):1300–5.

22. Small M, Vickers A, Anderson P, Kay S. The patient–physician partnership in asthma: real-world observations associated with clinical and patient-reported outcomes. Adv Ther. 2010;27(9):591–9.

23. Price D, Musgrave SD, Shepstone L, Hillyer EV, Sims EJ, Gilbert RF, et al. Leukotriene antagonists as first-line or add-on asthma-controller therapy. N Engl J Med. 2011;364(18):1695–707.

24. Hayashida M, Murayama N, Toyoshima K, Fujiwara H, Teraoka O, Yamamoto Y, et al. Persistence rate for clinic visit in children with asthma after initiating controller therapy. Arerugi. 2012;61(7):959–69.

25. Kim H, Oh SY, Kang MH, Kim KN, Kim Y, Chang N. Association between kimchi intake and asthma in Korean adults: the fourth and fifth Korea National Health and Nutrition Examination Survey (2007–2011). J Med Food. 2014;17(1):172–8.

26. Kwon JW, Han YJ, Oh MK, Lee CY, Kim JY, Kim EJ, et al. Emergency department visits for asthma exacerbation due to weather conditions and air pollution in Chuncheon, Korea: a case-crossover analysis. Allergy Asthma Immunol Res. 2016;8(6):512–21.

27. Chang C, Lee SM, Choi BW, Song JH, Song H, Jung S, et al. Costs attributable to overweight and obesity in working asthma patients in the United States. Yonsei Med J. 2017;58(1):187–94.

8

Clinical implications of CD4$^+$ T cell subsets in adult atopic asthma patients

Matthew Wiest[1,2†], Katherine Upchurch[1,2†], Wenjie Yin[1,2], Jerome Ellis[1], Yaming Xue[1], Bobby Lanier[3], Mark Millard[4], HyeMee Joo[1,2] and SangKon Oh[1,2*]

Abstract

Background: T cells play a central role in chronic inflammation in asthma. However, the roles of individual subsets of T cells in the pathology of asthma in patients remain to be better understood.

Methods: We investigated the potential signatures of T cell subset phenotypes in asthma using fresh whole blood from adult atopic asthma patients (n = 43) and non-asthmatic control subjects (n = 22). We further assessed their potential clinical implications by correlating asthma severity.

Results: We report four major features of CD4$^+$ T cells in the blood of atopic asthma patients. First, patients had a profound increase of CCR7$^+$ memory CD4$^+$ T cells, but not CCR7$^-$ memory CD4$^+$ T cells. Second, an increase in CCR4$^+$ CD4$^+$ T cells in patients was mainly attributed to the increase of CCR7$^+$ memory CD4$^+$ T cells. Accordingly, the frequency of CCR4$^+$CCR7$^+$ memory CD4$^+$ T cells correlated with asthma severity. Current common asthma therapeutics (including corticosteroids) were not able to affect the frequency of CCR4$^+$CCR7$^+$ memory CD4$^+$ T cell subsets. Third, patients had an increase of Tregs, as assessed by measuring CD25, Foxp3, IL-10 and CTLA-4 expression. However, asthma severity was inversely correlated only with the frequency of CTLA-4$^+$ CD4$^+$ T cells. Lastly, patients and control subjects have similar frequencies of CD4$^+$ T cells that express CCR5, CCR6, CXCR3, CXCR5, CD11a, or α4 integrin. However, the frequency of α4$^+$ CD4$^+$ T cells in patients correlated with asthma severity.

Conclusions: CCR4$^+$CCR7$^+$ memory, but not CCR4$^+$CCR7$^-$ memory, α4$^+$, and CTLA4$^+$ CD4$^+$ T cells in patients show significant clinical implications in atopic asthma. Current common therapeutics cannot alter the frequency of such CD4$^+$ T cell subsets in adult atopic asthma patients.

Keywords: Asthma, Atopic, CD4$^+$ T cell, CCR7, CCR4, Integrin, Alpha 4, CTLA-4, β-Agonist, Corticosteroid, Therapy

Background

Chronic inflammation in the lung with airway hyper-responsiveness is one of the major characteristics of asthma [1]. Asthma is a highly heterogeneous disease comprised of distinct clinical, immunological, and genetic phenotypes [2–4]; however, the pathogenesis of asthma has been classically characterized as elevated Th2-type inflammatory responses to antigen. These elevated Th2-type cells have also been found in the blood of

asthma patients, indicating that immune cells responsible for chronic inflammation in the lung circulate in the blood [5–8].

The normal response to a harmless allergen is tolerance, but asthmatic patients can respond with elevated Th2-type immune responses. Th2-type CD4$^+$ T cells secrete IL-4, IL-5, and IL-13, which play important downstream roles in asthma pathogenesis [9]. IL-4 induces IgE class-switching and expression of vascular cell adhesion molecule-1 on endothelial cells [10, 11]. IL-5 is crucial for the activation of eosinophils and their migration into the lung [12]. IL-13 is associated with various important events during the effector phase of asthma including airway hyper-responsiveness, mucus hyper-production, and airway remodeling [13, 14]. However, the high level

---

*Correspondence: bobkid.jo@gmail.com; sangkono@baylorhealth.edu
†Matthew Wiest and Katherine Upchurch contributed equally to this work
[1] Baylor Institute for Immunology Research, 3434 Live Oak St., Dallas, TX 75204, USA
Full list of author information is available at the end of the article

of clinical heterogeneity of asthma suggests that the pathogenesis of asthma must not be solely driven by Th2-type immune responses [15]. In almost all patients with asthma, one can find a counter-regulatory population, regulatory T cells (Tregs), that are capable of suppressing inflammatory responses [16–18]. In addition, CD8$^+$ T cells can also contribute to the etiopathology of asthmatic inflammation [19, 20]. Overall, T cells can play a central role in the initiation, progression, and exacerbation of asthma. However, the underlying mechanisms of the chronic inflammation in the lung and the levels of contribution by different T cell subsets remain to be fully elucidated.

Antigen-experienced T cells are phenotypically classified into effector and memory T cell populations, the latter being subdivided into CCR7$^-$ effector memory T cells (Tem) and CCR7$^+$ central memory T cells (Tcm) [21]. It has been previously reported that memory T cells are associated with chronic inflammatory diseases [22, 23]. However, the specific subpopulations of human memory T cells that are responsible for chronic allergic disorders, including asthma, have not been well characterized. This is partly due to variations in the phenotypes of pathogenic T cells in asthma patients. It is further exacerbated by patient-intrinsic factors, such as differences in offending allergens, as well as environmental changes, which can affect timing of allergen exposure (e.g., perennial vs. seasonal allergy). Furthermore, the number of memory T cells recoverable from lungs of asthma patients is extremely limited. Despite these complicating factors, it is imperative to find which T cell subsets, especially which subset of memory T cells, are associated with chronic inflammation in the lungs of asthma patients.

To this end, we hypothesized that T cells in atopic asthma patients display unique phenotypes and functions that can support chronic inflammation in the lung. We utilized fresh whole blood from atopic asthma patients and non-asthmatic control subjects as a source of T cells for investigation. Although T cells in the peripheral blood may not be the same as those in the lungs of asthma patients, their altered phenotypes and functions could also be associated with the pathogenesis of asthma [23–27]. We found that T cells in the blood of adult atopic asthma patients display several unique phenotypic and functional features. More importantly, some of the new features found in this study correlate with asthma severity, supporting the clinical relevance of these altered phenotypes and functions in atopic asthma patients. Further clinical data analysis concluded that corticosteroids do not affect these altered phenotypes or functions of T cells in atopic asthma. Data from this study could thus help us extend our knowledge of the pathophysiology of human asthma and potentially

contribute to the rational design of new therapeutic approaches for asthma in the future.

Methods

Patients and control subjects

Adult asthma patients (n = 43) were recruited in this study (Table 1). Clinical variables, including asthma control test (ACT) score, lung function, as defined by the forced expiratory volume in 1 s (% predicted FEV1), and frequency of symptoms (e.g., total number of symptoms per week and nighttime sleep disruptions) as defined by the expert panel report from the National Asthma Education and Prevention Program [28], were acquired. All patients showed positive responses to at least one allergen by a skin prick test, as measured by the assessment of hypersensitivity (wheal—a raised white bump surrounded by a small circle of itchy red skin) to allergens. Except for four patients, all patients were being treated with either short- or long-acting β-agonists at the time of blood draw. Non-asthmatic control subjects (n = 22) were also recruited. All subjects were enrolled under protocols approved by the Institutional Review Board of Baylor Scott & White Research Institute. Donors were excluded if they were pregnant, under the age of 18, or if they had any other chronic diseases.

Whole blood T cell analysis

Blood was drawn twice over a 1-week interval and average values from two separate experiments were used. Complete blood count (CBC) was performed with Coulter Ac·T$^{™}$ 5diff (Beckman Coulter). Whole blood (200 µL) was stained with the indicated antibodies and 50 µL of brilliant stain buffer (Becton–Dickinson: BD) to

Table 1 Information of atopic asthma patients and non-asthmatic control subjects recruited in this study

Characteristics	Asthma patients	Non-asthmatic controls
Total population, n	43	22
Inhaled corticosteroid (%)	25 (58)	
Oral corticosteroid (%)	7 (14)	
Leukotriene inhibitor (%)	22 (51)	
Untreated (%)	9 (21)	
Age (years)	51.9 (± 11.31)	47.59 (± 12.60)
Sex (M/F) (%M)	15/28 (35)	8/14 (36)
Height (in)	66.54 (± 3.31)	67.55 (± 3.41)
Weight (lbs)	188.8 (± 39.30)	162.0 (± 28.99)
Caucasian, n (%)	38 (88)	17 (77)
African American, n (%)	3 (7)	4 (18)
Asian, n (%)	1 (2)	1 (5)

All data are expressed as mean with SD (if applicable)

enhance brilliant violet fluorochrome stability. Red blood cells were lysed, and cells were fixed with lysing solution (BD). Stained cells were analyzed on an LSR Fortessa flow cytometer (BD), and the results were analyzed with Flow Jo (TreeStar). Detailed information for antibodies used in this study is summarized in Additional file 1: Table S1. To count cell numbers, 20 μL of CountBright absolute counting beads (Life Technologies) were added to each sample. Cell counts were calculated using the number of cell events (A) divided by the number of bead events (B) multiplied by the assigned number of counting beads added based on lot (C) divided by the volume of the sample (D):

$$\frac{A}{B} \times \frac{C}{D} = \text{concentration of sample.}$$

PBMC isolation and measurement of T cell cytokines

Peripheral blood mononuclear cells (PBMCs) were isolated by density gradient centrifugation using Ficoll-Plaque PLUS (GE Healthcare). PBMCs were plated at 5×10^5 cells/100 μL in 96-well U-bottom plates in RPMI 1640 (Invitrogen) supplemented with HEPES (Invitrogen), 1% non-essential amino acids, 2 mM L-glutamate (Sigma-Aldrich), 50 μg/mL penicillin, and 50 μg/mL streptomycin (Life Technologies). T cells were stimulated with αCD3/αCD28 human dynabeads (Life Technologies) at a 1:1, bead:cell ratio. The amounts of cytokines in diluted supernatants were measured by multiplex bead-based assay (Bio-Rad) after 36-h stimulation when the amount of cytokines reaches maximum levels. A 5-parameter curve fitting algorithm was applied for standard curve generation. Detection limits of the standard curve were 0.2 ng/mL < IL-10 ≤ 3.5 ng/mL, 0.2 ng/mL ≤ IFN-γ ≤ 15 ng/mL, 0.05 ng/mL ≤ IL-4 ≤ 5 ng/mL, 0.2 ng/mL ≤ IL-5 ≤ 1 ng/mL, and 0.2 ng/mL ≤ IL-13 ≤ 3 ng/mL. For intracellular staining, cells were stimulated with αCD3/αCD28 dynabeads for 5–6 h, with Golgiplug (BD) added 1–2 h after stimulation.

Statistical analysis

Statistical significance was determined using a non-parametric Mann–Whitney test. One-way analysis of variance (ANOVA) with the Tukey test was utilized for statistical significance where specified. Correlation analysis was performed with non-parametric Spearman correlation. Statistical significance analysis was performed with Prism 5 (GraphPad Software). Significance was set at P < 0.05.

Results

Atopic asthma patients have an increase of CCR7$^+$ memory CD4$^+$ T cells

We first investigated the frequency of naïve and memory T cells in the peripheral blood of adult atopic

asthma patients (n = 43) and non-asthmatic control subjects (n = 22) by staining whole blood with antibodies specific for surface molecules (Fig. 1a). As summarized in Fig. 1b, atopic asthma patients and control subjects had similar percentages of CD3$^+$, CD3$^+$CD4$^+$, CD3$^+$CD4$^+$CD45RA$^+$CD45RO$^-$ and CD3$^+$CD4$^+$CD8$^+$ T cells in their blood. However, atopic asthma patients had a greater percentage of CD45RA$^-$CD45RO$^+$ memory CD4$^+$ T cells than control subjects, as previously described [29]. CBC data show that total numbers of lymphocytes were not significantly different in the two groups (Table 2). However, atopic asthma patients had significantly more circulating eosinophils and neutrophils. Basophil numbers were also increased in patients, but the difference was not statistically significant. No significant difference was observed for red blood cell or platelet counts in the two groups.

Memory (CD45RA$^-$CD45RO$^+$) CD4$^+$ T cells were further analyzed based on their CCR7 expression (Fig. 1a). Compiled data from atopic asthma patients and control subjects indicated that atopic asthma patients have more CD45RA$^-$CD45RO$^+$CCR7$^+$ CD4$^+$ T cells than control subjects (Fig. 1c, left). The percentage of CD45RA$^-$CD45RO$^+$CCR7$^-$ CD4$^+$ T cells was similar in the two groups (Fig. 1c, right). The numbers of CD45RA$^-$CD45RO$^+$CCR7$^+$ (Fig. 1d, left) and CD45RA$^-$CD45RO$^+$CCR7$^-$ CD4$^+$ T cells per microliter of blood (Fig. 1d, right) also showed similar trends. There was no significant correlation between ages of patients recruited in this study and the frequency of CD45RA$^-$CD45RO$^+$, CD45RA$^-$CD45RO$^+$CCR7$^+$, or CD45RA$^-$CD45RO$^+$CCR7$^-$ CD4$^+$ and CD8$^+$ T cells (Additional file 2: Figure S1), confirming previously reported observations [30, 31]. Both atopic asthma patients and control subjects had similar frequencies of naïve (CD45RA$^+$CD45RO$^-$CCR7$^+$) and CD45RA$^+$CD45RO$^-$CCR7$^-$ CD4$^+$ T cells (Fig. 1e).

Therefore, we concluded that adult atopic asthma patients have an increase of circulating CD45RA$^-$CD45RO$^+$CCR7$^+$ T cells, but not CD45RA$^-$CD45RO$^+$CCR7$^-$ or CD45RA$^+$CD45RO$^-$ CD4$^+$ T cells.

The increase of CCR7$^+$ memory CD4$^+$ T cells is observed in atopic asthma subgroups and is resistant to common therapeutics

Due to the heterogeneity of asthma phenotypes and clinical variation, we next investigated whether the increase of CCR7$^+$ memory CD4$^+$ T cells is a common feature of different asthma subtypes. Atopic asthma patients were divided into two subgroups, based on their blood eosinophil counts. We found that patients with blood eosinophilia (eosinophil count > 450/μL blood) and

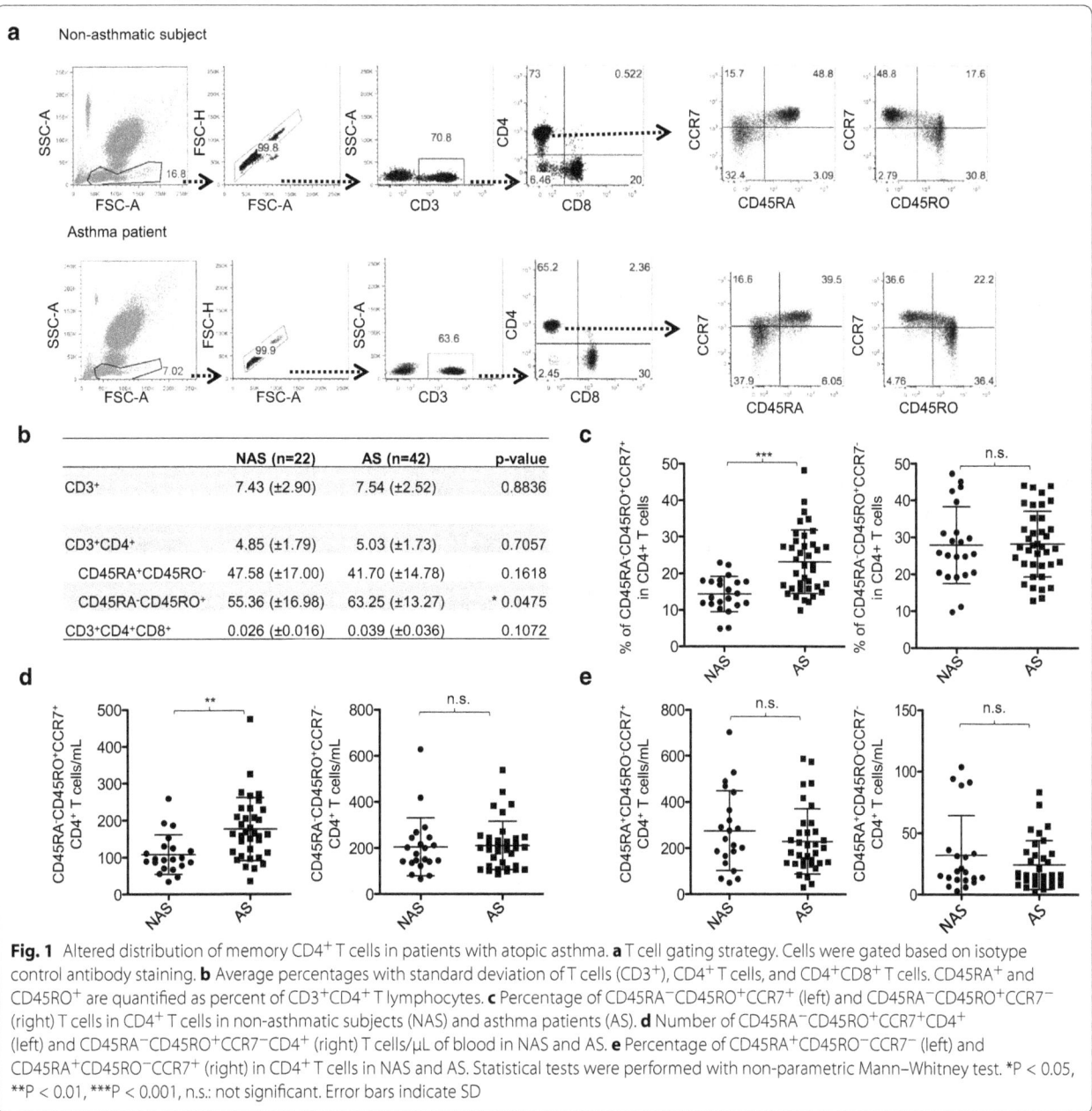

Fig. 1 Altered distribution of memory CD4$^+$ T cells in patients with atopic asthma. **a** T cell gating strategy. Cells were gated based on isotype control antibody staining. **b** Average percentages with standard deviation of T cells (CD3$^+$), CD4$^+$ T cells, and CD4$^+$CD8$^+$ T cells. CD45RA$^+$ and CD45RO$^+$ are quantified as percent of CD3$^+$CD4$^+$ T lymphocytes. **c** Percentage of CD45RA$^-$CD45RO$^+$CCR7$^+$ (left) and CD45RA$^-$CD45RO$^+$CCR7$^-$ (right) T cells in CD4$^+$ T cells in non-asthmatic subjects (NAS) and asthma patients (AS). **d** Number of CD45RA$^-$CD45RO$^+$CCR7$^+$CD4$^+$ (left) and CD45RA$^-$CD45RO$^+$CCR7$^-$CD4$^+$ (right) T cells/μL of blood in NAS and AS. **e** Percentage of CD45RA$^+$CD45RO$^-$CCR7$^-$ (left) and CD45RA$^+$CD45RO$^-$CCR7$^+$ (right) in CD4$^+$ T cells in NAS and AS. Statistical tests were performed with non-parametric Mann–Whitney test. *P < 0.05, **P < 0.01, ***P < 0.001, n.s.: not significant. Error bars indicate SD

non-eosinophilia (eosinophil count < 450/μL blood) had similar percentages of circulating CCR7$^+$ memory CD4$^+$ T cells, but both subgroups of patients had a higher percentage of CCR7$^+$ memory CD4$^+$ T cells than non-asthmatic control subjects (Fig. 2a). We next divided patients into three subgroups based on their % predicted FEV1 (mild: FEV1 > 80; moderate: FEV1 = 60–80; and severe: FEV1 < 60). As shown in Fig. 2b, all three subgroups of patients had higher percentages of CCR7$^+$ memory T cells than control subjects. There was no significant difference between the three subgroups of patients.

We further investigated whether prescribed therapeutics could impact the frequency of the CCR7$^+$ memory CD4$^+$ T cells. Patients treated with corticosteroids [either inhaled (N = 26) or oral corticosteroid (N = 7)] and patients who did not receive corticosteroid therapy (N = 14) within 2 weeks before blood draw had more CCR7$^+$ memory CD4$^+$ T cells than non-asthmatic control subjects (Fig. 2c, left). However, the two groups of patients (corticosteroid versus no corticosteroid) had similar percentages of CCR7$^+$ memory CD4$^+$ T cells. We further found that oral corticosteroid usage did not

Table 2 Complete blood counts, per microliter of blood

Cell types	Atopic asthma patients	Non-asthmatic controls	p-value
Lymphocytes	1473 ($\pm$ 389)	1353 ($\pm$ 332)	0.2347
Eosinophils	321 ($\pm$ 258)	105 ($\pm$ 38)	0.0005
Neutrophils	3953 ($\pm$ 1417)	2310 ($\pm$ 551)	0.0001
Basophils	33 ($\pm$ 17)	25 ($\pm$ 13)	0.0529
Monocytes	577 ($\pm$ 207)	410 ($\pm$ 233)	0.0057
RBC	4.03×10^6 ($\pm 0.442 \times 10^6$)	3.93×10^6 ($\pm 0.343 \times 10^6$)	0.3938
Platelets	215×10^3 ($\pm 69.1 \times 10^3$)	215×10^3 ($\pm 56.5 \times 10^3$)	0.9863

Data are expressed as mean cell number per microliter with SD. A Bonferroni correction was used for the multiple comparisons

significantly alter the percentage of such CD4$^+$ T cell subset (Fig. 2c, right). In addition, inhaled corticosteroid did not significantly alter the percentage of CCR7$^+$ memory CD4$^+$ T cells in patients (data not shown). Furthermore, leukotriene inhibitors did not alter the percentage of CCR7$^+$ memory CD4$^+$ T cells in the blood of adult atopic asthma patients (Fig. 2d).

We thus concluded that the increase of circulating CCR7$^+$ memory CD4$^+$ T cells is a common feature of adult atopic asthma patients. This feature was also

maintained throughout different atopic asthma subtypes examined in this study. In addition, corticosteroids or leukotriene inhibitors were not able to change the frequency of CCR7$^+$ memory CD4$^+$ T cells in patients.

Atopic asthma patients have an increase of CCR4$^+$ CD4$^+$ T cells, but this is mainly due to the increase of CCR7$^+$ memory CD4$^+$ T cells

Chemokine receptors expressed on T cells can contribute to T cell migration into local tissues as well as into lymph nodes. They are also indicative markers of T cell subsets—CXCR3 for Th1, CCR4 for Th2, CCR6 for Th17, and CXCR5 for follicular helper T cells (Tfh) [32]. CD4$^+$ T cells expressing CCR4 have thus been of particular interest in the pathogenesis of allergic asthma. As such, we analyzed the frequency of CD4$^+$ T cell subsets expressing CCR4 in atopic asthma patients and non-asthmatic control subjects.

Atopic asthma patients have a higher percentage of CCR4$^+$CD4$^+$ T cells (Fig. 3a), as has been previously described [33]. Such increases can also be seen in the percentage of CCR4$^+$CD45RA$^-$CD45RO$^+$ CD4$^+$ T cells (Fig. 3b). However, the difference between patients and control subjects was more significant when analyzing the percentage of CCR4$^+$CD45RA$^-$CD45RO$^+$CCR7$^+$ cells in CD4$^+$ T cells (Fig. 3c, left). There was

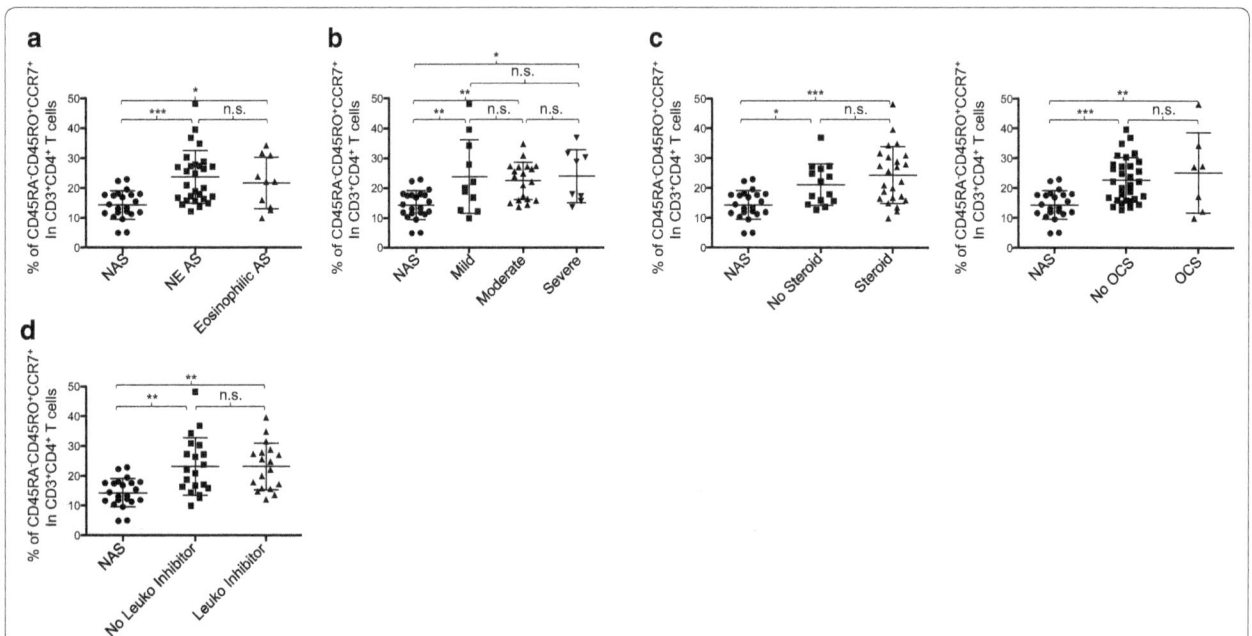

Fig. 2 The increase of CCR7$^+$ memory CD4$^+$ T cells is unaffected by common therapeutics. **a** Percentage of CD45RA$^-$CD45RO$^+$CCR7$^+$ cells in CD3$^+$CD4$^+$ T cells across non-asthmatic subjects (NAS) and asthma patients (AS) with (Eosinophilic AS) or without (NE AS) blood eosinophilia. **b** Percentage of CD45RA$^-$CD45RO$^+$CCR7$^+$ cells in CD4$^+$ T cells in atopic asthma of different severities based on % predicted FEV1 scores (mild: > 80%, moderate: 60–79%, severe: < 60%). Percentage of CD45RA$^-$CD45RO$^+$CCR7$^+$ cells in CD3$^+$CD4$^+$ T cells in NAS and AS treated with/without corticosteroids (**c**, left) oral corticosteroid (OCS) (**c**, right) and leukotriene inhibitor (**d**). Analysis based on one-way ANOVA with Tukey test. *P < 0.05, **P < 0.01, ***P < 0.001, n.s.: not significant. Error bars indicate SD

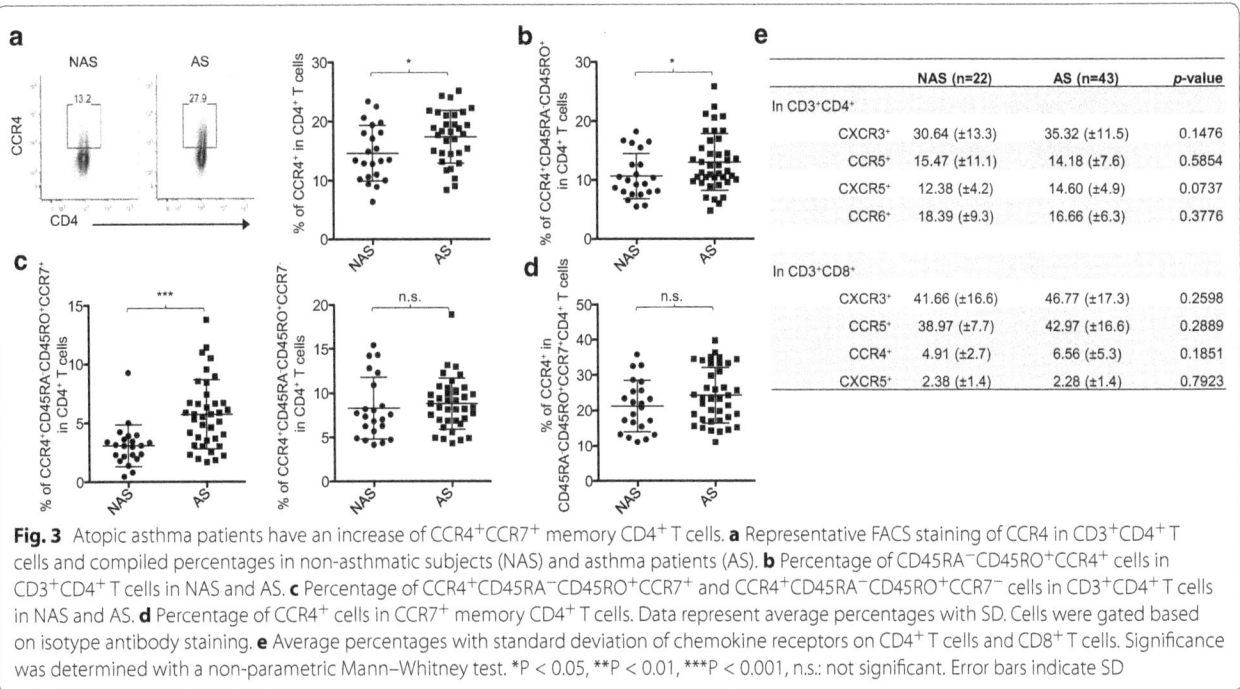

	NAS (n=22)	AS (n=43)	p-value
In CD3⁺CD4⁺			
CXCR3⁺	30.64 (±13.3)	35.32 (±11.5)	0.1476
CCR5⁺	15.47 (±11.1)	14.18 (±7.6)	0.5854
CXCR5⁺	12.38 (±4.2)	14.60 (±4.9)	0.0737
CCR6⁺	18.39 (±9.3)	16.66 (±6.3)	0.3776
In CD3⁺CD8⁺			
CXCR3⁺	41.66 (±16.6)	46.77 (±17.3)	0.2598
CCR5⁺	38.97 (±7.7)	42.97 (±16.6)	0.2889
CCR4⁺	4.91 (±2.7)	6.56 (±5.3)	0.1851
CXCR5⁺	2.38 (±1.4)	2.28 (±1.4)	0.7923

Fig. 3 Atopic asthma patients have an increase of CCR4⁺CCR7⁺ memory CD4⁺ T cells. **a** Representative FACS staining of CCR4 in CD3⁺CD4⁺ T cells and compiled percentages in non-asthmatic subjects (NAS) and asthma patients (AS). **b** Percentage of CD45RA⁻CD45RO⁺CCR4⁺ cells in CD3⁺CD4⁺ T cells in NAS and AS. **c** Percentage of CCR4⁺CD45RA⁻CD45RO⁺CCR7⁺ and CCR4⁺CD45RA⁻CD45RO⁺CCR7⁻ cells in CD3⁺CD4⁺ T cells in NAS and AS. **d** Percentage of CCR4⁺ cells in CCR7⁺ memory CD4⁺ T cells. Data represent average percentages with SD. Cells were gated based on isotype antibody staining. **e** Average percentages with standard deviation of chemokine receptors on CD4⁺ T cells and CD8⁺ T cells. Significance was determined with a non-parametric Mann–Whitney test. *P < 0.05, **P < 0.01, ***P < 0.001, n.s.: not significant. Error bars indicate SD

no significant difference in the percentage of CCR4⁺CD45RA⁻CD45RO⁺CCR7⁻ cells in CD4⁺ T cells between the two groups (Fig. 3c, right), which was consistent with the data in Fig. 1c. Interestingly, there was no significant difference in the percentage of CCR4⁺ cells in CCR7⁺ memory CD4⁺ T cells between the two groups (Fig. 3d). This indicates that the increase of CCR4⁺CD45RA⁻CD45RO⁺CCR7⁺ cells in CD4⁺ T cells (Fig. 3c) was mainly due to the increase of CCR7⁺ memory cell in CD4⁺ T cells in patients.

No significant difference was seen in CXCR5⁺, CXCR3⁺, CCR5⁺, or CCR6⁺ CD4⁺ T cells in the two groups (Fig. 3e). There was no significant difference of CXCR3⁺, CXCR5⁺, CCR4⁺, or CCR5⁺ CD8⁺ T cells in the two groups.

We thus concluded that adult atopic asthma patients have increased CCR4⁺ CD4⁺ T cells in their blood and this increase is mainly due to the increase of CCR4⁺CD45RA⁻CD45RO⁺CCR7⁺ CD4⁺ T cells.

The frequency of CCR4⁺ CD4⁺ T cells varies among atopic asthma subtypes, but it is not influenced by corticosteroid or leukotriene treatment

We next investigated whether the increase of circulating CCR4⁺ CD4⁺ T cells in patients could be a feature of asthma subtypes. Patients without blood eosinophilia showed a significantly higher percentage of CCR4⁺ CD4⁺ T cells (Fig. 4a, left). This difference was even more significant when the percentage of

CCR4⁺CD45RA⁻CD45RO⁺CCR7⁺ CD4⁺ T cells was compared (Fig. 4a, right). Patients with blood eosinophilia did not show a significant increase of either CCR4⁺ CD4⁺ or CCR4⁺CD45RA⁻CD45RO⁺CCR7⁺ CD4⁺ T cells compared to control subjects.

The percentage of CCR4⁺ in CD4⁺ T cells was significantly different between control subjects and patients with severe asthma based on the % predicted FEV1 (Fig. 4b, left). Patients with moderate to mild asthma did not show such difference. However, both moderate and severe patient subgroups had significantly greater percentages of CCR4⁺CD45RA⁻CD45RO⁺CCR7⁺ CD4⁺ T cells than control subjects (Fig. 4b, right). Furthermore, the percentages of CCR4⁺ CD45RA⁻CD45RO⁺CCR7⁺ CD4⁺ T cells (Fig. 4c) inversely correlated with % predicted FEV1 scores of all patients. We also found that the increase of CCR4⁺CD45RA⁻CD45RO⁺CCR7⁺ in CD4⁺ T cells was not significantly influenced by either corticosteroid (Fig. 4d) or leukotriene inhibitor treatment (Fig. 4e).

Taken together, we concluded that the frequency of CCR4⁺ CD4⁺ T cells, particularly CCR4⁺CD45RA⁻CD45RO⁺CCR7⁺ CD4⁺ T cells, varies among atopic asthma subtypes, but are not significantly influenced by corticosteroid or leukotriene inhibitor treatments. In addition, the percentage of circulating CCR4⁺CD45RA⁻CD45RO⁺CCR7⁺ CD4⁺ T cells in patients correlated with asthma severity, as measured with % predicted FEV1 scores. Either corticosteroid or

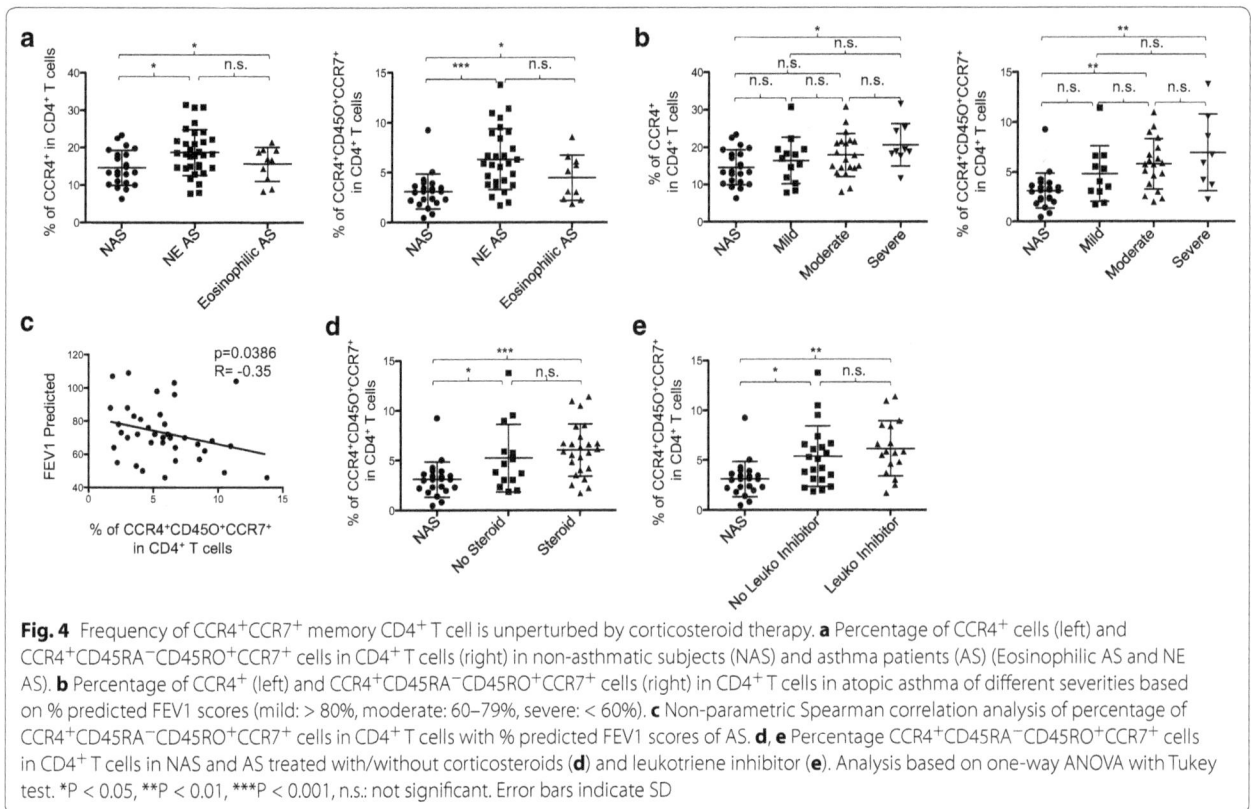

Fig. 4 Frequency of CCR4+CCR7+ memory CD4+ T cell is unperturbed by corticosteroid therapy. **a** Percentage of CCR4+ cells (left) and CCR4+CD45RA−CD45RO+CCR7+ cells in CD4+ T cells (right) in non-asthmatic subjects (NAS) and asthma patients (AS) (Eosinophilic AS and NE AS). **b** Percentage of CCR4+ (left) and CCR4+CD45RA−CD45RO+CCR7+ cells (right) in CD4+ T cells in atopic asthma of different severities based on % predicted FEV1 scores (mild: > 80%, moderate: 60–79%, severe: < 60%). **c** Non-parametric Spearman correlation analysis of percentage of CCR4+CD45RA−CD45RO+CCR7+ cells in CD4+ T cells with % predicted FEV1 scores of AS. **d, e** Percentage CCR4+CD45RA−CD45RO+CCR7+ cells in CD4+ T cells in NAS and AS treated with/without corticosteroids (**d**) and leukotriene inhibitor (**e**). Analysis based on one-way ANOVA with Tukey test. *P < 0.05, **P < 0.01, ***P < 0.001, n.s.: not significant. Error bars indicate SD

leukotriene inhibitor treatment did not alter the percentages of CD4+ T cells expressing the chemokine receptors tested in Fig. 3f (data not shown).

Increase of CRTH2+ CD4+ T cells in patients is also due to the increase of CCR7+ memory CD4+ T cells

CRTH2 is expressed on eosinophils, basophils and mast cells as well as Th2-type memory CD4+ T cells [34] and is also known to be associated with the pathogenesis of asthma [35]. Palikhe et al. have also reported that the increase of circulating CRTH2+ CD4+ T cells is a feature of severe asthma [5]. However, another study reported that CRTH2+ CD4+ T cells are unlikely to have a significant involvement in the pathogenesis of asthma in patients, although asthma patients have increased CRTH2+ CD4+ T cells in both blood and BAL fluid [36]. We thus investigated CRTH2 expression on the subsets of memory CD4+ T cells and further tested whether the frequency of the subsets of CRTH2+ memory CD4+ T cells is associated with any clinical readouts for assessing disease severity, including % predicted FEV1 scores.

We found that atopic asthma patients and control subjects had similar percentages of CRTH2+ cells in CD4+ T cells (Fig. 5a, left) and CRTH2+CD45RO+ memory cells in CD4+ T cells (Fig. 5a, right). However, patients had an increase of CRTH2+CD45RA−CD45RO+CCR7+

CD4+ T cells (Fig. 5b, left) without an increase of CRTH2+CD45RA−CD45RO+CCR7− CD4+ T cells (Fig. 5b, right). There was no significant difference in the percentage of CRTH2+ cells in CD45RA−CD45RO+CCR7+ CD4+ T cells (Fig. 5c). Therefore, the increase of CRTH2+CD45RA−CD45RO+CCR7+ CD4+ T cells in patients was mainly due to the increase of CCR7+ memory CD4+ T cells, which is in line with the data in Figs. 1, 2, 3, and 4.

Consistent with the higher percentage of CCR4+CD45RA−CD45RO+CCR7+ CD4+ T cells in patients without blood eosinophilia (Fig. 4a), atopic asthma patients without blood eosinophilia showed an increase of CRTH2+CD45RA−CD45RO+CCR7+ CD4+ T cells, compared to control subjects (Fig. 5d). In addition, the two groups of patients had similar percentages of circulating CRTH2+CD45RA−CD45RO+CCR7+ CD4+ T cells. Although patients had a higher percentage of CRTH2+CD45RA−CD45RO+CCR7+ cells in CD4+ T cells (Fig. 5b), such an increase was not seen when patients were divided into three subgroups based on the % predicted FEV1 scores (Fig. 5e). Furthermore, percentages of CRTH2+CD45RA−CD45RO+CCR7+ cells in CD4+ T cells or numbers of CRTH2+CD45RA−CD45RO+CCR7+ CD4+ T cells did not correlate with % predicted FEV1

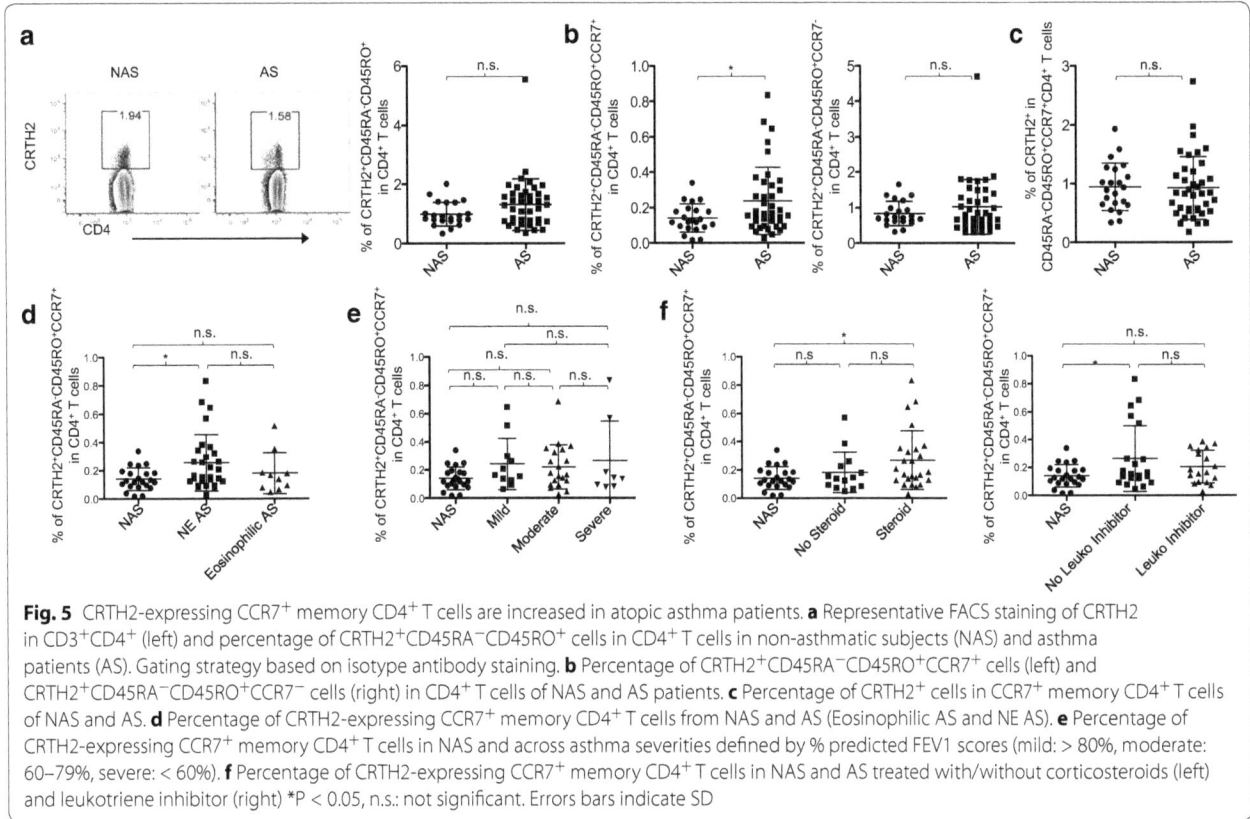

Fig. 5 CRTH2-expressing $CCR7^+$ memory $CD4^+$ T cells are increased in atopic asthma patients. **a** Representative FACS staining of CRTH2 in $CD3^+CD4^+$ (left) and percentage of $CRTH2^+CD45RA^-CD45RO^+$ cells in $CD4^+$ T cells in non-asthmatic subjects (NAS) and asthma patients (AS). Gating strategy based on isotype antibody staining. **b** Percentage of $CRTH2^+CD45RA^-CD45RO^+CCR7^+$ cells (left) and $CRTH2^+CD45RA^-CD45RO^+CCR7^-$ cells (right) in $CD4^+$ T cells of NAS and AS patients. **c** Percentage of $CRTH2^+$ cells in $CCR7^+$ memory $CD4^+$ T cells of NAS and AS. **d** Percentage of CRTH2-expressing $CCR7^+$ memory $CD4^+$ T cells from NAS and AS (Eosinophilic AS and NE AS). **e** Percentage of CRTH2-expressing $CCR7^+$ memory $CD4^+$ T cells in NAS and across asthma severities defined by % predicted FEV1 scores (mild: > 80%, moderate: 60–79%, severe: < 60%). **f** Percentage of CRTH2-expressing $CCR7^+$ memory $CD4^+$ T cells in NAS and AS treated with/without corticosteroids (left) and leukotriene inhibitor (right) *$P < 0.05$, n.s.: not significant. Errors bars indicate SD

scores or any other clinical variables, including ACT scores, FVC1%, FEV1/FVC1, frequency of β-agonist usages and night-time awakenings (data not shown). Data in Fig. 5f show that patients received corticosteroid therapy (left) and patients who were not treated with leukotriene inhibitor (right) have increased proportions of $CRTH2^+CD45RA^-CD45RO^+CCR7^+$ cells when compared to control subjects. Corticosteroid (Fig. 5f, left) treatments did not alter the proportion of $CRTH2^+CD45RA^-CD45RO^+CCR7^+$ cells in patients.

We thus concluded that adult atopic asthma patients had a minor increase of circulating $CRTH2^+$ $CD4^+$ T cells and this increase was also mainly due to the increase of central memory $CD4^+$ T cells. However, such an increase in $CRTH2^+CD45RA^-CD45RO^+CCR7^+$ $CD4^+$ T cells was not significantly associated with asthma severity and was not affected by corticosteroid treatment.

Patients have an increase of $CD4^+$ Tregs, but only $CTLA-4^+$ $CD4^+$ T cells show clinical relevance

Tregs exist in both healthy people and asthma patients [16, 37, 38]. The balance between Tregs and inflammatory Th2-type T cells could be a critical factor that determine immune tolerance or inflammation in the lung. Previous studies reported that Tregs in asthma patients

might not be fully functional [37–39]. However, another study showed that such Tregs can suppress allergic inflammatory responses [16]. To gain better insight into Tregs in adult atopic asthma patients we assessed the frequency of Tregs along with those expressing IL-10. We further tested whether the frequency of Tregs in patients was clinically relevant.

As shown in Fig. 6a, atopic asthma patients have significantly more $CD25^+$ $CD4^+$ T cells than non-asthmatic control subjects. In addition, significant increases of $Foxp3^+$ (Fig. 6b) and $CTLA-4^+$ $CD4^+$ T cells (Fig. 6c) in patients were also observed. When we further analyzed double-positive populations, we found that patients had greater proportions of both $Foxp3^+CD25^{high}$ (Fig. 6d) and $Foxp3^+CTLA-4^+$ (Fig. 6e) Tregs than control subjects. We also assessed IL-10 expression in $Foxp3^+$ $CD4^+$ T cells. While some patients had increases of $Foxp3^+IL-10^+$ $CD4^+$ T cells, there was no significant difference between patients and control subjects (Fig. 6f). Corticosteroid therapy did not significantly impact the percentage of $Foxp3^+IL-10^+$ $CD4^+$ T cells (Fig. 6g). We also found that there was no significant difference in the amounts of IL-10 secreted by T cells from the different populations cultured for 36 h with αCD3/αCD28 beads (Fig. 6h). However, patient T cells secreted more Th2 cytokines,

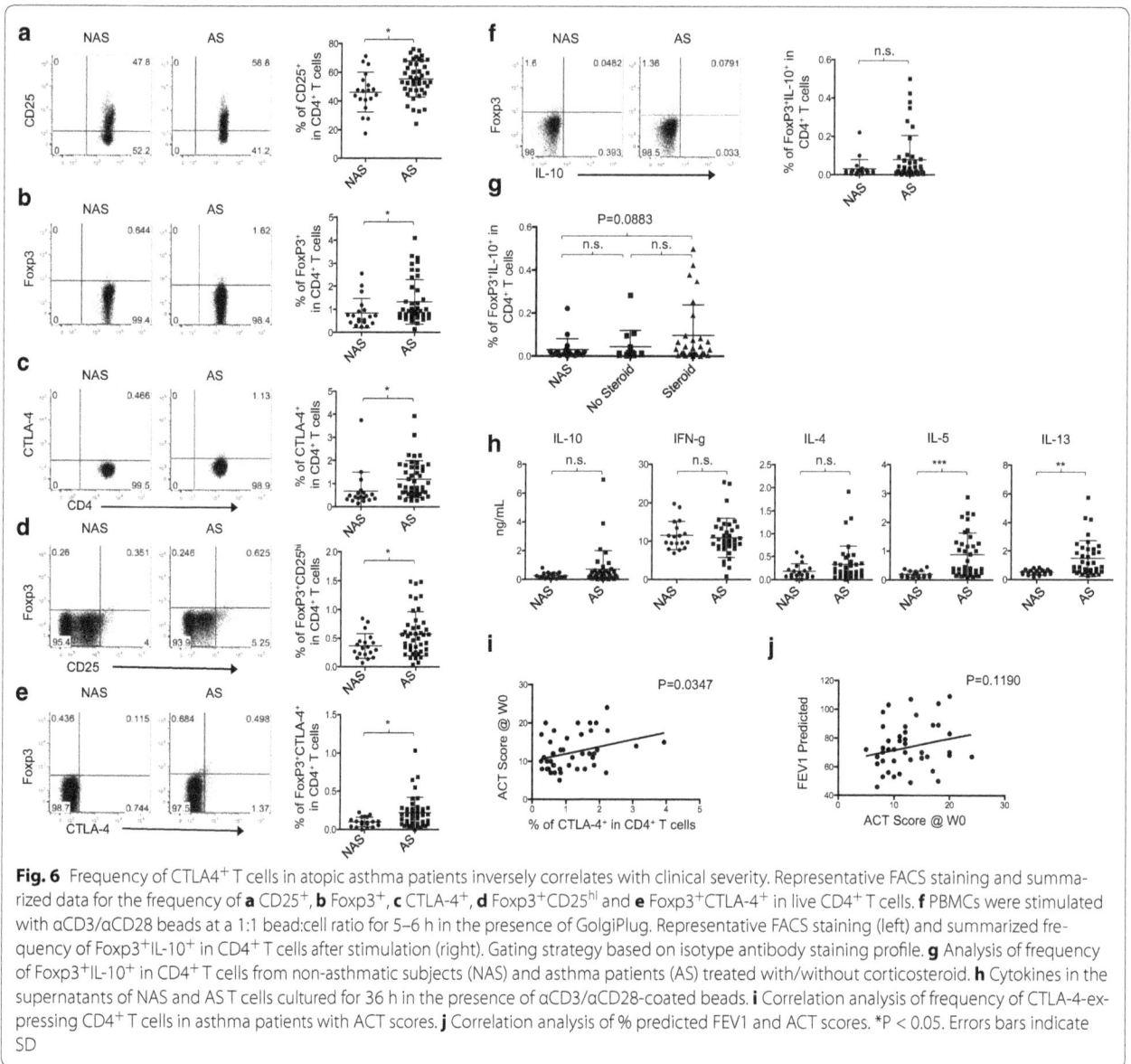

Fig. 6 Frequency of CTLA4+ T cells in atopic asthma patients inversely correlates with clinical severity. Representative FACS staining and summarized data for the frequency of **a** CD25+, **b** Foxp3+, **c** CTLA-4+, **d** Foxp3+CD25hi and **e** Foxp3+CTLA-4+ in live CD4+ T cells. **f** PBMCs were stimulated with αCD3/αCD28 beads at a 1:1 bead:cell ratio for 5–6 h in the presence of GolgiPlug. Representative FACS staining (left) and summarized frequency of Foxp3+IL-10+ in CD4+ T cells after stimulation (right). Gating strategy based on isotype antibody staining profile. **g** Analysis of frequency of Foxp3+IL-10+ in CD4+ T cells from non-asthmatic subjects (NAS) and asthma patients (AS) treated with/without corticosteroid. **h** Cytokines in the supernatants of NAS and AS T cells cultured for 36 h in the presence of αCD3/αCD28-coated beads. **i** Correlation analysis of frequency of CTLA-4-expressing CD4+ T cells in asthma patients with ACT scores. **j** Correlation analysis of % predicted FEV1 and ACT scores. *P < 0.05. Errors bars indicate SD

particularly IL-5 and IL-13, but not IFNγ. T cells from patients and control subjects secreted similar amounts of IL-21, IL-22, IL-17, and TNFα (data not shown). The percentage of Foxp3+IL-10+ cells in CD4+ T cells did not correlate with any of the clinical variables, including % predicted FEV1 and ACT scores (data not shown). However, the percentage of CTLA4+ cells in CD4+ T cells correlated with ACT scores (Fig. 6i), but not % predicted FEV1 (data not shown). This was not surprising because ACT scores do not always correlate with FEVs (Fig. 6j), as previously described [40].

We thus concluded that adult atopic asthma patients have an increase of circulating CD4+ T cells that are CD25+, FoxP3+, and CTLA-4+, FoxP3+CD25high, or

FoxP3+CTLA-4+. In addition, the percentage of CD4+ T cells expressing surface CTLA-4 inversely correlates with asthma severity, as determined by the ACT scores. There was no significant correlation between the percentage of IL-10-expressing Tregs and clinical measurements.

Altered expression of integrins on CD4+ and CD8+ T cells in atopic asthma patients

In addition to chemokine receptors, cell surface integrins expressed on T cells are also linked to T cell migration into lungs and could thus be involved in the pathophysiology of asthma [41–45]. We thus investigated whether T cells in atopic asthma patients have altered expressions of the integrins α4, β7, and CD11a that could be associated with asthma pathogenesis. The lack of α4 integrin not only impedes lymphocyte migration to lung and airways, but also prevents upregulation of vascular cell adhesion molecule-1 (VCAM-1) in inflamed lung vasculature [41, 46]. β7 along with α4 can also contribute to T cell and eosinophil accumulation in BAL and to airway inflammation in the absence of CCL19 and CCL21 [44, 45]. CD11a is an α chain of LFA-1 that is crucial for migration of leukocytes across the endothelial barrier into the surrounding tissues [47, 48].

Representative flow cytometry data show that patients and control subjects had similar percentages of α4$^+$ (Fig. 7a, left) and CD11a$^+$ CD4$^+$ T cells (Fig. 7a, right). Summarized data of α4$^+$ and CD11a$^+$ CD4$^+$ T cells are shown in Fig. 7b. Both patients and control subjects also had similar percentages of CD11a$^+$ CD8$^+$ T cells (Fig. 7b). Interestingly, however, the percentages and numbers of α4$^+$ CD4$^+$ T cells inversely correlated with the ACT scores (Fig. 7c). There was an increase of α4$^+$ CD8$^+$ T cells in patients (Fig. 7d), but the frequency of α4$^+$ CD8$^+$ T cells did not correlate with any of the clinical

variables assessed, including ACT and % predicted FEV1 scores (data not shown). We also found decreases of β7$^+$ CD4$^+$ (Fig. 7e) and CD8$^+$ T cells (Fig. 7f) in patients, compared to control subjects.

In conclusion, atopic asthma patients and non-asthmatic control subjects have a similar frequency of α4$^+$ CD4$^+$ T cells. However, their frequency of α4$^+$ CD4$^+$ T cells in patients inversely correlated with the ACT scores. Atopic asthma patients also have significantly lower percentages of CD4$^+$ and CD8$^+$ T cells that expressed β7 integrin, but not CD11a.

Discussion

A persistent allergic inflammation in the lower airway may require an abundant presence of memory T cells [22, 23, 49] that can readily respond to allergens that are intermittently available throughout the year. In both murine models of allergic asthma and asthma patients, CD4$^+$ memory T cells are involved in recurrent episodes of inflammation [23–25, 50]. Accordingly, we found a significant increase of circulating CD45RA$^-$CD45RO$^+$

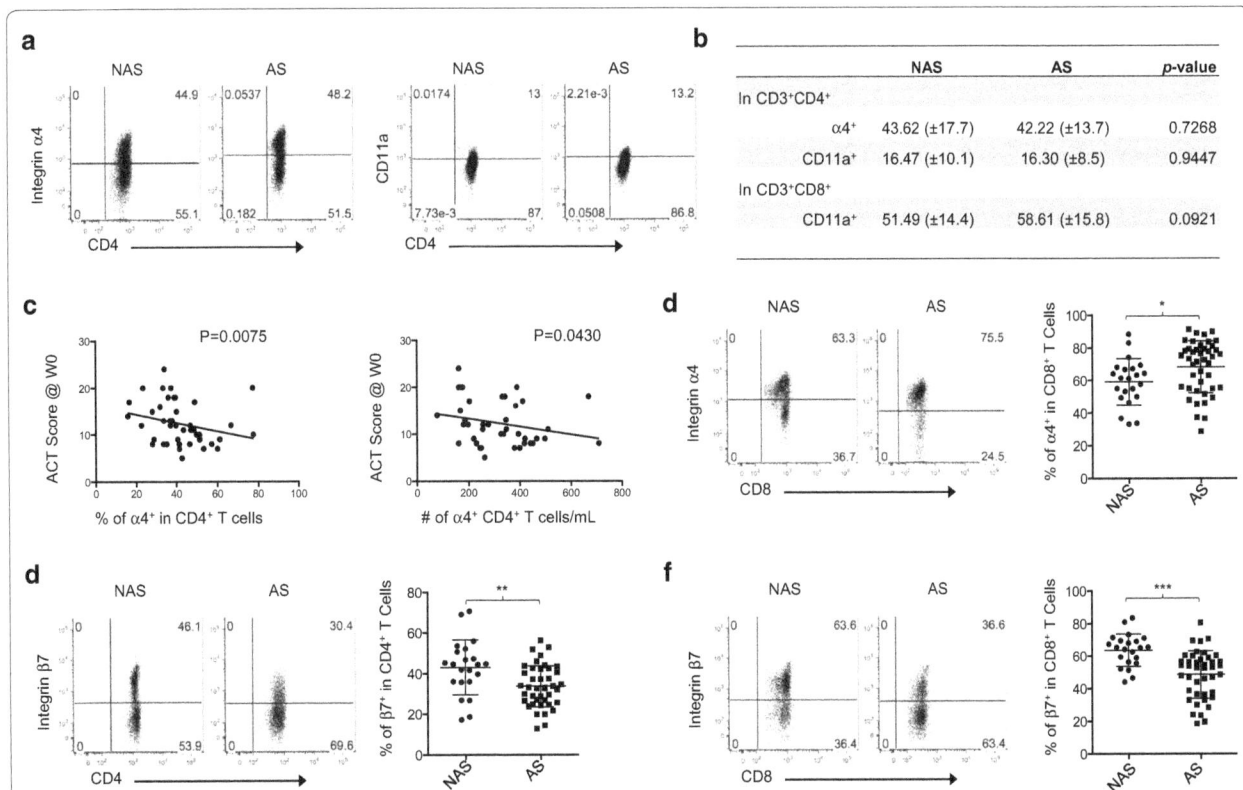

Fig. 7 Frequency of α4$^+$ CD4$^+$ T cells in atopic asthma patients correlates with clinical severity. **a** Representative FACS analysis of whole blood staining for α4 and CD11a in CD4$^+$ T cells in non-asthmatic subjects (NAS) and asthma patients (AS). Gates based on isotype antibody staining pattern. **b** Frequency analysis of integrin-expressing cells in CD4$^+$ and CD8$^+$ T cells in NAS and AS. **c** Correlation analysis of the frequency and number of α4-expressing CD4$^+$ T cells in AS with ACT score. **d** Representative FACS data of whole blood staining (left) and compiled frequency of α4$^+$ in CD8$^+$ T cells (right) in NAS and AS. Representative FACS data of whole blood staining and compiled frequencies of β7-expressing CD4$^+$ T cells (**e**) and CD8$^+$ T cells (**f**) in NAS and AS. *P < 0.05, **P < 0.01, ***P < 0.001. Error bars indicate SD

memory CD4$^+$ T cells in atopic asthma patients, compared to non-asthmatic control subjects. In this study, however, we further found that atopic asthma patients have a significant increase in memory CD4$^+$ T cells that express CCR7, but not CCR7$^-$ memory CD4$^+$ T cells.

Both Tem and Tcm circulate in the blood. In contrast to Tem, CCR7$^+$ Tcm cells can migrate to the lymph nodes and can quickly proliferate in response to infiltrating antigen-presenting cells (APCs). Thus, Tcm cells are also considered reactive memory cells [21, 51, 52]. They also can acquire an effector-like phenotype with the secretion of cytokines and chemokines [21, 52]. It is therefore possible that such long-lived CD4$^+$ Tcm cells found in the blood of asthma patients could play an important role in the chronic inflammation in the lower airway in response to a variety of allergens that are intermittently available year-round. It was also important to note that the absolute numbers of CD4$^+$ Tcm cells were also greater in atopic asthma patients than non-asthmatic control subjects. Therefore, the increase of CD4$^+$ Tcm cells in atopic asthma patients was not due to a decrease of CD4$^+$ Tem cells in their blood.

The roles of CCR4$^+$ T cells in the pathogenesis of asthma are still controversial in both a murine model of asthma and asthma patients [29, 33, 43, 53–57]. The increase of CCR4$^+$ CD4$^+$ T cells in asthma patients has been previously reported [29, 33]. However, data from other studies indicate that the proportion of CCR4$^+$ CD4$^+$ T cells in peripheral blood or in the lungs does not always correlate with the severity of asthma [43, 57]. In our study, we found that atopic asthma patients have more circulating CCR4$^+$ CD4$^+$ T cells and this was mainly due to the increase of CD4$^+$ Tcm cells. In line with this, the difference in the frequency of CCR4$^+$ CD4$^+$ T cells between atopic asthma patients and control subjects was even greater when we compared them in Tcm cells. The inverse correlation between the frequency of CCR4$^+$ CD4$^+$ Tcm cells and asthma severity further support that CCR4$^+$ CD4$^+$ Tcm cells could play an important role in the pathogenesis of atopic asthma. This increase of CCR4$^+$ CD4$^+$ Tcm cells can be seen across atopic asthma subtypes and severities. It was also important to note that current therapy (i.e. corticosteroids, β-agonists, leukotriene inhibitors, and combinations thereof) was not capable of reducing the frequency of either total CD4$^+$ Tcm or CCR4$^+$ CD4$^+$ Tcm cells in atopic asthma patients. A previous study reported that corticosteroid treatment slightly decreased the percentage of CCR4$^+$ total T cells, but it was performed with patients that had mild and stable asthma [58]. Our findings raise a fundamental question concerning the mechanisms responsible for the increased numbers of CCR4$^+$ CD4$^+$ Tem cells in atopic asthma patients. Nonetheless, our data might also be highlighting the possible reasons behind the ineffectiveness of current therapies (i.e., corticosteroids).

In line with the increase of CCR4$^+$ T cells in patients, T cells from atopic asthma patients secreted more of IL-5 and IL-13 than T cells from non-asthmatic control subjects. Our data also show that there was no significant difference in the frequencies of CXCR3$^+$ (for Th1), CXCR5$^+$ (for Th21), or CCR6$^+$ (for Th17) CD4$^+$ T cells in the blood of patients and control subjects. Consistent with the similar frequencies of T cells expressing such chemokine receptors, T cells from patients and control subjects also secreted similar amounts of IFNγ, IL-21, IL-17, TNFα and IL-22.

Atopic asthma patients have a higher percentage of CRTH2$^+$ cells, but this is only in the CD4$^+$ Tcm cell compartment. Such increase in patients was not observed when we analyze the frequency of CRTH2$^+$ cells in total CD4$^+$ T cells or in total memory CD4$^+$ T cells. This might explain inconsistent results from previous studies of the frequency of CRTH2$^+$ cells in asthma patients [5, 35]. However, the increase of CRTH2$^+$ CD4$^+$ Tcm in patients was less significant than the increase of CCR4$^+$ CD4$^+$ Tcm cells. In addition, the frequency of CRTH2$^+$ CD4$^+$ T cells or CRTH2$^+$ CD4$^+$ Tcm cells did not show a significant correlation with any clinical variables, including ACT and % predicted FEV1 scores.

Consistent with the previously published data, we found that patients have an increased frequency of CD4$^+$ Tregs as assessed by measuring the frequency of CD25$^{+/high}$, Foxp3$^+$, CTLA4$^+$, Foxp3$^+$CD25^{high}, and Foxp3$^+$CTLA-4$^+$ CD4$^+$ T cells [39]. Such increases in patients could be a natural process to counteract ongoing inflammatory responses, although corticosteroid treatment might also increase Treg frequency [59, 60]. However, the percentages of Foxp3$^+$IL-10$^+$ CD4$^+$ T cells in the two groups of subjects were similar, and this is in line with the data from a previous study [61]. Only a few patients showed increased frequency of Foxp3$^+$IL-10$^+$ CD4$^+$ T cells compared to other patients. The amounts of IL-10 secreted from T cells also showed a similar pattern to what was observed for the frequency of Foxp3$^+$IL-10$^+$ CD4$^+$ T cells. This suggests that Tregs in asthma patients might not be fully functional, as previously reported [37–39]. We were not able to test the suppressive function of Tregs due to the limited amounts of blood samples collected from patients. The frequency of Foxp3$^+$IL-10$^+$ CD4$^+$ T cells did not correlate with asthma severity (data not shown). Interestingly, we found that the frequency of CTLA4$^+$ T cells correlated with the ACT scores. This suggested that fractions of Tregs in patients might still display certain levels of suppressive functions via the action of CTLA4, an inhibitory molecule, even though they may not be fully functional [39].

Integrins play key roles in adhesion of leukocytes to walls of blood vessels associated with inflammation and in migration of leukocytes to inflamed tissues [62, 63]. Integrins present on leukocyte surface belong to a large family of heterodimeric glycoproteins, which in the active conformation are composed of 2 noncovalently associated α and β subunits. Currently, 18 α and 8 β subunits are identified, which are associated in a restricted manner to create 24 heterodimers for specific ligand binding [64]. Among those, both $\alpha4$ and CD11a, an α chain of LFA-1, are known to play important roles in leukocyte migration to lung [46–48, 65, 66]. A previous study also reported that IL-5 could increase VCAM-1 expression that can facilitate $\alpha4^+$ leukocyte migration to inflamed lung and airways [42]. One could thus expect an increase of $\alpha4^+$ CD4$^+$ T cells in asthma patients. Interestingly, however, patients and control subjects have similar frequencies of circulating $\alpha4^+$ CD4$^+$ T cells. However, we found that the frequency of $\alpha4^+$ CD4$^+$ T cells significantly correlated with asthma severity, as assessed with the ACT scores. In contrast to $\alpha4^+$ and CD11a$^+$ CD4$^+$ T cells, patients have significant reductions in the percentages of $\beta7^+$ CD4$^+$ and CD8$^+$ T cells. The clinical relevance of the decrease of $\beta7^+$ T cells in asthma is not clear at this moment. $\beta7$ is generally known to play an important role in lymphocyte migration into guts [67, 68], and T cells in the lungs of asthmatic and non-asthmatic control subjects express only low level of $\alpha4\beta7$ [43]. However, others have also reported that $\beta7$ along with $\alpha4$ can contribute to T cell and eosinophil accumulation in BAL and to airway inflammation in the absence of CCL19 and CCL21 [44, 45].

Conclusions

This study reports for the first time that an increase of long-lived CD4$^+$ Tcm cells along with CCR4$^+$ CD4$^+$ Tcm cells is one of the major features of circulating blood T cells in adult atopic asthma patients. Our data also demonstrate that such T cell subpopulations seem to be resistant to current common therapeutics, including corticosteroids. Although atopic asthma patients have an increase of Tregs, these cells may not be fully functional, although CTLA-4 could contribute to their suppressive function. This study also provides evidence that the frequency of $\alpha4^+$ CD4$^+$ T cells is clinically relevant in adult atopic asthma patients. Therefore, this study extends our knowledge on the pathogenesis of human atopic asthma and further guides us toward the rational design of therapeutics for atopic asthma in the future.

Abbreviations
ACT: asthma control test; AS: asthma patient; FEV1: forced expiratory volume in 1 s; NAS: non-asthmatic; Tcm: central memory T cells; Tem: effector memory T cells.

Authors' contributions
MW and KU carried out experiments and analyzed data. WY and JE helped with experiments and data analysis. BL and MM provided clinical samples. KU, HJ, MM, and SO designed this study and analyzed the data. MW, KU, HJ, and SO wrote this manuscript. All authors read and approved the final manuscript.

Author details
[1] Baylor Institute for Immunology Research, 3434 Live Oak St., Dallas, TX 75204, USA. [2] Institute for Biomedical Studies, Baylor University, Waco, TX, USA. [3] Texas Allergy Experts, Fort Worth, TX, USA. [4] Martha Foster Lung Care Center, Baylor University Medical Center, Dallas, TX, USA.

Acknowledgements
We thank the Biobank & Project Management Core and the Flow Cytometry Core at Baylor Institute for Immunology Research (BIIR). We also thank Dr. Jacob Turner and Jacob Cardenas (Biostatics Core at BIIR). We also thank Shiying Bian (BIIR) as well as staff members and nurses in Drs. Lanier's and Millard's clinics for the recruitment of control and patient donors and for drawing blood samples.

Competing interests
The authors declare that they have no competing interests.

Funding
This study was supported by the Baylor Health Care System Foundation, Genentech (S. Oh), American Asthma Foundation (15-0038) (S. Oh) and NIAID, NIH (1R21AI101810-01) (S. Oh).

References
1. Fahy JV, Dickey BF. Airway mucus function and dysfunction. N Engl J Med. 2010;363:2233–47.
2. Busse WW, Lemanske RF Jr, Gern JE. Role of viral respiratory infections in asthma and asthma exacerbations. Lancet. 2010;376:826–34.
3. Martinez FD. Gene by environment interactions in the development of asthma. Clin Exp Allergy. 1998;28(Suppl 5):21–5 (discussion 26–28).
4. Lima JJ, Blake KV, Tantisira KG, Weiss ST. Pharmacogenetics of asthma. Curr Opin Pulm Med. 2009;15:57–62.
5. Palikhe NS, Laratta C, Nahirney D, Vethanayagam D, Bhutani M, Vliagoftis H, Cameron L. Elevated levels of circulating CD4(+) CRTh2(+) T cells characterize severe asthma. Clin Exp Allergy. 2016;46:825–36.
6. Grob M, Schmid-Grendelmeier P, Joller-Jemelka HI, Ludwig E, Dubs RW, Grob PJ, Wuthrich B, Bisset LR. Altered intracellular expression of the chemokines MIP-1alpha, MIP-1beta and IL-8 by peripheral blood CD4$^+$ and CD8$^+$ T cells in mild allergic asthma. Allergy. 2003;58:239–45.

7. Francis JN, Sabroe I, Lloyd CM, Durham SR, Till SJ. Elevated CCR6+CD4+ T lymphocytes in tissue compared with blood and induction of CCL20 during the asthmatic late response. Clin Exp Immunol. 2008;152:440–7.

8. Raedler D, Ballenberger N, Klucker E, Bock A, Otto R, Prazeres da Costa O, Holst O, Illig T, Buch T, von Mutius E, Schaub B. Identification of novel immune phenotypes for allergic and nonallergic childhood asthma. J Allergy Clin Immunol. 2015;135:81–91.

9. Barrett NA, Austen KF. Innate cells and T helper 2 cell immunity in airway inflammation. Immunity. 2009;31:425–37.

10. Gould HJ, Sutton BJ. IgE in allergy and asthma today. Nat Rev Immunol. 2008;8:205–17.

11. Paul WE, Zhu J. How are T(H)2-type immune responses initiated and amplified? Nat Rev Immunol. 2010;10:225–35.

12. Takatsu K, Nakajima H. IL-5 and eosinophilia. Curr Opin Immunol. 2008;20:288–94.

13. Ingram JL, Kraft M. IL-13 in asthma and allergic disease: asthma phenotypes and targeted therapies. J Allergy Clin Immunol. 2012;130:829–42 **(quiz 843–824)**.

14. Wills-Karp M. Interleukin-13 in asthma pathogenesis. Immunol Rev. 2004;202:175–90.

15. Lloyd CM, Saglani S. T cells in asthma: influences of genetics, environment, and T-cell plasticity. J Allergy Clin Immunol. 2013;131:1267–74 **(quiz 1275)**.

16. Akdis M, Verhagen J, Taylor A, Karamloo F, Karagiannidis C, Crameri R, Thunberg S, Deniz G, Valenta R, Fiebig H, et al. Immune responses in healthy and allergic individuals are characterized by a fine balance between allergen-specific T regulatory 1 and T helper 2 cells. J Exp Med. 2004;199:1567–75.

17. Noval Rivas M, Chatila TA. Regulatory T cells in allergic diseases. J Allergy Clin Immunol. 2016;138:639–52.

18. Donma M, Karasu E, Ozdilek B, Turgut B, Topcu B, Nalbantoglu B, Donma O. CD4(+), CD25(+), FOXP3 (+) T regulatory cell levels in obese, asthmatic, asthmatic obese, and healthy children. Inflammation. 2015;38:1473–8.

19. Miyahara N, Swanson BJ, Takeda K, Taube C, Miyahara S, Kodama T, Dakhama A, Ott VL, Gelfand EW. Effector CD8+ T cells mediate inflammation and airway hyper-responsiveness. Nat Med. 2004;10:865–9.

20. Wells JW, Choy K, Lloyd CM, Noble A. Suppression of allergic airway inflammation and IgE responses by a class I restricted allergen peptide vaccine. Mucosal Immunol. 2009;2:54–62.

21. Sallusto F, Geginat J, Lanzavecchia A. Central memory and effector memory T cell subsets: function, generation, and maintenance. Annu Rev Immunol. 2004;22:745–63.

22. Wang YH, Voo KS, Liu B, Chen CY, Uygungil B, Spoede W, Bernstein JA, Huston DP, Liu YJ. A novel subset of CD4(+) T(H)2 memory/effector cells that produce inflammatory IL-17 cytokine and promote the exacerbation of chronic allergic asthma. J Exp Med. 2010;207:2479–91.

23. Lloyd CM, Hessel EM. Functions of T cells in asthma: more than just T(H)2 cells. Nat Rev Immunol. 2010;10:838–48.

24. Machura E, Mazur B, Pieniazek W, Karczewska K. Expression of naive/memory (CD45RA/CD45RO) markers by peripheral blood CD4+ and CD8+ T cells in children with asthma. Arch Immunol Ther Exp (Warsz). 2008;56:55–62.

25. Abdulamir AS, Hafidh RR, Abubakar F, Abbas KA. Changing survival, memory cell compartment, and T-helper balance of lymphocytes between severe and mild asthma. BMC Immunol. 2008;9:73.

26. Corrigan CJ, Kay AB. T cells and eosinophils in the pathogenesis of asthma. Immunol Today. 1992;13:501–7.

27. Corrigan CJ, Hamid Q, North J, Barkans J, Moqbel R, Durham S, Gemou-Engesaeth V, Kay AB. Peripheral blood CD4 but not CD8 t-lymphocytes in patients with exacerbation of asthma transcribe and translate messenger RNA encoding cytokines which prolong eosinophil survival in the context of a Th2-type pattern: effect of glucocorticoid therapy. Am J Respir Cell Mol Biol. 1995;12:567–78.

28. National Asthma E, Prevention P. Expert panel report 3 (EPR-3): guidelines for the diagnosis and management of asthma-summary report 2007. J Allergy Clin Immunol. 2007;120:S94–138.

29. Kurashima K, Fujimura M, Myou S, Ishiura Y, Onai N, Matsushima K. Asthma severity is associated with an increase in both blood CXCR3+ and CCR4+ T cells. Respirology. 2006;11:152–7.

30. Saule P, Trauet J, Dutriez V, Lekeux V, Dessaint JP, Labalette M. Accumulation of memory T cells from childhood to old age: central and effector memory cells in CD4(+) versus effector memory and terminally differentiated memory cells in CD8(+) compartment. Mech Ageing Dev. 2006;127:274–81.

31. Haynes L, Maue AC. Effects of aging on T cell function. Curr Opin Immunol. 2009;21:414–7.

32. Geginat J, Paroni M, Facciotti F, Gruarin P, Kastirr I, Caprioli F, Pagani M, Abrignani S. The CD4-centered universe of human T cell subsets. Semin Immunol. 2013;25:252–62.

33. Vijayanand P, Durkin K, Hartmann G, Morjaria J, Seumois G, Staples KJ, Hall D, Bessant C, Bartholomew M, Howarth PH, et al. Chemokine receptor 4 plays a key role in T cell recruitment into the airways of asthmatic patients. J Immunol. 2010;184:4568–74.

34. Nagata K, Tanaka K, Ogawa K, Kemmotsu K, Imai T, Yoshie O, Abe H, Tada K, Nakamura M, Sugamura K, Takano S. Selective expression of a novel surface molecule by human Th2 cells in vivo. J Immunol. 1999;162:1278–86.

35. Campos Alberto E, Maclean E, Davidson C, Palikhe NS, Storie J, Tse C, Brenner D, Mayers I, Vliagoftis H, El-Sohemy A, Cameron L. The single nucleotide polymorphism CRTh2 rs533116 is associated with allergic asthma and increased expression of CRTh2. Allergy. 2012;67:1357–64.

36. Mutalithas K, Guillen C, Day C, Brightling CE, Pavord ID, Wardlaw AJ. CRTH2 expression on T cells in asthma. Clin Exp Immunol. 2010;161:34–40.

37. Joller N, Lozano E, Burkett PR, Patel B, Xiao S, Zhu C, Xia J, Tan TG, Sefik E, Yajnik V, et al. Treg cells expressing the coinhibitory molecule TIGIT selectively inhibit proinflammatory Th1 and Th17 cell responses. Immunity. 2014;40:569–81.

38. Hartl D, Koller B, Mehlhorn AT, Reinhardt D, Nicolai T, Schendel DJ, Griese M, Krauss-Etschmann S. Quantitative and functional impairment of pulmonary CD4+CD25hi regulatory T cells in pediatric asthma. J Allergy Clin Immunol. 2007;119:1258–66.

39. Lin YL, Shieh CC, Wang JY. The functional insufficiency of human CD4+CD25 high T-regulatory cells in allergic asthma is subjected to TNF-alpha modulation. Allergy. 2008;63:67–74.

40. Melosini L, Dente FL, Bacci E, Bartoli ML, Cianchetti S, Costa F, Di Franco A, Malagrino L, Novelli F, Vagaggini B, Paggiaro P. Asthma control test (ACT): comparison with clinical, functional, and biological markers of asthma control. J Asthma. 2012;49:317–23.

41. Xu B, Aoyama K, Kusumoto M, Matsuzawa A, Butcher EC, Michie SA, Matsuyama T, Takeuchi T. Lack of lymphoid chemokines CCL19 and CCL21 enhances allergic airway inflammation in mice. Int Immunol. 2007;19:775–84.

42. Sanmugalingham D, De Vries E, Gauntlett R, Symon FA, Bradding P, Wardlaw AJ. Interleukin-5 enhances eosinophil adhesion to bronchial epithelial cells. Clin Exp Allergy. 2000;30:255–63.

43. Campbell JJ, Brightling CE, Symon FA, Qin S, Murphy KE, Hodge M, Andrew DP, Wu L, Butcher EC, Wardlaw AJ. Expression of chemokine receptors by lung T cells from normal and asthmatic subjects. J Immunol. 2001;166:2842–8.

44. Abonia JP, Hallgren J, Jones T, Shi T, Xu Y, Koni P, Flavell RA, Boyce JA, Austen KF, Gurish MF. Alpha-4 integrins and VCAM-1, but not MAdCAM-1, are essential for recruitment of mast cell progenitors to the inflamed lung. Blood. 2006;108:1588–94.

45. Hallgren J, Gurish MF. Mast cell progenitor trafficking and maturation. Adv Exp Med Biol. 2011;716:14–28.

46. Banerjee ER, Jiang Y, Henderson WR Jr, Scott LM, Papayannopoulou T. Alpha4 and beta2 integrins have nonredundant roles for asthma development, but for optimal allergen sensitization only alpha4 is critical. Exp Hematol. 2007;35:605–17.

47. Gupta A, Espinosa V, Galusha LE, Rahimian V, Miro KL, Rivera-Medina A, Kasinathan C, Capitle E, Aguila HA, Kachlany SC. Expression and targeting of lymphocyte function-associated antigen 1 (LFA-1) on white blood cells for treatment of allergic asthma. J Leukoc Biol. 2015;97:439–46.

48. Hogg N, Smith A, McDowall A, Giles K, Stanley P, Laschinger M, Henderson R. How T cells use LFA-1 to attach and migrate. Immunol Lett. 2004;92:51–4.

49. Mineev VN, Trofimov VI, Nesterovich II, Emanuel VL, Lugovaia AV. Disturbance of apoptosis of peripheral blood lymphocytes in different variants of bronchial asthma. Ter Arkh. 2008;80:43–9.

50. Mojtabavi N, Dekan G, Stingl G, Epstein MM. Long-lived Th2 memory in experimental allergic asthma. J Immunol. 2002;169:4788–96.

51. Mueller SN, Gebhardt T, Carbone FR, Heath WR. Memory T cell subsets, migration patterns, and tissue residence. Annu Rev Immunol. 2013;31:137–61.

52. Pepper M, Jenkins MK. Origins of CD4(+) effector and central memory T cells. Nat Immunol. 2011;12:467–71.

53. Mikhak Z, Fukui M, Farsidjani A, Medoff BD, Tager AM, Luster AD. Contribution of CCR4 and CCR8 to antigen-specific T(H)2 cell trafficking in allergic pulmonary inflammation. J Allergy Clin Immunol. 2009;123(67–73):e63.

54. Conroy DM, Jopling LA, Lloyd CM, Hodge MR, Andrew DP, Williams TJ, Pease JE, Sabroe I. CCR4 blockade does not inhibit allergic airways inflammation. J Leukoc Biol. 2003;74:558–63.

55. Kawasaki S, Takizawa H, Yoneyama H, Nakayama T, Fujisawa R, Izumizaki M, Imai T, Yoshie O, Homma I, Yamamoto K, Matsushima K. Intervention of thymus and activation-regulated chemokine attenuates the development of allergic airway inflammation and hyperresponsiveness in mice. J Immunol. 2001;166:2055–62.

56. Schuh JM, Power C, Proudfoot AE, Kunkel SL, Lukacs NW, Hogaboam CM. Airway hyperresponsiveness, but not airway remodeling, is attenuated during chronic pulmonary allergic responses to Aspergillus in CCR4−/− mice. FASEB J. 2002;16:1313–5.

57. Gluck J, Rymarczyk B, Rogala B. Chemokine receptors expression on CD3+ blood cells in bronchial asthma. Adv Med Sci. 2016;61:11–7.

58. Kurashima K, Fujimura M, Myou S, Kasahara K, Tachibana H, Amemiya N, Ishiura Y, Onai N, Matsushima K, Nakao S. Effects of oral steroids on blood CXCR3+ and CCR4+ T cells in patients with bronchial asthma. Am J Respir Crit Care Med. 2001;164:754–8.

59. Dao Nguyen X, Robinson DS. Fluticasone propionate increases CD4CD25 T regulatory cell suppression of allergen-stimulated CD4CD25 T cells by an IL-10-dependent mechanism. J Allergy Clin Immunol. 2004;114:296–301.

60. Karagiannidis C, Akdis M, Holopainen P, Woolley NJ, Hense G, Ruckert B, Mantel PY, Menz G, Akdis CA, Blaser K, Schmidt-Weber CB. Glucocorticoids upregulate FOXP3 expression and regulatory T cells in asthma. J Allergy Clin Immunol. 2004;114:1425–33.

61. Han D, Wang C, Lou W, Gu Y, Wang Y, Zhang L. Allergen-specific IL-10-secreting type I T regulatory cells, but not CD4(+)CD25(+)Foxp3(+) T cells, are decreased in peripheral blood of patients with persistent allergic rhinitis. Clin Immunol. 2010;136:292–301.

62. Hogg N, Patzak I, Willenbrock F. The insider's guide to leukocyte integrin signalling and function. Nat Rev Immunol. 2011;11:416–26.

63. Evans R, Patzak I, Svensson L, De Filippo K, Jones K, McDowall A, Hogg N. Integrins in immunity. J Cell Sci. 2009;122:215–25.

64. Hynes RO. Integrins: bidirectional, allosteric signaling machines. Cell. 2002;110:673–87.

65. Banerjee ER, Jiang Y, Henderson WR Jr, Latchman Y, Papayannopoulou T. Absence of alpha 4 but not beta 2 integrins restrains development of chronic allergic asthma using mouse genetic models. Exp Hematol. 2009;37(715–727):e713.

66. Bai TR, Bates JH, Brusasco V, Camoretti-Mercado B, Chitano P, Deng LH, Dowell M, Fabry B, Ford LE, Fredberg JJ, et al. On the terminology for describing the length-force relationship and its changes in airway smooth muscle. J Appl Physiol. 1985;2004(97):2029–34.

67. Strauch UG, Mueller RC, Li XY, Cernadas M, Higgins JM, Binion DG, Parker CM. Integrin alpha E(CD103)beta 7 mediates adhesion to intestinal microvascular endothelial cell lines via an E-cadherin-independent interaction. J Immunol. 2001;166:3506–14.

68. Petrovic A, Alpdogan O, Willis LM, Eng JM, Greenberg AS, Kappel BJ, Liu C, Murphy GJ, Heller G, van den Brink MR. LPAM (alpha 4 beta 7 integrin) is an important homing integrin on alloreactive T cells in the development of intestinal graft-versus-host disease. Blood. 2004;103:1542–7.

9

Loss of bronchoprotection to Salbutamol during sputum induction with hypertonic saline: implications for asthma therapy

Hongyu Wang[1,2], Melanie Kjarsgaard[1,2], Terence Ho[1,2], John D. Brannan[3] and Parameswaran Nair[1,2]* ⓘ

Abstract

Background: Sputum induction with hypertonic saline in obstructive airway diseases is generally safe. However, saline induces bronchoconstriction in some patients despite pre-medication with Salbutamol. Our objectives were to investigate the predictors of failure of Salbutamol to protect against saline-induced-bronchoconstriction in patients with asthma and COPD and to evaluate implications for asthma therapy.

Methods: Retrospective survey on a database of 3565 patients with obstructive airway diseases who had sputum induced with hypertonic saline. The effect of baseline FEV_1, bronchitis and concomitant medication on saline-induced-bronchoconstriction ($\geq 15\%$ drop in FEV_1) were examined by logistic regression analysis. A subgroup had this re-examined 8–12 weeks after decreasing long-acting-beta-2-agonist dose or after adding Montelukast, which included an assessment of mast cell activity in sputum.

Results: 222 (6.2%) patients had saline-induced-bronchoconstriction despite pre-treatment with inhaled Salbutamol. Baseline airflow obstruction ($FEV_1\%$ predicted $< 60\%$ OR 3.29, $p < 0.001$) and long-acting-beta-agonist use (OR 2.02, $p = 0.001$), but not bronchitis, were predictors of saline-induced-bronchoconstriction, which decreased when long-acting-beta-agonist dose was decreased. Refractoriness to subsequent bronchodilation was associated with mast cell activity and was attenuated by Montelukast.

Conclusion: Sputum induction with saline provides information on bronchitis and additional physiological data on tolerance to beta-agonists and mast cell activity that may have implications for clinical therapy.

Keywords: Hypertonic saline, Sputum induction, Bronchoconstriction, Long-acting beta-agonists, Asthma, COPD

Background

Hypertonic saline nebulization is a relatively non-invasive procedure to collect sputum for airway diseases even in the presence of moderate to severe airflow obstruction [1]. Occasionally, despite pre-medication with Salbutamol, saline-induced bronchoconstriction (SIB) occurs. This may be related to baseline airflow obstruction, increased airway hyperresponsiveness (AHR), or lowered

sensitivity to β_2-agonists [2–5]. The loss of bronchoprotection is considered to be primarily due to β_2-receptor downregulation and desensitization [3], and the refractoriness to subsequent bronchodilation with Salbutamol (i.e. recovery time) is considered to be mediated partly by leukotrienes and thus reflecting mast cell activity [6].

The objectives of this retrospective cross-sectional survey were to determine predictors of SIB in a large cohort of patients with airway disease and to illustrate the wealth of information on airway physiology that could be obtained during the process of sputum induction. As proof of principle, we also evaluated the effect

*Correspondence: parames@mcmaster.ca
[1] Firestone Institute for Respiratory Health, St. Joseph's Healthcare, 50 Charlton Avenue East, Hamilton, ON L8N 4A6, Canada
Full list of author information is available at the end of the article

of LABA-dose reduction and leukotriene antagonism on SIB in a non-randomised observational study.

Methods

Data were collected from a computerized database of induced sputum cell counts from January, 2004 to January, 2008 at the Firestone Institute for Respiratory Health in Hamilton, Ontario. The database contained the following information: age, gender, post-bronchodilator spirometry, FEV_1 after each concentration increment of saline (3, 4, 5%, each for 7 min), and after subsequent administration of Salbutamol, sputum cell counts, referring physician diagnosis, indication for the test, and current relevant medications. Three groups of patients were included in the analysis: current asthma with or without associated chronic airflow limitation, possible asthma (when the referring physician was not certain of the diagnosis), and non-asthmatic COPD. A diagnosis of asthma was based on previous evidence of reversible airflow limitation (an increase in $FEV_1 \geq 15\%$ and ≥ 200 ml from the pre-bronchodilator value) or airway hyper responsiveness (a provocative concentration of methacholine causing a $> 20\%$ fall in $FEV_1 < 8$ mg/ml). COPD was indicated by a post-bronchodilator $FEV_1/VC < 70\%$, and history of cigarette smoking or smoker's inclusions within macrophages.

FEV_1 and FEV_1/VC were measured according to ATS standards 10 min after subjects received 200 µg of Salbutamol. Sputum was induced and processed according to previously published methods [7]. Saline-induced bronchoconstriction was defined as a $\geq 15\%$ drop in FEV_1 from pre-saline values at any of the concentrations of saline. Prior to induction, subjects did not withhold

their regular medications, including long-acting bronchodilators, as per our protocol. Metachromatic cells were stained using toluidine blue in a subset of patients who also had their tryptase measured in cell-free sputum supernatant by ELISA. Methacholine provocation test results (by the tidal breathing method; [8]) were available for 56 subjects, where bronchodilating medications were withheld as per guidelines [9]. Two subsets of patients with SIB were re-evaluated 8–12 weeks after either reducing their dose of LABA by half ($n = 36$) or after treating them with Montelukast 10 mg daily ($n = 20$), as part of their routine clinical management. The study was approved by the Research Ethics Board of St. Joseph's Healthcare, Hamilton. Descriptive statistics were used to summarize the baseline characteristics of the patients. Multivariate logistic regression was used in forward and backward stepwise approach to determine predictors of SIB (PASW Statistics 18, SPSS, Chicago, IL).

Results

3565 patients had sputum induced for the assessment of bronchitis (Table 1), of whom 222 (6.2%) had a $\geq 15\%$ fall in FEV_1. Overall, the predictors of Salbutamol failing to protect against SIB were the use of LABA (OR 2.02, 95% CI 1.32–3.01, $p = 0.001$), high doses of ICS (OR 1.85, 95% CI 1.11–3.09, $p = 0.02$), and baseline airflow obstruction ($FEV_1/VC < 70\%$; OR 2.08, 95% CI 1.40–3.10, $p < 0.001$) and FEV_1 predicted $< 60\%$ (OR 3.29, 95% CI 2.06–5.26, $p < 0.001$). The presence or type of bronchitis were not predictors (Table 2). In the subset of patients who had a concurrent methacholine test ($n = 56$), a PC_{20} methacholine of < 2 mg/ml was significantly associated with SIB

Table 1 Baseline characteristics of patients

	Patients, no. (%)			
	All patients n = 3565	Asthma n = 2013	Possible asthma n = 157	Non-asthmatic COPD n = 1395
$FEV_1 \downarrow > 15\%$ (%)	222 (6.2)	152 (7.5)	22 (14.0)	48 (3.4)
Male sex (n, %)	1569 (44.0)	708 (40.3)	100 (63.7)	761 (54.5)
Age year (mean, SD)	54 (17)	47 (17)	44 (13)	66 (11)
ICS (n, %)	1957 (54.9)	1661 (82.5)	102 (65)	194 (13.9)
LABA (n, %)	2426 (68)	1381 (68.6)	51 (32.5)	994 (71.3)
OCS (n, %)	174 (4.9)	135 (6.7)	8 (5.1)	31 (2.2)
NB (n, %)	328 (16.6)	106 (5.3)	15 (9.6)	207 (14.8)
EB (n, %)	592 (13.8)	534 (26.5)	20 (12.7)	37 (2.7)
FEV_1 % (mean, SD)	62.5 (45.5)	68.7 (33.6)	78.4 (22.5)	59.8 (40.8)
FEV_1/VC % (mean, SD)	64.4 (37.0)	68.7 (43.7)	72.2 (24.6)	54.6 (34.5)

ICS inhaled corticosteroid, *NB* neutrophilic bronchitis, *EB* eosinophilic bronchitis, *OCS* oral corticosteroid, regular or intermittent, *LABA* long-acting β-agonist

Eosinophilic bronchitis (EB) was defined as percentage of sputum eosinophils $\geq 3\%$. Neutrophilic bronchitis (NB) was defined as a total cell count ≥ 15 million cells/g of sputum and proportion of neutrophils $\geq 64\%$

Table 2 Predictors of saline-induced bronchoconstriction

	All patients, n = 3565			
	No.	FEV$_1$ fall > 15%, no. (%)	OR (95% CI)	p value
High ICS dose	785	84 (10.7)	1.85 (1.11–3.09)	0.019
LABA use	2426	142 (10.0)	2.02 (1.32–3.10)	0.001
FEV$_1$ <60% predicted	596	93 (15.6)	3.29 (2.06–5.26)	<0.001
FEV$_1$/VC <70%	1165	149 (12.8)	2.08 (1.40–3.10)	<0.001

ICS inhaled corticosteroid, *LABA* long-acting β-agonist

(OR 7.50, 95% CI 2.04–22.66, with p = 0.002 by Fisher's exact test).

Of the 36 asthmatics who had their dose of LABA halved, 25 (69%) did not demonstrate SIB during a second sputum induction done 8–12 weeks after the dose adjustment. Sputum mast cell activity was measured in 20 subjects who demonstrated refractoriness to bronchodilation after saline induction (mean time for FEV$_1$ to return to within 5% of pre-induction baseline was 38 ± 6 min), and this revealed that metachromatic cells (2.2 ± 0.8% vs. 0%) and tryptase (5.6 ± 1.8 vs. 0.8 ± 1.4 pg/ml) were both increased when compared to reference values [7]. In 14 (70%) of these patients, the addition of Montelukast for 8–12 weeks resulted in reduced SIB and a faster recovery of FEV$_1$ (mean time 17 ± 8 min).

Discussion

We confirmed previous observations that baseline airflow limitation and airway hyperresponsiveness to a direct stimulus such as methacholine can predict the loss of bronchoprotection to Salbutamol during saline induction [2], but also established that LABA use is a risk factor in a mixed population of obstructive airway diseases. LABA appears to cause these effects by way of receptor tolerance, [10–13]. β-receptor tolerance of airway smooth muscle cells can manifest as reduced bronchodilation, whereas for mast cells may manifest with an increased propensity to release inflammatory mediators [14]. For those on high-dose LABA, we found that reducing the dose by half led to the resolution of SIB in almost 70% of subjects. This suggests that it is important to recognize this phenomenon and to reduce the dose of LABA rather than increasing it in those patients with asthma who may have tolerance either to its bronchodilator or bronchoprotective effects.

Although we did not observe the cellular nature of bronchitis in our study to be a predictor of tolerance to SIB, there is evidence to suggest that the tolerance to bronchoprotection occurs more readily to indirect rather than to direct bronchoconstrictive agents suggesting that

airway inflammation may contribute to this phenomenon. One possible explanation that may account for these previous findings is airway mast cell activity that we do not routinely assess in quantitative sputum cell counts. This is supported by a study demonstrating that regular short-acting β-agonist leads to higher sputum levels of tryptase and metachromatic cells (mostly basophils), and an enhanced early and late asthmatic response [14]. Our findings corroborate a role for mast cells, as we showed less SIB and a more rapid recovery of FEV$_1$ after SIB with the use of Montelukast in those with elevated sputum tryptase and metachromatic cells.

The major limitation of this study is the retrospective design of this study, which prevents the establishment of a causal relationship. LABA dose was not available for all patients and this study was not powered to detect differences between Formoterol and Salmeterol. Non-respiratory medications which may impact relevant pathways, including β-adrenergic blockers (e.g. eye drops, tablets) were not recorded within this retrospective survey. Finally, the interventions were not evaluated in a placebo, controlled, randomised trial design thus limiting interpretation of the efficacy that we observed.

Conclusions

In summary, we report two clinically relevant findings regarding airway pathophysiology that could be gleaned during the process of sputum induction using hypertonic saline: first, failure of Salbutamol to protect against saline-induced bronchoconstriction should raise suspicion of tolerance to the bronchoprotective effect of β-agonists. Such patients may benefit from reducing the dose or frequency of use of LABA. Second, a prolonged recovery time (refractoriness) of FEV$_1$ following saline bronchoconstriction may indicate mast cell activity and may suggest that these are patients who may respond to mast-cell directed therapy or therapy directed against products of mast cells such as leukotriene receptor antagonists. It would be relevant to examine this phenomenon in relation to the mast cell signatures that have recently been reported using transcriptomic analysis of sputum [15, 16]. It is important to test both LABA dose reduction to improve β-agonist sensitivity and mast-cell targeted therapy to improve refractoriness to hyperosmolar stimuli induced bronchoconstriction in placebo-controlled randomised clinical trials.

Abbreviations
SIB: saline-induced bronchoconstriction; AHR: airway hyperresponsiveness; LABA: long-acting β-agonist; ICS: inhaled corticosteroid; EB: eosinophilic bronchitis; NB: neutrophilic bronchitis.

Loss of bronchoprotection to Salbutamol during sputum induction with hypertonic saline: implications...

81

Authors' contributions

PN, JB and HW designed the study and edited the manuscript. HW, MK and TH collected and analyzed the data, and wrote the manuscript. All authors read and approved the final manuscript.

Author details

[1] Firestone Institute for Respiratory Health, St. Joseph's Healthcare, 50 Charlton Avenue East, Hamilton, ON L8N 4A6, Canada. [2] Department of Medicine, McMaster University, Hamilton, ON, Canada. [3] John Hunter Hospital, Newcastle, NSW, Australia.

Acknowledgements

Not applicable.

Competing interests

PN holds membership on advisory boards for AstraZeneca, Teva, Roche, and Sanofi Aventis, and received honoraria from these companies as well as Novartis and Boehringer Ingelheim for lectures given at symposia. He has also consulted with Knopp, Theravance, 4D Therapeutics, and Inflamax. The other authors declare no competing interests or conflicts of interest.

Funding

This research did not receive any specific grant from funding agencies in the public, commercial, or not-for-profit sectors. PN is supported by the Frederick E. Hargreave Teva Innovation Chair in Airway Diseases. This had no impact on the study design, data collection and analysis, or contents of the manuscript.

References

1. Vlachos-Mayer H, Leigh R, Sharon RF, Hussack P, Hargreave FE. Success and safety of sputum induction in the clinical setting. Eur Respir J. 2000;16(5):997–1000.
2. ten Brinke A, de Lange C, Zwinderman AH, Rabe KF, Sterk PJ, Bel EH. Sputum induction in severe asthma by a standardized protocol. Am J Respir Crit Care Med. 2001;164(5):749–53.
3. Barnes PJ. Beta-adrenergic receptors and their regulation. Am J Respir Crit Care Med. 1995;152(3):838–60.
4. Haney S, Hancox RJ. Tolerance to bronchodilation during treatment with long-acting beta-agonists, a randomised controlled trial. Respir Res. 2005;6(1):1–7.
5. Jabbal S, Manoharan A, Lipworth BJ. Bronchoprotective tolerance with indacaterol is not modified by concomitant tiotropium in persistent asthma. Clin Exp Allergy. 2017;163:44–7.
6. Zuhlke IE, Kanniess F, Richter K, Nielsen-Gode D, Bohme S, Jorres RA, et al. Montelukast attenuates the airway response to hypertonic saline in moderate-to-severe COPD. Eur Respir J. 2003;22(6):926–30.
7. Pizzichini E, Pizzichini MMM, Efthimiadis AE, Evans S, Morris MM, Squillace D, et al. Indices of airway inflammation in induced sputum: reproducibility and validity of cell and fluid-phase measurements. Am J Respir Crit Care Med. 1996;154:308–17.
8. Cockcroft DW, Berscheid BA. Standardization of inhalation provocation tests. Chest. 1982;82(5):572–5.
9. Coates AL, Wanger J, Cockcroft DW, Culver BH, the Bronchoprovocation Testing Task Force, Carlsen KH, Diamant Z, et al. ERS technical standard on bronchial challenge testing: general considerations and performance of methacholine challenge tests. Eur Respir J. 2017;49(5):1601526.
10. Jones SL, Cowan JO, Flannery EM, Hancox RJ, Herbison GP, Taylor DR. Reversing acute bronchoconstriction in asthma: the effect of bronchodilator tolerance after treatment with formoterol. Eur Respir J. 2001;17(3):368–73.
11. Hancox RJ, Aldridge RE, Cowan JO, Flannery EM, Herbison GP, McLachlan CR, et al. Tolerance to beta-agonists during acute bronchoconstriction. Eur Respir J. 1999;14(2):283–7.
12. Haney S, Hancox RJ. Rapid onset of tolerance to beta-agonist bronchodilation. Respir Med. 2005;99(5):566–71.
13. Lipworth BJ, Aziz I. A high dose of albuterol does not overcome bronchoprotective subsensitivity in asthmatic subjects receiving regular salmeterol or formoterol. J Allergy Clin Immunol. 1999;103(1):88–92.
14. Swystun VA, Gordon JR, Davis EB, Zhang X, Cockcroft DW. Mast cell tryptase release and asthmatic responses to allergen increase with regular use of salbutamol. J Allergy Clin Immunol. 2000;106(1):57–64.
15. Hekking P-P, Loza MJ, Pavlidis S, de Meulder B, Lefaudeux D, Baribaud F, et al. Pathway discovery using transcriptomic profiles in adult-onset severe asthma. J Allergy Clin Immunol. 2017;141(4):1280–90.
16. Berthon BS, Gibson PG, Wood LG, MacDonald-Wicks LK, Baines KJ. A sputum gene expression signature predicts oral corticosteroid response in asthma. Eur Respir J. 2017;49(6):1700180.

10

4-month omalizumab efficacy outcomes for severe allergic asthma: the Dutch National Omalizumab in Asthma Registry

S. M. Snelder[1*], E. J. M. Weersink[2] and G. J. Braunstahl[1]

Abstract

Background: Omalizumab is licensed as add-on therapy for patients with severe allergic asthma. Response is in most studies scored by the physician's global evaluation of treatment effectiveness (GETE). A good clinical and validated parameter for treatment response is currently missing. Also, there are no established criteria for identifying patients who will respond to omalizumab based on pre-treatment characteristics. The Dutch National Omalizumab in Asthma Registry was developed in 2011 to better evaluate inclusion criteria and measure treatment response after 4 months.

Methods: This is a "real world" prospectively designed, observational data registry in which the outcomes of patients who received omalizumab between 2012 and 2015 were evaluated. Data were collected from all centers in the Netherlands comprising demographic features, criteria for starting treatment, GETE, FEV1, oral corticosteroid use and ACQ.

Results: 65.5% of the 403 patients had a good or excellent response to omalizumab after 16 weeks according to the treating physician GETE. 64.5% fulfilled all the criteria for prescribing omalizumab at baseline. The mean ACQ improved from 2.96 at baseline to 1.83 at 16 weeks (p < 0.001). 75.3% of the responders showed more than 0.5 points improvement in the ACQ. The mean FEV1 increased from 71.58 to 79.06 (p < 0.001). There was no relationship between patients with a FEV1 <80 and ≥80% at baseline and response (p = 0.981). Most of the responders had a considerable improvement of FEV1 either/or ACQ or OCS use (88.3%). While 86.7% of the responders had an improvement of either ACQ or FEV1. 75.4% of the responders had an improvement of ACQ, while 50.4% had an improvement of FEV1. Finally 11.7% of the patients with no improvement of FEV1, ACQ or OCS use were considered to have a good response.

Conclusions: This registry of 403 inadequately controlled severe allergic asthma patients in the Netherlands showed a good or excellent response of 65.5% to omalizumab after 16 weeks, in accordance with previous studies. The assumption that careful registration would lead to higher response rates could not be supported by the data from this registry. Improvement of ACQ appears to be a useful additional assessment tool to measure response in omalizumab treated patients.

Keywords: Allergic asthma, Omalizumab, ACQ, FEV1

Background

Omalizumab (Xolair®) is a subcutaneously administrated humanized anti-immunoglobulin E (IgE) monoclonal antibody that targets circulating free IgE and prevents its interaction with the high-affinity IgE receptor (FCƐR1).

It is licensed in the European Union as add-on therapy for patients aged 6 years and older with either allergic asthma or chronic idiopatic urticaria [1, 2]. Since 2006, omalizumab has been prescribed for inadequately controlled severe allergic asthma in the Netherlands. Randomized studies demonstrated a significantly greater improvement in asthma control in patients treated with add-on omalizumab than patients treated with placebo [3–6].

*Correspondence: S.Snelder@Franciscus.nl
[1] Franciscus Gasthuis & Vlietland, Kleiweg 500, 3045 PM Rotterdam, The Netherlands
Full list of author information is available at the end of the article

Response is in most studies scored by the physician's global evaluation of treatment effectiveness (GETE). The physicians GETE is a composite measure that encompasses multiple aspects of evaluation of response, including patient interviews, review of medical notes, spirometry and diaries of symptoms and rescue medication [7]. As GETE is a subjective parameter for response we want to search for a more objective parameter. Other often used measurements for improvement are the asthma control questionnaire (ACQ) [8], asthma control test (ACT) [9], asthma quality-of-life questionnaire (AQLQ) [10], mini-AQLQ [11], asthma symptom score, FEV1 and exacerbation rate [3, 4, 12]. A single good parameter for response is missing.

EU indication for prescribing omalizumab is: severe persistent (IgE-mediated) allergic asthma, positive skin test or in vitro reactivity to a perennial aeroallergen, frequent daytime symptoms or night-time awakenings, multiple documented severe asthma exacerbations despite daily high-dose ICS plus a LABA and in patients >12 years reduces lung function (FEV1 <80%) [1]. Criteria for prescribing omalizumab in Australia are the same as in the EU, except that the FEV1 had to be documented less than 80% on more than three occasions in the previous 3 months [13]. In the USA a FEV1 <80% is not a criteria for prescribing [14].

At present, there are no established criteria for identifying patients who will respond to omalizumab based on pre-treatment characteristics [15]. Initially, omalizumab was started in some patients that did not strictly fulfill the criteria for omalizumab prescription [12]. In 2011, the Dutch reimbursement authority required more data about starting criteria and treatment response which lead to the formation of Dutch National Omalizumab in Asthma Registry. The organization and monitoring was in the hands of the Dutch Organization of Chest Physicians (NVALT). The assumption was that a stricter registration policy would lead to higher response rates and therefore be more cost-effective. Moreover, several clinical parameters were monitored to see which ones would best objectively relate to treatment response.

Methods

This is a "real world" prospectively designed, observational data registry in which the outcomes of patients who received omalizumab between 2012 and 2015 were evaluated. Data were collected from all centers in the Netherlands where omalizumab was prescribed for the treatment of severe allergic asthma. The survey questionnaire was approved by the national board of Chest Physicians (NVALT) and comprised the following start criteria: severe allergic asthma, age >6 years, a positive skin test or in vitro activity to a relevant perennial aeroallergen,

a FEV1 less than 80%, more than two severe exacerbations and substantial symptoms despite treatment with inhaled corticosteroids (ICS) and long-acting B2-agonists (LABAs). In addition, inhalation technique and compliance were checked and optimized, and smoking stopped (or at least tried). Patients gave informed consent to participate in the survey. The data were centrally collected and analyzed by three independent physicians.

Response evaluation

Response was defined as a physician-rating GETE of excellent or good. Non-response was defined as a physician-rating GETE of moderate, poor or worsening. Response evaluation was left to the discretion of the treating physician. However, it was strongly recommended to measure ACQ-6 and FEV1 at baseline, at 2 and 4 months. Also, when patients were on maintenance therapy with oral corticosteroids the average daily dose was registered. The ACQ-6 includes both patient-reported symptoms and use of rescue medication [8]. ACQ scores range from 0 (completely controlled) to 6 (extremely poorly controlled). A decrease in ACQ score of more than 0.5 points is considered to be the minimal clinically important improvement [11].

A sub-analysis was performed between patients with FEV1 ≥80% and FEV1 <80% at baseline.

Statistical analysis

The unpaired Student's t test was used for continuous variables with normal distributions, and Chi square test/Fisher's Exact test for categorical variables. A p value <0.05 (two-sided) is considered a statistically significant difference. Correlation was measured using the Spearman Rank correlation coefficient. Statistical analyses were performed using SPSS version 18.0 (SPSS Inc., Chicago, Illinois, USA).

Results

403 patients had a full data set and could be evaluated. Baseline characteristics are shown in Table 1. The mean age was 47. 62.8% of the patients were female. The mean IgE was 619.9 with a range from 3 to 10,800. 69.2% had a FEV1 <80% of predicted. 64.5% of the patients fulfilled all of the criteria for prescribing omalizumab at baseline (Table 2).

65.5% of the patients had a good or excellent response to omalizumab after 16 weeks according to the treating physician GETE. Table 3 shows if the patients fullfilled the criteria for prescribing omalizumab and if they had good response to omalizumab. As shown in Table 4, the mean ACQ improved from 2.96 at baseline to 1.83 at 16 weeks (p < 0.001). 75.3% of the responders showed more than 0.5 points improvement in the ACQ score

Table 1 Baseline characteristics

Variable	Value
Total no patients	403
Age	
Mean (SD)	47 (15.6)
Gender (%)	
Male	149 (37.0)
Female	253 (62.8)
Body weight, kg	
Mean (SD)	78.6 (17.4)
Baseline IgE level, IU/mL	
Mean (SD)	619. 9 (1036.4)
Range	3–10,800
Severe allergic asthma (%)	
Yes	380 (94.3)
No	12 (3.0)
Positive skin-prick test/RAST (%)	
Yes	363 (90.3)
No	26 (6.5)
FEV1 <80 (%)	
Yes	279 (69.2)
No	116 (28.8)
More than 2 exacerbations (%)	
Yes	384 (95.3)
No	11 (2.7)
Maximum dose ICS and LABAs (%)	
Yes	394 (99)
No	4 (1)
Smoking (%)	
Tried to quit smoking	101 (25.1)
Didn't try to quit smoking	29 (7.2)

Table 2 Fulfilled all the criteria for prescribing omalizumab at baseline vs response

	Response		
	Yes	No	Total
Criteria fulfilled yes	173	87	260
Criteria fulfilled no	91	52	143
Total	264	139	403
	$p = 0.558$		

after 16 weeks. The mean FEV1 increased from 71.58 to 79.06 (p < 0.001). 50.4% of the responders had an improvement of ≥5% of FEV1 %pred. There was no relation between FEV1 <80%pred and ≥80%pred at baseline and response after 4 months (p = 0.981). Table 4 shows that the maintenance OCS use was lower at 16 weeks (66.5% none at baseline vs 72.2% none at 16 weeks)

Table 3 Criteria for prescribing omalizumab fulfilled and good response

	Fulfilled/good response	Not fulfilled/ good response
Severe allergic asthma	380/250	12/5
Age >6 years	403/263	0/0
A positive skin test or RAST	364/241	26/12
FEV1 <80	279/183	116/77
>2 exacerbations	384/250	11/7
Maximum dose LABAs and ICS	394/257	4/3

Table 4 ACQ, FEV1 and OCS at baseline vs 16 weeks

	Baseline	16 weeks
ACQ		
n	334	307
Mean (SD)	2.96 (1.12)	1.83 (1.12)
		$p < 0.001$
FEV1		
n	338	287
Mean (SD)	71.58 (19.6)	79.06 (20.06)
		$p < 0.001$
OCS		
n	364	334
None (%)	242 (66.5)	241 (72.2)
1–5 mg (%)	45 (12.4)	46 (13.8)
6–9 mg (%)	15 (4.1)	12 (3.6)
>10 mg (%)	61 (16.8)	35 (10.5)
		$p < 0.001$

p < 0.001. The response remained stable over the years 2012–2015, p = 0.690.

Figure 1a shows that most of the responders had an improvement of either FEV1 or ACQ or OCS (88.6%). While 86.7% of the responders had an improvement of either FEV1 or ACQ. It also shows that ACQ alone (75.4%) appears to be a better measurement for a response than either improvement of the FEV1 (50.4%) or OCS use (16.7%). Figure 1b shows that 60.4% of the non-responders had neither an improvement of ACQ nor FEV1 nor OCS. 66.5% of the patients who fulfilled all of the criteria at baseline had a good or excellent response (Table 2). There is no relationship between fulfilling all the criteria and response (p = 0.558).

11.7% of the patients with no improvement of the ACQ, FEV1 or OCS had a good response. There was a sufficient degree of correlation between improvement of ACQ and response according to GETE [r = 0.458, p < 0.001(=7.92E−18)] and a weak correlation between improvement of FEV1 and response according to GETE [r = 0.292, p < 0.001(=4.98E−7)].

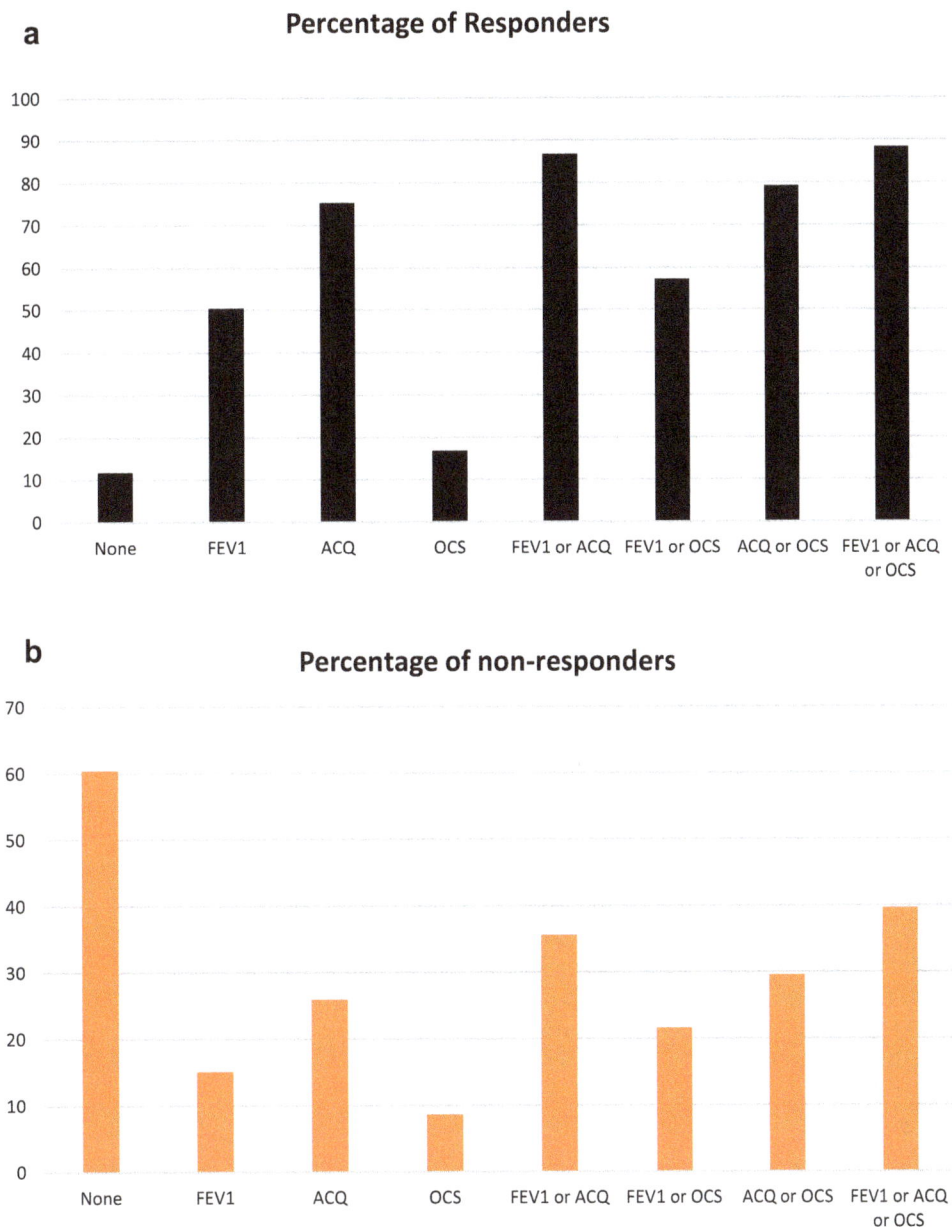

Fig. 1 a Percentage of responders versus an improvement of FEV1, ACQ or OCS. **b** Percentage of non-responders versus an improvement of FEV1, ACQ or OCS

Discussion

65.5% of the 403 patients with inadequately controlled severe allergic asthma had a good or excellent response to omalizumab after 16 weeks. 75.3% of the responders had more than 0.5 points improvement of the ACQ. Overall the ACQ improved, FEV1 increased and there was lower use of OCS at 16 weeks. 50.4% of the responders had an improvement of more than 5% of the FEV1. More patients who had a good or excellent response had an improvement of the ACQ (75.3%) than

an improvement of FEV1 (50.4%) or OCS use (16.7%). This suggests that the ACQ may be the best measurement for response.

We found a response rate of 65.5%, which is in accordance with previous data from randomized controlled trials and real world data. Bousquet et al. found a response of 62.0% at 16 weeks [3]. Niven et al. found a response of 70% [5]. Schumann et al. had a response of 78.8% in their prospective multicenter study [16]. Brusselle et al. even showed that more than 82% had good/excellent

GETE [17]. The eXpeRience registry showed a response of 69.9% after 16 weeks by GETE [12]. The assumption that careful registration would lead to higher response rates could not be proven in this study. In fact, only 64.5% fulfilled all of the criteria for prescribing omalizumab at baseline. There is no relationship between fulfilling all the criteria and response (p = 0.558). The main reason for not strictly following the rules was a FEV1 >80 (28.8% of the total population), followed by missing of a positive skin test or in vitro activity to a perennial aeroallergen (Table 1).

Schumann et al. described that the ACQ score significantly decreased from 3.58 ± 1.28 to 2.01 ± 1.05 after 16 weeks (−43.7%), treatment responders showed greater and highly significant improvements of symptoms compared with non-responders even after 16 weeks (−46.9%, p < 0.0001 vs −36.1%, p < 0.05) [16]. This is in agreement with our findings and underlines the importance of using ACQ in response evaluation. According to FEV1 they described that patients who did respond to omalizumab treatment had higher absolute FEV1 values at baseline (2.11 L vs 1.87 L) and showed a higher expressed increase in % predicted of FEV1 compared with non-responders (15.6% vs 13.7%) [16]. We didn't find a relationship between patients with a FEV1 <80 and ≥80% at baseline and response (p = 0.981).

There was a significant lowering of OCS use at 16 weeks, these results are in line with the eXpeRience registry [18]. The evaluation period of 4 months was too short to say something about exacerbations.

Despite our positive findings, it is important to recognize the limitations of our study. First as with all observational studies, is the lack of a control group and the open-label design. Other limitations of observational studies are that the results should be interpreted with due consideration that factors other than the treatment of interest may have contributed to the findings. Finally, the data quality relied heavily on the accuracy and completeness of available clinical records.

Conclusions

This registry of 403 inadequately controlled severe allergic asthma patients in the Netherlands showed a good or excellent response of 65.5% to omalizumab after 16 weeks. Overall the ACQ improved, FEV1 increased and there was lower use of OCS at 16 weeks. This is in accordance with previous data from randomized controlled trials and real word data. 75.3% of the responders had more than 0.5 points improvement of the ACQ. There was no relationship between patients with a FEV1 <80 and ≥80% at baseline and the response. Improvement of ACQ appears to be a useful assessment tool to measure response in omalizumab treated patients.

Abbreviations

GETE: global evaluation of treatment effectiveness; ACQ: asthma control questionnaire; FEV1: forced expiratory volume in 1 s; ACT: asthma control test; AQLQ: asthma quality-of-life questionnaire.

Authors' contributions

GJB and EJMW collected the patient data from all centers in the Netherlands. SMS analysed and interpreted the patient data and was a major contributor in writing the manuscript. All authors read and approved the final manuscript.

Author details

[1] Franciscus Gasthuis & Vlietland, Kleiweg 500, 3045 PM Rotterdam, The Netherlands. [2] Academisch Medisch Centrum, Amsterdam, The Netherlands.

Acknowledgements

Not applicable.

Competing interests

G-J Braunstahl has received grant/research support for consultations and/or speaking at conferences from Novartis, ALK-Abello, Meda Pharma, GSK, Takeda, AstraZeneca and MSD.

E.J.M. Weersink has received grant/research support for consultations and/or speaking at conferences from Novartis, GSK, AstraZeneca, Chiesi and TEVA.

References

1. European Medicine Agency. Xolair powder and solvent for solution for injection: summary of product characteristics. 2012. http://www.ema.europa.eu/docs/en_GB/document_library/EPAR_-_Product_Information/human/000606/WC500057298.pdf. Accessed 23 Dec 2016.
2. Maurer M, Rosen K, Hsieh HJ, Saini S, Grattan C, Gimenez-Arnau A, et al. Omalizumab for the treatment of chronic idiopathic or spontaneous urticaria. N Engl J Med. 2013;368(10):924–35.
3. Bousquet J, Siergiejko Z, Swiebocka E, Humbert M, Rabe KF, Smith N, et al. Persistency of response to omalizumab therapy in severe allergic (IgE-mediated) asthma. Allergy. 2011;66(5):671–8.
4. McKeage K. Omalizumab: a review of its use in patients with severe persistent allergic asthma. Drugs. 2013;73(11):1197–212.
5. Niven R, Chung KF, Panahloo Z, Blogg M, Ayre G. Effectiveness of omalizumab in patients with inadequately controlled severe persistent allergic asthma: an open-label study. Respir Med. 2008;102(10):1371–8.
6. Hanania NA, Alpan O, Hamilos DL, Condemi JJ, Reyes-Rivera I, Zhu J, et al. Omalizumab in severe allergic asthma inadequately controlled with standard therapy: a randomized trial. Ann Intern Med. 2011;154(9):573–82.
7. Bousquet J, Rao S, Manga V. Global evaluation of treatment effectiveness (GETE) is an accurate predictor of response to omalizumab in patients with severe allergic asthma: a pooled analysis. Eur Respir J. 2014;44:3483.
8. Juniper EF, O'Byrne PM, Guyatt GH, Ferrie PJ, King DR. Development and validation of a questionnaire to measure asthma control. Eur Respir J. 1999;14(4):902–7.

9. Schatz M, Sorkness CA, Li JT, Marcus P, Murray JJ, Nathan RA, et al. Asthma Control Test: reliability, validity, and responsiveness in patients not previously followed by asthma specialists. J Allergy Clin Immunol. 2006;117(3):549–56.

10. Juniper EF, Guyatt GH, Epstein RS, Ferrie PJ, Jaeschke R, Hiller TK. Evaluation of impairment of health related quality of life in asthma: development of a questionnaire for use in clinical trials. Thorax. 1992;47(2):76–83.

11. Juniper EF, Svensson K, Mork AC, Stahl E. Measurement properties and interpretation of three shortened versions of the asthma control questionnaire. Respir Med. 2005;99(5):553–8.

12. Braunstahl GJ, Chen CW, Maykut R, Georgiou P, Peachey G, Bruce J. The eXpeRience registry: the 'real-world' effectiveness of omalizumab in allergic asthma. Respir Med. 2013;107(8):1141–51.

13. Australian Public Assessment Report for Omalizumab (rch). Proprietary Product Name: Xolair Sponsor: Novartis Pharmaceuticals Australia Pty Ltd. https://www.tga.gov.au/sites/default/files/auspar-omalizumab-rch-160622.pdf. Accessed 27 Jun 2017.

14. Prescribing information Xolair. https://www.accessdata.fda.gov/drugsatfda_docs/label/2016/103976s5225lbl.pdf. Accessed 27 Jun 2017.

15. Bousquet J, Rabe K, Humbert M, Chung KF, Berger W, Fox H, et al. Predicting and evaluating response to omalizumab in patients with severe allergic asthma. Respir Med. 2007;101(7):1483–92.

16. Schumann C, Kropf C, Wibmer T, Rudiger S, Stoiber KM, Thielen A, et al. Omalizumab in patients with severe asthma: the XCLUSIVE study. Clin Respir J. 2012;6(4):215–27.

17. Brusselle G, Michils A, Louis R, Dupont L, Van de Maele B, Delobbe A, et al. "Real-life" effectiveness of omalizumab in patients with severe persistent allergic asthma: the PERSIST study. Respir Med. 2009;103(11):1633–42.

18. Braunstahl GJ, Chlumsky J, Peachey G, Chen CW. Reduction in oral corticosteroid use in patients receiving omalizumab for allergic asthma in the real-world setting. Allergy Asthma Clin Immunol. 2013;9(1):47.

11

Airway autoimmune responses in severe eosinophilic asthma following low-dose Mepolizumab therapy

Manali Mukherjee[1,4], Hui Fang Lim[2], Sruthi Thomas[1,4], Douglas Miller[1], Melanie Kjarsgaard[1,4], Bruce Tan[3], Roma Sehmi[1], Nader Khalidi[1] and Parameswaran Nair[1,4]*

Abstract

Background: Anti-interleukin (IL)-5 monoclonal antibodies as an eosinophil-depleting strategy is well established, with Mepolizumab being the first biologic approved as an adjunct treatment for severe eosinophilic asthma.

Case presentation: A 62-year old woman diagnosed with severe eosinophilic asthma showed poor response to Mepolizumab therapy (100 mg subcutaneous dose/monthly) and subsequent worsening of symptoms. The treatment response to Mepolizumab was monitored using both blood and sputum eosinophil counts. The latter was superior in assessing deterioration in symptoms, suggesting that normal blood eosinophil count may not always indicate amelioration or adequate control of the ongoing eosinophil-driven disease process. This perplexing situation of persistent airway eosinophilia and increased steroid insensitivity despite an anti-eosinophil therapy can be explained if the administered dose of the mAb was inadequate in comparison to the target antigen. The resultant immune complexes could act as 'cytokine depots', protecting the potency of the 'bound' IL-5, thereby sustaining the eosinophilic inflammation within the target tissue. Molecular analysis of the sputum indicated the development of a polyclonal autoimmune response as well as an increase in group 2 innate lymphoid cells, two novel observations in severe eosinophilic asthma, which were associated with indices of disease severity and progression. This case highlights the possibility of a previously unrecognised autoimmune-mediated worsening of asthma perhaps triggered by immune complexes formed due to inadequate dosing of administered monoclonal antibodies in the target tissue.

Conclusions: While anti-IL5 mAb therapy is an exciting novel option to treat patients with severe asthma, there is the rare possibility of worsening of asthma as observed in this case study, due to local autoimmune mechanisms precipitated by potential inadequate airway levels of the monoclonal antibody.

Keywords: Mepolizumab, Autoantibodies, Autoimmune, Eosinophilic asthma, IL-5, Sputum, Immune complex

Background

The past decade has witnessed the development of several anti-cytokine monoclonal antibody therapies (mAb) for asthma, with Mepolizumab, an IgG_1 mAb against IL-5, being the first biologic approved for severe eosinophilic asthma [1]. We report a worrying scenario of asthma worsening, following 100 mg subcutaneous (s.c) Mepolizumab therapy in a patient with severe eosinophilic asthma. In this article we draw attention to two factors: (i) enumerating eosinophils in sputum is more useful to monitor treatment response than in blood; (ii) low-dose mAb therapy might lead to increased inflammation triggered by in vivo immune complex (IC) formation between drug and the target cytokine (IL-5), when the latter is in excess to the former in the target tissue. This is more likely to affect patients whose asthma is severe enough to require maintenance systemic corticosteroids to control their airway eosinophilia.

*Correspondence: parames@mcmaster.ca
[4] Firestone Institute for Respiratory Health, 50 Charlton Avenue East, Hamilton, ON L8N 4A6, Canada
Full list of author information is available at the end of the article

Case presentation

A 62-year old non-atopic woman, with seven pack-year smoking history, and adult-onset asthma (diagnosed at 21 years) whose symptoms worsened at the age of 55 was seen in our clinic on February 22nd, 2010 with severe airway hyper-responsiveness (PC_{20} methacholine <0.03 mg/mL), mild airflow obstruction (FEV_1 2.04 L, 75% predicted, FEV_1/VC 75%), and chronic rhinosinusitis with polyposis. The eosinophilic nature of her asthma was confirmed by peripheral blood counts (peaked at 0.8×10^9/L in 2010) and sputum cellularity (eosinophils >3% of total cell count with free granules on multiple occasions). She did not have mutations for PDGFR-FIP1L1, c-kit, JAK2, or BCR-Abl or abnormal lymphocyte population or T cell receptor rearrangements. Her routine chemistry, total serum IgE, and tryptase were normal, as were her stool microscopy, antifungal precipitins, and autoantibody profile including cytoplasmic and perinuclear anti-neutrophil cytoplasmic antibodies. Computed tomography of thorax was unremarkable. She had two sinus polypectomies that did not improve her respiratory symptoms significantly. She has been prednisone-dependent since 2008. Methotrexate, hydroxyurea, and imatinib were not effective to wean her off prednisone (Fig. 1). The patient was known to be compliant with her medications, and her inhaler technique was deemed adequate.

By 2013, she required a daily dose of 2500 mcg fluticasone propionate, long-acting beta-2 agonists,

muscarinic antagonists, and 20 mg prednisone to maintain an FEV_1 of 1.76 L (65% of predicted), blood eosinophils 0.03×10^9 cells/L, and 4% sputum eosinophils (Fig. 1a). With four exacerbations in the preceding year, she was enrolled into a double-blinded placebo controlled Mepolizumab clinical trial (#MEA115575) (in which she received the active drug), followed by an open-label extension (#MEA115661). In the double-blinded trial, her FEV_1 was 1.76 L at the start of the study (Feb-13) that dropped to 0.9 L at the end of the study (Aug-13), with no demonstrable steroid-sparing effect (Fig. 1a). In the open-label extension, she received nine monthly infusions of 100 mg s.c Mepolizumab, without an improvement in her FEV_1, and two interim courses of intravenous solumedrol to manage her deteriorating symptoms. The anti-eosinophil effect of Mepolizumab was apparent from her depleting blood eosinophil levels and her sputum eosinophils being maintained below 3% until September 2013 (Fig. 1a). The initial drop in her FEV_1 was therefore not eosinophil-driven, indicating the presence of alternative mechanisms. Furthermore, her lung function continued to deteriorate with increasing airway eosinophilia (not reflected in blood), and prednisone requirement that now doubled from a pre-study dose of 20–40 mg daily (Fig. 1b). The patient did not develop any circulating anti-Mepolizumab antibodies that could explain this.

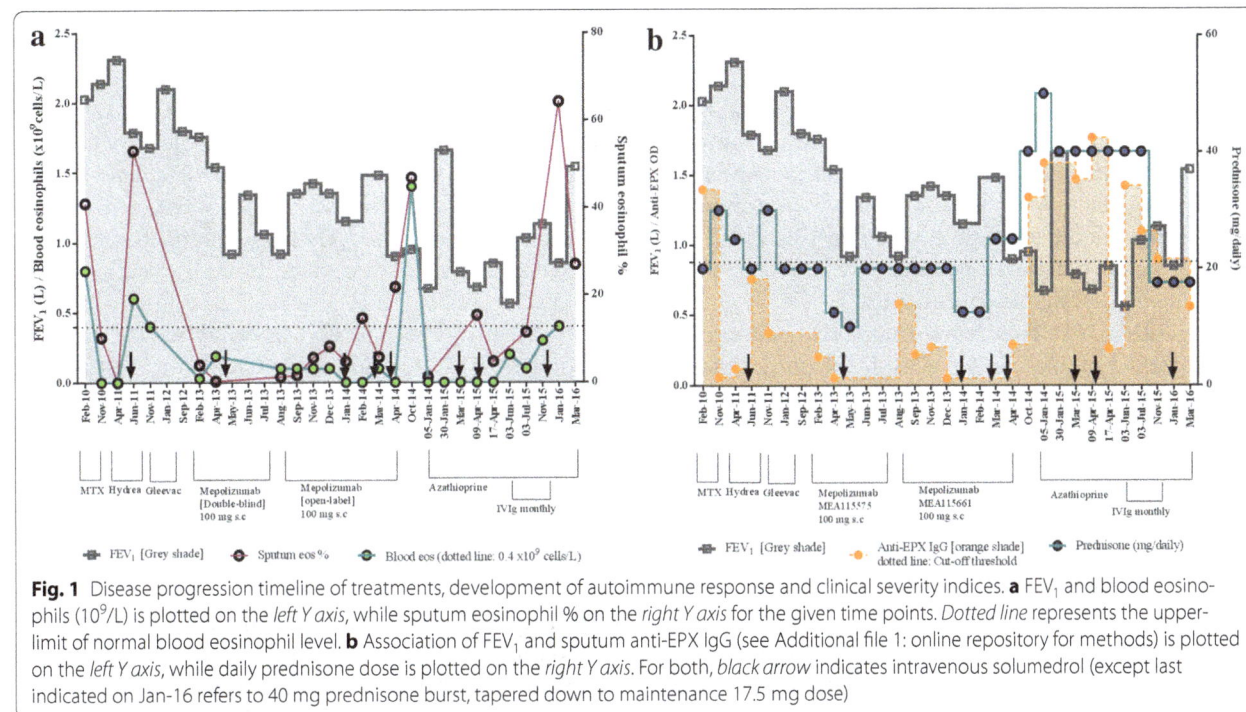

Fig. 1 Disease progression timeline of treatments, development of autoimmune response and clinical severity indices. **a** FEV_1 and blood eosinophils (10^9/L) is plotted on the *left Y axis*, while sputum eosinophil % on the *right Y axis* for the given time points. *Dotted line* represents the upper-limit of normal blood eosinophil level. **b** Association of FEV_1 and sputum anti-EPX IgG (see Additional file 1: online repository for methods) is plotted on the *left Y axis*, while daily prednisone dose is plotted on the *right Y axis*. For both, *black arrow* indicates intravenous solumedrol (except last indicated on Jan-16 refers to 40 mg prednisone burst, tapered down to maintenance 17.5 mg dose)

Discussion and molecular insights

Mepolizumab is an effective therapy to reduce blood and sputum eosinophils in severe prednisone-dependent asthma, with a good safety profile and low incidence of circulating anti-drug antibodies [1–3]. However, the magnitude of clinical efficacy may be lower regarding prednisone-sparing effect with 100 mg of the drug administered subcutaneously compared to 750 mg intravenously. This may be due to inadequate concentrations of the drug in the airway. We are unable to confirm this as the mAb pharmacokinetics in the airway of asthmatics has not been established. It is plausible, in the event of inadequate dosing in the airways of patients with high IL-5 concentration, drug-antigen IC clusters can form (Additional file 1: Figure S1 in the online repository). Being an IgG$_1$ humanised mAb, the IL-5/Mepolizumab ICs, can precipitate, bind complement and elicit further inflammation and tissue injury. In the complexed form, a neutralising mAb protects the active-site of the cytokine from in vivo degradation [4]. This increases the bioavailability of IL-5 to its target receptors present on tissue-resident cells like ILC2s and eosinophil progenitors (EoPs). Enumeration of both these cell types was recently reported to be significantly higher in severe asthmatic airways [5].

This case study offered us a unique opportunity to investigate this hypothesis of an IC-mediated worsening of patient symptoms in the event of inadequate mAb dosing. Due to unavailability of a biopsy sample, tissue deposition of ICs could not be performed. An attempt to quantify complement consumption in the sputum to assess local IC formations was inconclusive. The assay performance with sputum supernatants was unreliable in comparison to other biological samples like nasal polyp extracts performed alongside. Nevertheless, a series of molecular investigations were undertaken to answer this perplexing situation of persistent airway eosinophilia (but normal blood eosinophil) while on treatment with Mepolizumab, deteriorating lung function and subsequent increase in steroid-insensitivity.

Our molecular studies demonstrated that sputum IL-5 levels peaked at the end of her Mepolizumab therapy (Fig. 2). This increase in IL-5 during an anti-IL5 therapy, along with demonstrable sputum eosinophils, can be explained by IL-5/Mepolizumab ICs acting as 'cytokine depots.' Early studies in murine models from the 1990s report that cytokine: anti-cytokine complexes exhibit increased in vivo half-lives, functional potency, and downstream biological activity of the bound cytokine [4]. This increase in in vivo potency/downstream biological activity by cytokine: anti-cytokine mAb complexes has been demonstrated for several cytokines viz., IL-2 [6], IL-4 [7], IL-6 [8], IL-7 [9]. Indeed, by using a sandwich

ELISA (see Additional file 1: online repository for methods), we could detect IL-5 bound to immunoglobulins immunoprecipitated from the sputum supernatant induced at the Aug-2013 visit, post 6 infusions (Visit 9, #MEA115575), otherwise undetectable in prior samples (Additional file 1: Figure S2).

We enumerated IL-5$^+$ ILC2 cells by flow cytometry in both blood and sputum. There was a dramatic increase in circulating IL5$^+$ ILC2 s after six injections of Mepolizumab (Aug-13, Fig. 2). By Apr-14, sputum IL5$^+$ ILC2 s was demonstrable despite further nine infusions of s.c 100 mg Mepolizumab (Fig. 2). A recent study investigated the cause of rare eosinophilia post-low dose IL-2 therapy in HCV-induced vasculitis. This was shown to be an IL-2/anti-IL-2 mAb (IC)-mediated mechanism where the increased bioavailability of the bound IL-2 favoured interactions with IL-2R expressed by ILC2 s, stimulating in situ IL-5 production [10]. Further, ICs formed between an allergen, and its specific IgG can be intercepted by FcγRIII expressed on antigen-presenting cells, which leads to an increase in Th2 signalling through upregulation of IL-33 [11]. In fact, this can be extrapolated to any IC with IgG, since the up-regulation of IL-33 is mediated by the Fc:FcR binding and not the complexed antigen. IL-33 has been shown to activate resident ILC2 s (expressing the IL-33 receptor) to produce Th2 cytokines [11]. Therefore, an IC-mediated increase in Th2 signalling could lead to the observed airway eosinophilia via activation of IL-5 producing ILC2s, subsequent lung-homing and differentiation of EoPs, in situ.

Initial depletion of IL-5 by targeted therapy might have suppressed autoantigen-specific regulatory cells, thereby compromising the local tolerance, as per observations in a model of experimental autoimmune neuritis [12]. Being a retrospective case study, we were unable to enumerate regulatory cells pre- and post therapy (via flow cytometry) to gauge any effect of anti-IL-5 targeted therapy on regulatory lymphocyte population/activity. However, compared to data collated from 15 healthy volunteer sputum (mean IL-10 levels: 2.9 ± 1.3 pg/mL, upper 90% percentile 5.88 pg/mL), the study patient had low levels of IL-10 in sputum, that varied between 0.29 and 0.59 pg/mL in all the samples tested between Aug-2013 and Jun-2015. This was indicative of a 'local' micro-environment with compromised immune-regulation. Indeed, laboratory investigations, as early as 2010, showed that the patient had a propensity towards local autoimmune response [13]. We could detect high titres of anti-eosinophil peroxidase (EPX) IgG and anti-nuclear antibodies (ANAs, Figs. 1b, 2; see Additional file 1: online repository for methods) in the sputum, otherwise undetectable in circulation. Incidentally, there was also an increase documented for sputum B-cell activity (B-cell activating factor

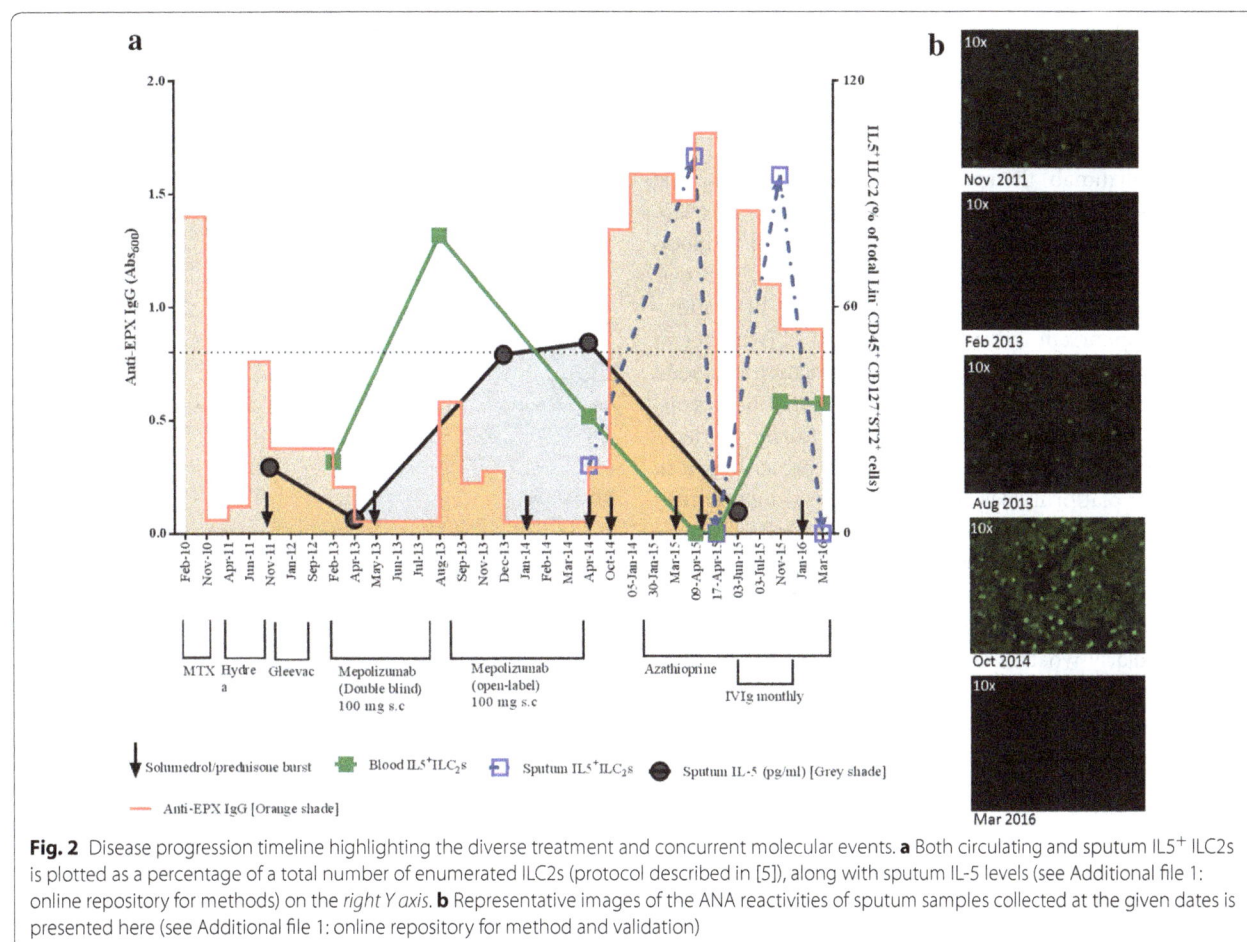

Fig. 2 Disease progression timeline highlighting the diverse treatment and concurrent molecular events. **a** Both circulating and sputum IL5+ ILC2s is plotted as a percentage of a total number of enumerated ILC2s (protocol described in [5]), along with sputum IL-5 levels (see Additional file 1: online repository for methods) on the *right Y axis*. **b** Representative images of the ANA reactivities of sputum samples collected at the given dates is presented here (see Additional file 1: online repository for method and validation)

(BAFF) levels: pre-Mepolizumab, Feb-13—19.2 pg/mL to post-Mepolizumab, Oct-14: 228 pg/mL). We speculate that increase in activated ILC2s contributed to the local B-cell activity since the former has recently been reported to activate and promote survival of B-cells in vitro [14]. The concurrent increase in eosinophils and autoantibodies would allow spontaneous IgG-mediated eosinophil degranulation in the airways, an event that is known to be steroid-unresponsive [15]. Increased frequency of a steroid-unresponsive event could explain the increase in maintenance prednisone dose to 40 mg (Fig. 1b).

To target the lymphocytes, the patient was then treated with daily 150 mg azathioprine without any continual clinical improvement. At an all-time low FEV_1 of 0.56 L (23% predicted), she was started on intravenous immunoglobulins (IVIgs, 2 g/kg weight, over 3 days, monthly) as an autoantibody mopping-up strategy. Post six monthly infusions (Nov-15) her sputum autoantibody titres reduced steadily, and FEV_1 improved to 1.13 L (Fig. 2), suggesting a plausible underlying autoimmune-type anomaly. Indeed, the autoantibody levels correlated with the deteriorating lung-function (FEV_1) over the

entire timeline of the case study (r = −0.55, P = 0.01, Fig. 1b).

At the last IVIg infusion, the prednisone dose was reduced to 17.5 mg to assess a steroid-sparing effect. The lowered dose was unable to suppress the local inflammatory mediators that allowed 'lung-homing' of lymphocytes and increased IL5+ ILC2s, driving an in situ eosinophilopoeisis evident by the concomitant increase in sputum eosinophils (Nov-15 Fig. 2). The exacerbation (Jan-16) was treated with a prednisone burst. In the absence of the steroid-unresponsive IgG-induced degranulation post-IVIg (Nov-15), an ILC2-mediated increase in sputum eosinophilia recently shown to be steroid-responsive [16], could be curbed by a prednisone burst. Thereafter, the patient was maintained at 17.5 mg of daily prednisone (Fig. 1b). Her recent FEV_1 in Mar-16 was recorded to be 1.54 L (Fig. 1b). She continues to be hyperresponsive (PC_{20} methacholine <0.03 mg/mL), contributing to her daily symptoms and poor asthma control, ACQ of 1.5). She is being considered for therapy with additional IVIg and/or intravenous reslizumab (an IgG_4 anti-IL5 mAb, weight-adjusted dosing) or anti-IL4Rα mAb (Dupulimab).

Conclusion

To our knowledge this is the first case report of an anti-IL-5 therapy leading to worsening of clinical symptoms in eosinophilic severe asthma. In summary, we provide evidence that normal blood eosinophil counts post low-dose Mepolizumab therapy does not confirm that the eosinophil-driven disease process is adequately controlled. Indeed, sputum was demonstrated to be superior to blood in monitoring response to therapy. Although a direct evidence of in vivo IC-mediated injury could not be demonstrated, a concurrent increase in sputum IL-5 (whether in a free-form or bound) and IL5$^+$ ILC2 population provided indirect evidence of possible ICs acting as 'cytokine depots', supporting in situ eosinophilopoiesis. And finally, we demonstrated that Mepolizumab, at the current prescribed dose and delivery platform, may precipitate steroid-insensitivity by triggering steroid-unresponsive auto-inflammatory mechanisms, especially in patients who are predisposed to it. Further studies are necessary to understand the airway pharmacokinetics of novel mAbs, effective dosing strategies particularly whether they have to be guided by antigen-concentrations or body weight, and the appropriate therapy for patients with inadequate or worsening clinical responses with the monoclonal antibodies.

Abbreviations

mAb: monoclonal antibody; IC: immune complex; FEV$_1$: forced expiratory volume in 1 s; s.c.: subcutaneous; EPX: eosinophil peroxidase; IP-Igs: immunoprecipitated immunoglobulin; IVIg: intravenous immunoglobulin; ANA: anti-nuclear antibody; BAFF: B-cell-activating factor of the TNF family; BAL: broncho-alveolar lavage; IL: interleukin; Ig: immunoglobulin; ILC2: innate lymphoid cells of group 2.

Authors' contributions

PN, NK, and HFL provided clinical care to the patient; MM performed the immunological experiments and prepared the first draft of the manuscript. RS supervised ILC$_2$ enumerations. BT assisted with complement assays. The other authors assisted with the clinical care and laboratory measurements. All authors have reviewed the final draft. PN provides an overall guarantee for the data in the manuscript. All authors read and approved the final manuscript.

Author details

[1] Department of Medicine, McMaster University & St. Joseph's Healthcare, Hamilton, ON, Canada. [2] Department of Respiratory Medicine, National University of Singapore, Singapore, Singapore. [3] Department of Otolaryngology, Northwestern University, Feinberg School of Medicine, Chicago, IL, USA. [4] Firestone Institute for Respiratory Health, 50 Charlton Avenue East, Hamilton, ON L8N 4A6, Canada.

Acknowledgements

The authors would like to acknowledge Ms. Katherine Radford and Dr. Steven Smith for their assistance with measurements in sputum.

Competing interests

PN is supported by the Frederick E. Hargreave Teva Innovation Chair in Airway Diseases. He has received consultancy fees from AstraZeneca, Boehringer Ingelheim, Sanofi, Teva, and Roche; research support from GlaxoSmithKline, AstraZeneca, and Novartis; and lecture fees from Roche, AstraZeneca, and Novartis. NK has received funding from GSK for a clinical trial. Rest of the contributing authors do not have any competing interests to declare for this work.

Ethics approval

Ethics for the Mepolizumab trial in which the reported subject received active drug was approved from the local Hospital Research Ethics Board (HiREB), St. Joseph's Hospital, Hamilton, ON [REB Number: RP#12-3748]. The molecular experiments investigating autoimmune responses were approved by the same committee (HIREB Project #422).

Funding

No additional funding was obtained. The manuscript was completed as a component of routine clinical and related academic research work.

References

1. FDA approves Nucala to treat severe asthma. US Food and Drug Administration: US Department of Health and Human Services; 2015. http://www.fda.gov/NewsEvents/Newsroom/PressAnnouncements/ucm471031.htm. Accessed 10 Sept 2016.
2. Bel E, Wenzel S, Thompson P, Prazma C, Keene O, Yancey S, et al. Oral glucocorticoid-sparing effect of Mepolizumab in eosinophilic asthma. N Engl J Med. 2014;371:1189–97.
3. Nair P, Pizzichini M, Kjarsgaard M. Mepolizumab for prednisone-dependent asthma with sputum eosinophilia. N Engl J Med. 2009;360:985–93.
4. Finkelman FD, Madden KB, Morris SC, Holmes JM, Boiani N, Katona IM, et al. Anti-cytokine antibodies as carrier proteins. Prolongation of in vivo effects of exogenous cytokines by injection of cytokine-anti-cytokine antibody complexes. J Immunol. 1993;151:1235–44.
5. Smith SG, Chen R, Kjarsgaard M, Huang C, Oliveria JP, O'Byrne PM, et al. Increased numbers of activated group 2 innate lymphoid cells in the airways of patients with severe asthma and persistent airway eosinophilia. J Allergy Clin Immunol. 2016;137(1):75–86.e8.
6. Wilson MS, Pesce JT, Ramalingam TR, Thompson RW, Cheever A, Wynn TA. Suppression of murine allergic airway disease by IL-2: anti-IL-2 monoclonal antibody-induced regulatory t cells. J Immunol. 2008;181:6942–54.
7. Sato TA, Widmer MB, Finkelman FD, Madani H, Jacobs CA, Grabstein KH, et al. Recombinant soluble murine IL-4 receptor can inhibit or enhance IgE responses in vivo. J Immunol. 1993;150:2717–23.
8. Martens E, Dillen C, Heremans H, Damme JV, Billiau A. Increased circulating interleukin-6 (IL-6) activity in endotoxin-challenged mice pretreated with anti-IL-6 antibody is due to IL-6 accumulated in antigen-antibody complexes. Eur J Immunol. 1993;23:2026–9.
9. Martin CE, van Leeuwen EMM, Im SJ, Roopenian DC, Sung Y-C, Surh CD. IL-7/anti-IL-7 mAb complexes augment cytokine potency in mice through association with IgG-Fc and by competition with IL-7R. Blood. 2013;121:4484–92.
10. Van Gool F, Molofsky AB, Morar MM, Rosenzwajg M, Liang H-E, Klatzmann D, et al. Interleukin-5-producing group 2 innate lymphoid cells control eosinophilia induced by interleukin-2 therapy. Blood. 2014;124:3572–6.
11. Tjota MY, Williams JW, Lu T, Clay BS, Byrd T, Hrusch CL, et al. IL-33-dependent induction of allergic lung inflammation by FcγRIII signaling. J Clin Investig. 2013;123:2287–97.
12. Tran GT, Hodgkinson SJ, Carter NM, Verma ND, Plain KM, Boyd R, et al. IL-5 promotes induction of antigen-specific CD4+ CD25+ T regulatory cells that suppress autoimmunity. Blood. 2012;119:4441–50.
13. Mukherjee M, Bulir D, Radford K, Helpard B, Kjarsgaard M, Jacobsen EA, et al. Pathogenic autoantibodies in patients with severe asthma and sputum eosinophils. J Allergy Clin Immunol. 2016;137:AB409.
14. Kasjanski R, Kato A, Poposki JA, Bochner BS, Cao Y, Norton JE, et al. Group 2 innate lymphoid cells directly induce b cell activation in humans. J Allergy Clin Immunol. 2016;137:AB1.
15. Weiler CR, Kita H, Hukee M, Gleich GJ. Eosinophil viability during immunoglobulin-induced degranulation. J Leukoc Biol. 1996;60:493–501.
16. Walford HH, Lund SJ, Baum RE, White AA, Bergeron CM, Husseman J, et al. Increased ILC2s in the eosinophilic nasal polyp endotype are associated with corticosteroid responsiveness. Clin Immunol. 2014;155:126–35.

12

Common allergies in urban adolescents and their relationships with asthma control and healthcare utilization

Hyekyun Rhee[1]*[iD], Tanzy Love[2], Donald Harrington[2] and Annette Grape[1]

Abstract

Background: Urban adolescents suffer a disproportionate burden of asthma morbidity, often in association with allergies. Literature is limited on comparing various types of allergies regarding prevalence and associations with asthma morbidity in urban dwelling adolescents. The purpose of this study was to examine the prevalence of common allergies reported by urban adolescents and to assess their relationships to healthcare utilization and asthma control.

Methods: Study participants included 313 urban adolescents (12–20 years of age) with persistent asthma who were recruited from three states in the United States. Self-report data were collected on nine indoor and outdoor allergies, healthcare utilization, and asthma exacerbation. Logistic regressions and zero-inflated Poisson regressions were conducted to examine the relationships between allergies and asthma morbidity.

Results: The mean age of participants was 14.58 ($\pm$ 1.97) and 52% were female, and 79% were black. Seventy-three percent (n = 229) reported one or more allergies. Dust mite and grass allergies were most common, each reported by 50%. The prevalence of pest allergies (cockroach and mouse) was 27.5% and 19%, respectively. Those with pest allergies were more likely to report ED visits (cockroach- Odds Ratio (OR) = 2.16, 95% CI 1.18–3.94, p = .01; mouse- OR = 2.13, 95% CI 1.09–4.07, p = .02), specialist visits (cockroach-OR = 2.69, 95% CI 1.60–4.54, p < .001; mouse-OR = 2.06, 95% CI 1.15–3.68, p = .01) and asthma exacerbation (cockroach-OR = 2.17, 95% CI 1.26–3.74, p < .001; mouse- OR = 2.30, 95% CI 1.26–4.18, p = .01). Cockroach allergies were associated with 2.2 times as many nights in the hospital (95% CI 1.053–3.398, p = 0.036) and 2.2 times as many specialist visits (95% CI 1.489–3.110, p < 0.001), and mouse allergy was associated with 1.6 times as many ED visits (95% CI 1.092–2.257, p = 0.015) compared to those without pest allergies.

Conclusions: Concomitant occurrence of allergies is ubiquitous among urban adolescents with asthma. Only pest allergies, of those examined, appear to have implications for poorly controlled asthma, exacerbation and acute healthcare utilization. To reduce asthma burden in urban adolescents, identification and management of high-risk adolescents with pest allergen sensitization and exposure are warranted.

Keywords: Urban adolescents, Asthma, Allergies, Cockroach, Mouse, Healthcare utilization

*Correspondence: hyekyun_rhee@urmc.rochester.edu
[1] University of Rochester School of Nursing, 601 Elmwood Ave. Box SON, Rochester, NY 14642, USA
Full list of author information is available at the end of the article

Background

Asthma is a leading chronic pediatric health condition affecting approximately 6.2 million children under age 18 years in the United States (US) [1]. Current asthma is reported in 10% of adolescents (2.5 million) age 12–17 years [1], and the alarming rates of asthma and its increasing morbidity in urban young people are particularly concerning [2–5]. The disproportionate burden of asthma morbidity in urban children has been attributed to their exposure and heightened sensitivity to certain indoor allergens such as cockroaches or mice [2, 6]. Exposure to some indoor and outdoor allergens has been identified as a major culprit in the development and exacerbation of asthma in pediatric patients [7]. Evidence has consistently shown that children with severe asthma tend to report greater allergic burden [8–11]. Similarly, a large epidemiologic study reported a major impact of allergen exposures and sensitivity on symptom severity and acute healthcare utilization in children with asthma [6].

Despite the wealth of literature elucidating the intricate links between inhalant or food allergen sensitization and asthma morbidity in pediatric populations, the majority of evidence is based on either young children or mixed age groups of young children and adolescents. Little is known about common allergies and their relationships with asthma morbidity specifically among adolescents. Furthermore, a number of studies target only specific allergens (e.g., cockroach or mice), yet there is limited literature comparing various types of allergies and their associations with asthma morbidity. Thus, the purpose of this study was to examine the prevalence of a broad spectrum of indoor/outdoor allergies among urban adolescents and to assess their relationships to asthma control and healthcare utilization.

Methods

Settings and sample

Subjects were recruited from US metropolitan cities including Buffalo, New York, Baltimore, Maryland and Memphis, Tennessee. Recruitment strategies included clinician referrals (n = 106), self-referrals responding to school or community outreach (n = 94), study flyers (n = 40), or word of mouth (n = 69). Eligible criteria included (1) age between 12–20; (2) physician-diagnosed asthma that has required healthcare utilization (preventive or acute) within 12 months prior to enrollment; (3) persistent asthma as defined by the National Asthma Education and Prevention Program (NAEPP) guidelines [12]; (4) primary residence located in the participating inner cities based on zip codes or school districts; and (5) ability to understand spoken and written English. Those with other comorbid conditions requiring daily

medication (e.g., diabetes, cancer, arthritis, cystic fibrosis, etc.) reported by parents or guardians were excluded.

Data collection and measurements

The study protocol was reviewed and approved by each Institutional Review Board of the academic institutions in participating cities. Informed consent was obtained from parents and older adolescents ($\geq$ 18 years old), and assent was obtained from adolescents, ages 17 or younger. Data were collected during in-person appointments in the project office, public libraries or in the home. Parents completed a sociodemographic form and forms reporting allergies and current medications. Adolescents ages 18 years or older completed these forms for themselves. Adolescents provided data on asthma control, exacerbation and healthcare utilization.

Allergy information sheet

The form assessed nine specific allergies (cat, dog, mouse, ragweed, tree, grass, cockroach, dust mite, and any food) plus other allergies reported by the subjects. Parents were also asked if their adolescent had ever had allergy tests (either skin or blood) or ever received allergy shots.

Healthcare utilization and asthma exacerbation

Adolescents were asked whether they had, in the previous 3 months, had asthma related asthma/allergy specialty visits, acute office visits, Emergency Department (ED) visits, or hospital admission. If so, they reported the number of visits and the nights in the hospital. Oral steroid use was also assessed; subjects who used oral steroids for at least 3 consecutive days in the past 12 months were categorized as having asthma exacerbation.

Asthma control

Four impairment-based criteria (symptoms, nocturnal awakening, activity limitations and rescue inhaler use in the past 4 weeks) were assessed on a 4-point scale as indicated by the NAEPP guidelines. Based on the criteria, subjects were classified into three categories, well-controlled, not well-controlled, and very poorly controlled. In addition, a total score was computed with higher scores indicating poorer asthma control. We also estimated odds ratios between better or worse control of the teens' asthma. Instead of using the NAEPP's three categories of asthma control which resulted in fewer than 15% of subjects having well-controlled asthma, we used the mean to dichotomize the control total score into less than 7.6 (controlled) vs. 7.6 or greater (uncontrolled).

Data analysis

Healthcare utilization responses were dichotomized into users and non-users of each healthcare service. Logistic regression was fit for each model to predict the probability of utilization and asthma exacerbation with allergy status as a predictor adjusting for subject age and sex. Multiple linear regressions were fit to predict the asthma control (total score) associated with subject allergy status adjusted for age and sex. Estimates of the odds ratio or slope and 95% confidence intervals were calculated along with p-values for the strength of the effect. The Hosmer–Lemeshow goodness-of-fit test was performed to check the predictive power of the logistic regression models. Residual analysis was examined for linear and logistic models to look for outliers, influential points, and over-dispersion. No substantial departures from the assumptions were found in these models.

To examine the counts of each type of healthcare utilization outcome, zero-inflated poisson (ZIP) regression was fit for each outcome to predict both the probability of utilization and the change in amount of utilization from allergy status as a predictor while adjusting for subject age and sex. Estimates of the increase in utilization and 95% confidence intervals were calculated and reported with p-values. Residual analysis was examined for each model to look for outliers, influential points, and unusual patterns. No substantial departures from the assumptions were found in these models. To test for differences in allergy effect between those with a sensitivity test ("tested" group) and those without ("never-test" group), we also fit ZIP regression with interactions between allergens and test status. In these models, we estimated the difference between the subjects reporting an allergy in the tested and never-tested groups.

Results

Sample characteristics

A total of 313 adolescents from Buffalo NY (n = 123), Baltimore MD (n = 100), and Memphis TN (n = 90) participated in the study. Table 1 summarizes the demographic characteristics of the sample. No significant site differences were found on sociodemographic factors except for the number of non-black participants. The Buffalo subsample had a greater number of white adolescents (32%) than Baltimore and Memphis (5 and 1% respectively) ($\chi^2 = 50.3$, p < .0001).

The majority of the sample (74%) reported an asthma diagnosis before the age of 6. According to the NAEPP criteria, uncontrolled asthma was reported by 85.3% (n = 266), of which 42% (n = 112) were very poorly controlled. The majority of the sample (75%) reported being on at least one controller medication. The most common type of controller medication was inhaled corticosteroids (ICS) followed by the combination of ICS and long acting bronchodilator, 52% and 21% respectively. Almost

Table 1 Sociodemographic characteristics of the sample and descriptive statistics of outcome measures (N = 313)

Sex	
Male, n (%)	153 (49)
Female, n (%)	160 (51)
Race	
White, n (%)	45 (14.4)
Nonwhite	
Black or African American, n (%)	246 (78.6)
Multi race, n (%)	19 (6.1)
Others, n (%)	3 (0.9)
Hispanic/latino, n (%)	26 (8.3)
Age, mean (SD)	14.69 (1.96)
12–14, n (%)	149 (47.6)
15–17, n (%)	146 (46.6)
18–20, n (%)	15 (4.8)
Annual household income	
≤ $10,000, n (%)	93 (29.7)
> $10,000 and ≤ $30,000, n (%)	86 (27.5)
> $30,000 and ≤ $70,000, n (%)	80 (25.6)
> $70,000, n (%)	45 (14.4)
Healthcare utilization	
Hospitalization nights, mean (SD), range	0.18 (0.80), 0–7
ED visit, mean (SD), range	0.50 (1.62), 0–20
Acute office visit, mean (SD), range	0.75 (1.38), 0–10
Specialist visit, mean (SD), range	0.67 (1.59), 0–12
Asthma exacerbation, n (%)	83 (26)
Asthma control score, mean (SD), range	7.6 (2.8), 4–16

all participants (97%) reported having a short-acting bronchodilator.

Prevalence of self-reported allergies

Dust mites and grasses were the most commonly reported allergies, followed by trees and ragweed (see Fig. 1). Thirty-percent reported some type of food-related allergies. Peanut was the most common food allergen (16%) followed by seafood (10%). At least one type of allergy (maximum of 12 allergies) was reported by 73% (n = 229), of which 87% (n = 200) reported two or more allergies. The average number of allergies per subject was 3.36 (range 0–12). No site or gender differences were found in the types of allergies, except for mice for which Baltimore had significantly higher prevalence than Buffalo or Memphis, 33% vs. 13% or 12%, respectively ($\chi^2 = 12.5$, p < .001). Despite the extensiveness of self-reported allergies, only 60% had reported having been tested for inhalant and food allergen sensitization, and 15% (n = 46) had ever received immunotherapy (i.e., allergy shots). Figure 1 also shows the prevalence of each of the allergies only in the subsample of adolescents who

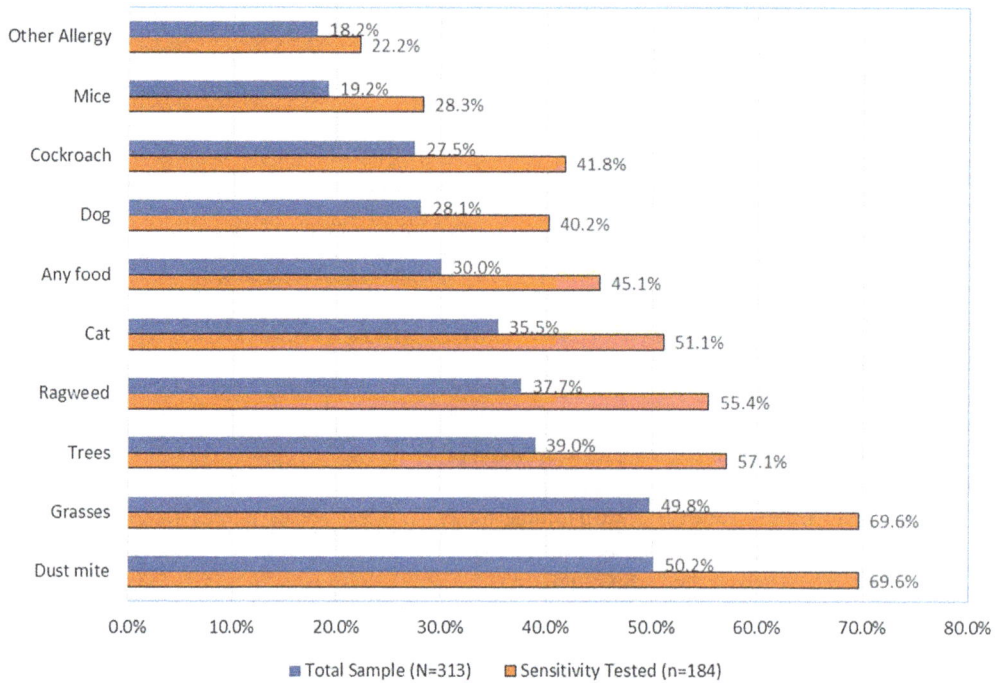

Fig. 1 Self-reported common allergies in inner-city adolescents

had ever been tested for sensitivity. Overall, the prevalence of each allergy within the subsample (n = 184) is substantially higher than that of the total sample. Sensitivity to dust mites or grasses was most common, reported by nearly 70% of tested adolescents.

Allergies predicting healthcare utilization, exacerbation and asthma control

No significant age differences were found on healthcare utilization although older adolescents reported better controlled asthma (0.18 points average lower score per year of age, p = 0.023). Females were more likely to report ED visits (OR = 1.82, p = 0.044), but not significantly different than males in using other healthcare services. Because of the sex and age differences in these outcome measures, these two demographic variables were included in the subsequent prediction models as covariates. Also, cat and dog allergies were grouped into "pets", and trees, ragweed and grasses into "plants" for subsequent prediction models.

Healthcare utilization was significantly predicted by self-report allergies related to cockroaches, mice, dust mites and plants (Fig. 2) after adjusting for age and sex. Both cockroach and mouse allergies were associated with an increase in the probability of ED visits, specialist visits, and asthma exacerbation. Those with cockroach allergy were two times more likely to visit an ED

or experience exacerbation, and 2.7 times more likely to use an asthma specialist than those without the allergy. Similarly, the odds of ED visits, specialist visits or exacerbation among those with mouse allergy was 2 to 2.3 times higher than those without the allergy. Dust mite and plant allergies were each separately associated with increased odds of specialist visits by 2.5 times compared to counterparts without these allergies. Pet or food allergies did not predict healthcare utilization, asthma exacerbation or asthma control. Asthma control was predicted by only pest allergies. Based on linear regression models, the control score for subjects with cockroach and mouse allergies were 1.02 (95% CI 0.34–1.70, p = .003) and 0.95 (95% CI 0.18–1.73, p = .017) points higher on average, respectively, indicating poorer asthma control compared to those without such allergies. Figure 2 shows that those with cockroach or mouse allergies are two times more likely to have the total score indicating uncontrolled asthma. Total number of allergies also predicted specialist visits and exacerbation. Each additional number of allergy increased the probability of specialist visits (OR = 1.1, p = 0.001) and asthma exacerbation (OR = 1.1, p = 0.003).

The average count of each of healthcare utilization for adolescents with and without each of the allergies examined is shown in Fig. 3. The asterisks on each case indicate significant group differences in the number of visits between the groups, after adjusting for age and sex. The

Common allergies in urban adolescents and their relationships with asthma control and healthcare...

97

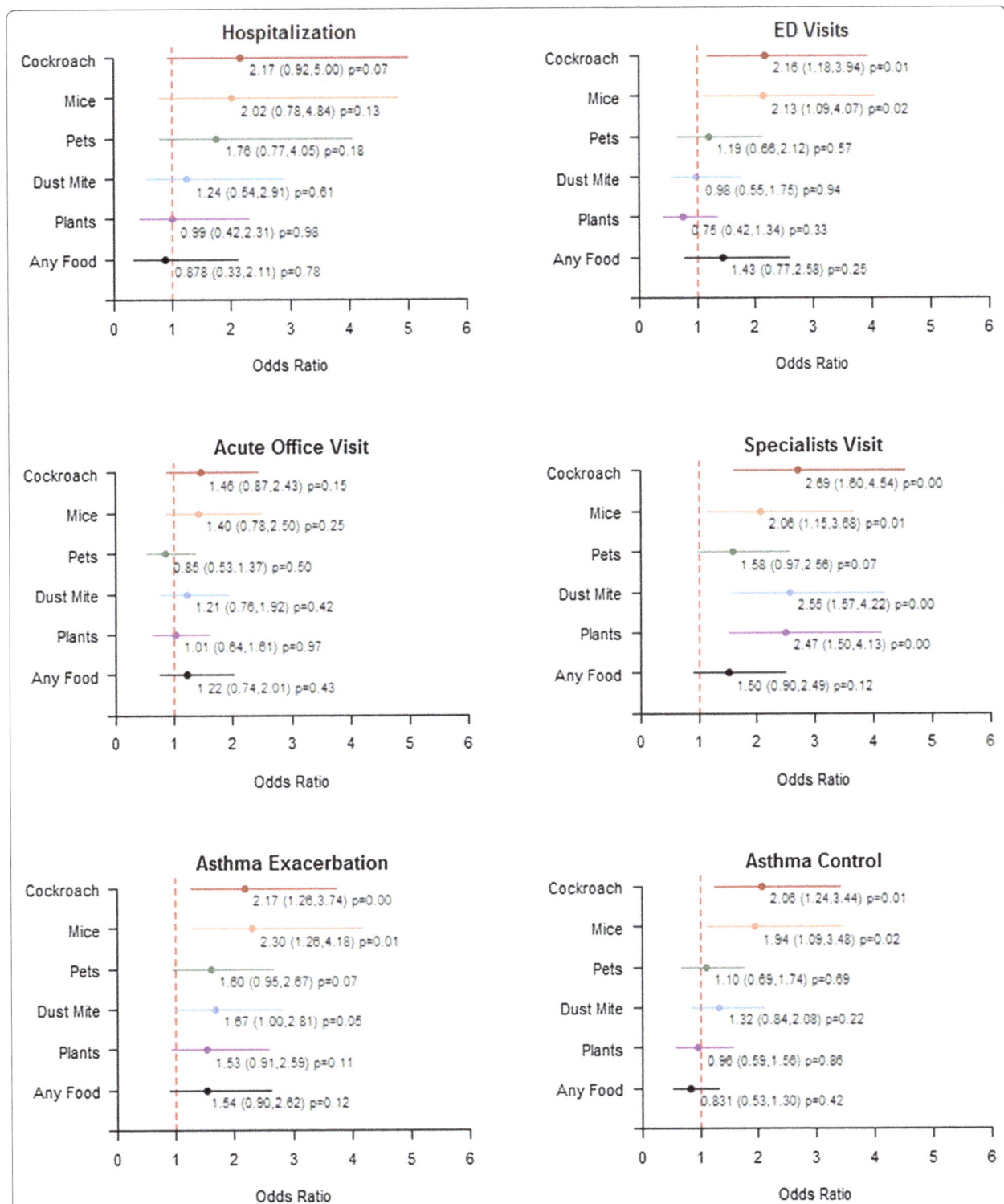

Fig. 2 Healthcare utilization, exacerbation, and uncontrolled asthma associated with each type of allergy. Odds ratio (95% CIs) for dichotomous outcome measures after adjusting for age and sex. Odds ratios greater than 1 indicate an increased chance of healthcare utilization, exacerbation, or uncontrolled asthma control predicted by each allergy

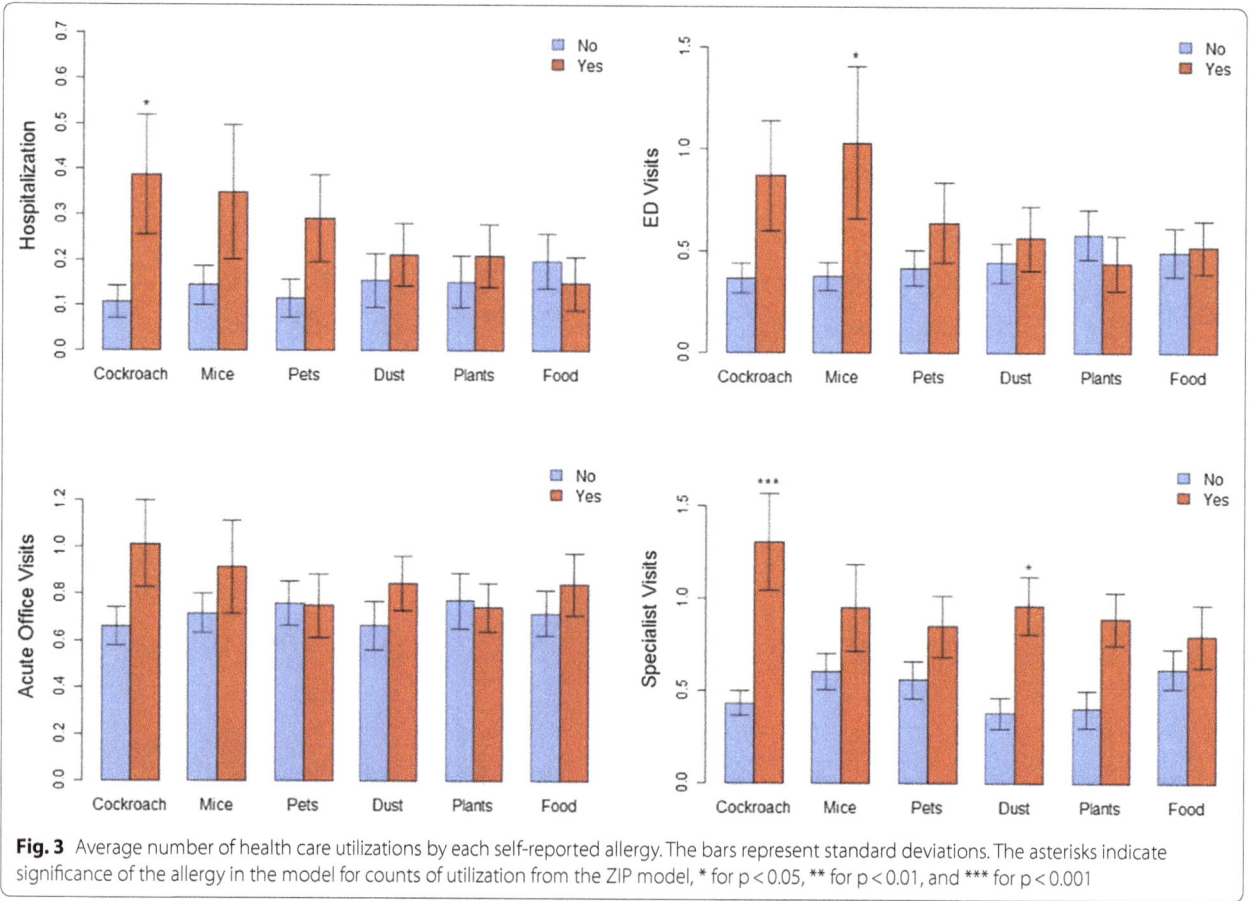

Fig. 3 Average number of health care utilizations by each self-reported allergy. The bars represent standard deviations. The asterisks indicate significance of the allergy in the model for counts of utilization from the ZIP model, * for p < 0.05, ** for p < 0.01, and *** for p < 0.001

Table 2 Models for the healthcare utilization multiplier predicted by each allergy after adjusting for age and sex (N = 313)

Types of allergies	Hospitalization exp (b)[a] (95% CI)	ED visits exp (b)[a] (95% CI)	Acute office visits exp (b)[a] (95% CI)	Specialist visits exp (b)[a] (95% CI)
Cockroach	2.151 (1.053, 3.398) p = 0.0357	1.368 (0.955, 1.960) p = 0.087	1.395 (0.990, 1.964) p = 0.057	2.152 (1.489, 3.110) p < 0.001
Mice	1.079 (0.536, 2.174) p = 0.832	1.570 (1.092, 2.257) p = 0.0148	1.076 (0.725, 1.596) p = 0.716	1.029 (0.698, 1.518) p = 0.885
Pets	1.723 (0.805, 3.689) p = 0.161	1.233 (0.852, 1.783) p = 0.267	1.146 (0.811, 1.619) p = 0.441	1.178 (0.837, 1.658) p = 0.348
Dust mite	1.017 (0.532, 1.945) p = 0.959	1.149 (0.785, 1.682) p = 0.474	1.216 (0.856, 1.727) p = 0.275	1.543 (1.021, 2.333) p = 0.040
Plants	1.687 (0.839, 3.391) p = 0.142	0.876 (0.605, 1.270) p = 0.486	0.976 (0.692, 1.376) p = 0.889	1.210 (0.803, 1.822) p = 0.362
Any food	0.689 (0.307, 1.548) p = 0.363	0.681 (0.455, 1.020) p = 0.063	1.052 (0.735, 1.506) p = 0.782	0.928 (0.647, 1.333) p = 0.687
Number of Allergies	1.031 (0.949, 1.121) p = 0.467	0.984 (0.937, 1.033) p = 0.517	1.066 (1.014, 1.120) p = 0.0124	1.090 (1.036, 1.147) p = 0.001

[a] Multiplicative regression coefficients from the zero-inflated Poisson regression: values greater than 1 indicate an increased number of healthcare utilizations predicted for teens with the allergy while values less than 1 indicate a prediction of lower healthcare utilization with the allergy

change in the number of instances of healthcare utilization predicted by each allergy status was examined in the ZIP models reported in Table 2. Cockroach allergies were associated with 2.2 times as many nights in the hospital (p = 0.036) and 2.2 times as many specialist visits (p < 0.001). Mouse and dust mite allergies were associated

Table 3 Models for the healthcare utilization multiplier predicted by each sensitivity after adjusting for age and sex only for the subsample with a prior sensitivity test (n = 184)

Types of allergies	Hospitalization exp (b)[a] (95% CI)	ED visits exp (b)[a] (95% CI)	Acute office visits exp (b)[a] (95% CI)	Specialist visits exp (b)[a] (95% CI)
Cockroach	1.422 (0.322, 6.285) p = 0.642	0.942 (0.517, 1.716) p = 0.845	1.155 (0.746, 1.789) p = 0.518	2.292 (1.465, 3.585) p < 0.001
Mice	0.470 (0.162, 1.368) p = 0.166	1.036 (0.581, 1.848) p = 0.904	0.730 (0.439, 1.212) p = 0.223	0.798 (0.506, 1.258) p = 0.331
Pets	0.807 (0.167, 3.899) p = 0.789	1.037 (0.584, 1.841) p = 0.902	1.064 (0.672, 1.686) p = 0.792	1.001 (0.673, 1.489) p = 0.996
Dust mite	0.220 (0.032, 1.533) p = 0.126	1.283 (0.587, 2.804) p = 0.532	1.562 (0.853, 2.863) p = 0.149	1.507 (0.885, 2.568) p = 0.131
Plants	1.464 (0.327, 6.552) p = 0.619	0.700 (0.384, 1.277) p = 0.245	0.895 (0.541, 1.481) p = 0.667	1.236 (0.714, 2.139) p = 0.449
Any food	0.912 (0.298, 2.791) p = 0.871	0.785 (0.440, 1.402) p = 0.413	1.142 (0.716, 1.819) p = 0.578	1.037 (0.696, 1.545) p = 0.857
Number of allergies	1.020 (0.868, 1.198) p = 0.811	0.955 (0.883, 1.033) p = 0.247	1.095 (1.019, 1.178) p = 0.014	1.092 (1.028, 1.159) p = 0.004

[a] Multiplicative regression coefficients from the zero-inflated Poisson regression: values greater than 1 indicate an increased number of healthcare utilizations predicted for teens with the sensitivity while values less than 1 indicate a prediction of lower healthcare utilization with that sensitivity

with 1.6 times as many ED visits (p = 0.015) and 1.5 times as many specialist visits (p = 0.040), respectively. Total number of allergies also predicted the instances of specialist visits and acute office visits. Each additional allergy was associated with both 1.1 times as many acute office visits (p = 0.012) and specialist visits (p = 0.001).

Sensitivity test status was reported by 309 subjects; 184 have had a sensitivity test ("tested" group) and 125 have not ("never-tested" group). Almost all of the subjects reporting an allergy had been given a sensitivity test (for instance, of 155 teens reporting a dust mite allergy, 128 (82.5%) were in the tested group), making the inference in Table 2 nearly exclusively about the subjects with sensitivity testing. Nonetheless, for each of those models, we checked for differences in the allergy effect on healthcare utilization, depending on their sensitivity test status. In doing so, we used a regression model adding an interaction term between test status (tested vs. untested) and allergy report (yes vs. no) after removing an outlier with 20 recent ED visits. None of the odds of healthcare utilization changed significantly depending on sensitivity test status, but the estimated count of visits was significantly different for five models. For four significant comparisons, the estimated increase in acute office visits and specialist visits was even more pronounced for the "tested" group than the "never-tested" group: expected acute office visits increased for the subjects with dust mite allergy within the "tested" group (337%, p < 0.001), and expected specialist visits also substantially elevated for the subjects with cockroach, mouse, or pet allergy within the "tested" group (376% p = 0.014, 428% p = 0.049, and 1000% p < 0.001, respectively) compared to the "never-tested" group. Only one comparison contradicted the increased healthcare utilization for the subjects with an allergy: among those reporting mouse allergy, there was a 2/3 reduction in the expected number of ED visits for the "tested" group (p = 0.024) compared to the "never-tested" group.

Subsequently, we repeated the ZIP models for each of allergies with only the "tested" group (n = 184) (Table 3). Overall, the effect sizes of sensitivities predicting each type of healthcare utilization were similar to those in the ZIP models with the entire sample (see Table 2) with only two exceptions including cockroach sensitivity predicting hospitalization and mouse sensitivity predicting ED visits for which effect sizes became smaller and statistically nonsignificant. The number of specialist visits remained significantly higher with each additional sensitivity and for those with cockroach sensitivity. Particularly, the number of specialist visits was 50.7% higher in those with dust mite sensitivity, and this effect was significant even after the "never-tested" group (n = 125) were added as shown in Table 2.

Discussion

This study demonstrates the ubiquitous prevalence of a wide range of self-reported allergies among urban adolescents with asthma, and their associations with asthma morbidity. Dust mites were identified as the most common allergen, reported by more than a half of this population, and the prevalence was strikingly higher, nearly 70%, among adolescents who had been tested for sensitivity. The rate of dust mite allergy in our study is substantially greater than the 35% reported in a previous large study of inner-city children [6]. The difference might be due in part to differences in data sources between our finding and the earlier report, self-report vs. skin testing, respectively. In our study, the self-reported allergy information was based on prior sensitivity testing as well as their experience of allergic reaction to dust mites, thus resulting in a higher rate. Nonetheless, given that the high proportion of adolescents (> 82%) reporting dust mite allergy had been tested for sensitivity, our estimate of mite allergy may closely align with that of sensitivity testing.

We found that allergies to cockroaches and mice were linked to poor asthma control and more frequent ED visits, hospitalization, or specialist visits. Similarly, Busse et al. [6] identified cockroach allergen as a dominant and sole factor of other allergens linked to greater asthma morbidity and urgent healthcare use in young inner-city children. In their study, sensitivity to cockroaches was found in about 37% of the inner-city children; that is slightly higher than our 31% based on self-report. In many urban dwellings, cockroach and mouse infestation is widespread [2, 6, 13], which is often linked to suboptimal living conditions with compromised structural integrity (e.g., cracks and holes in the wall, water leaks) of the house [14, 15]. Cockroach allergens were detected in over 85% of inner-city houses [2], and even when there was no apparent exposure to cockroaches at home, children can become sensitized to the pest from exposures at other places. African American children, 6–16 years of age, are 2.5 times more likely to have cockroach sensitivity than their white counterparts [16]. This alarming rate underscores the importance of a pest-reduction intervention targeting the broader urban community instead of individual houses. Regional differences in the rates of mouse allergy in our study could be due in part to differences in the types of housing. Compared to other sites, Baltimore's predominant use of multifamily dwellings with shared walls and/or floors/ceilings may provide an ideal environment for the widespread infestation of cockroaches and mice.

The prevalence of self-reported food allergies in our adolescent sample was 30%, a rate slightly higher than that of a previous report in younger children with asthma, 24% [10]. However, our food allergy rate is considerably higher than the prevalence of self-reported food sensitization, 17%, in the general population based on a large U.S. national survey [11]. Similar to the previous reports [11], we found peanut to be the most common food allergen in adolescents with asthma. This is the first study documenting the extent of peanut allergy in adolescents with asthma. In contrast to the previous study [11], in which food allergy was associated with the increased risk of ED visits and asthma exacerbations, we found no significant associations between food allergy and urgent healthcare utilization or exacerbation. This discrepancy may have been in part due to the differences in the sample in the two studies. While the earlier report was based on the general population of all ages, our sample is limited only to urban adolescents. Another reason might have to do with asthma severity. Liu et al. study [11] included those of a wide range of severity, and revealed that food allergy became more prevalent in those with higher levels of asthma severity, thus resulting in ED visits more often. In contrast, all of our participants had persistent asthma and over 85% had not-well controlled or very poorly controlled asthma based the NAEPP classification. The lack of variability due to the relative homogeneity regarding disease severity might have prevented us from detecting any differences in healthcare utilization associated with food allergy. Also, without assessment of specific serum IgE levels, our study is unable to quantify the varying degrees of food sensitivity. If only severe food allergy is linked to asthma morbidity, possible mild cases of food allergy in many of our sample might have contributed to non-significant relationships between the allergy and asthma morbidity in this study.

Plant-based allergies (grasses, trees, and ragweed) were highly prevalent in our urban adolescent sample. Consistent with other studies [17, 18], we found no associations between plant allergies and asthma morbidity, except that those with a plant-based allergy were more likely to receive specialist care for asthma. Pet allergies were also common: however, unlike a previous study demonstrating positive associations between pet allergies and asthma severity [19], we found no relationships between pet allergies and asthma morbidity.

It is noteworthy that the magnitude and directions of associations between certain allergies and healthcare utilization differed by sensitivity testing status. We demonstrated that dust mite allergy was associated with substantially increased urgent office visits due to asthma among the tested group compared to their untested counterparts. Likewise, the positive associations between pest allergies and specialist visits appeared more pronounced among the tested group than their untested counterparts. These findings may simply reflect common clinical practice that sensitivity testing is more often indicated when a patient is presented with severe or uncontrolled asthma necessitating frequent acute office visits or specialist care. When we considered only the subgroup with prior sensitivity testing, however, the relationships between those pest allergies and acute healthcare utilization (ED and hospital admission) became weak and non-significant. This may have been due in part to diminished power (sample size) or the possibility that the pest allergies reported by those never tested for sensitivity could be more strongly linked to the acute healthcare utilization than the tested adolescents. The latter speculation is somewhat supported by our finding that the association between mouse allergy and ED visits was negative among those who were tested, indicating fewer ED visits associated with mouse allergy by the tested subjects than those untested. This seemingly counterintuitive finding might have been reflecting the influence of intervening effects, such as treatments (e.g., immunotherapy) or modifications of the home environment to eliminate the pest that were offered to those who tested positive to mouse allergen, resulting in fewer acute asthma episodes requiring emergency care. On the other hand, the untested patients with mouse allergy were left untreated, continuing to suffer greater morbidity represented by more frequent ED visits. Such implication underscores the importance of conducting sensitivity testing for asthma patients reporting pest allergies or living in pest-infested areas to adequately address the issue and ultimately improve asthma outcomes. Future research is warranted to investigate the implications of sensitivity testing for treatment choices and its impact on asthma outcomes in urban adolescents.

This study has several limitations that warrant caution. First, this study relies on self-report data rather than sensitivity testing. Therefore, we cannot rule out the possibility of reporting bias in our prevalence estimation, particularly for about 40% of participants who had never been tested for sensitivity. Those untested adolescents might not be aware of their sensitivity status unless they had prior allergic reactions to certain inhalants or foods, resulting in underreporting allergies. Second, because of the absence of information about specific IgE levels, we were unable to assess how varying degrees of allergic sensitivity play a role in the relationships between certain allergies and asthma morbidity. Third, although this study is based on a relatively large number of urban adolescents representing three discrete regions in the U.S., the sample is by no means representative of urban adolescents in other parts of the country. Moreover, selection bias toward those with higher asthma severity may have occurred as a large proportion (34%) of the sample were referred by clinicians. Future research using a representative sample of urban adolescents is needed to minimize the selection bias. Finally, this study was based on cross-sectional survey data, which limits our ability to making inference about causal links between allergies of various types and asthma morbidity.

Despite the identified limitations, this study offers important insight into the relative prevalence of self-reported allergies of various types in urban adolescents with asthma and the relationships between each type of allergy and asthma morbidity. In general, allergies appear to increase the likelihood of asthma-related healthcare utilization in urban adolescents. Particularly, pest allergies are linked to uncontrolled asthma and exacerbation as well as frequent use of acute healthcare services. Our findings underscore the importance of identifying and eliminating cockroaches and mice that have particular implications for asthma morbidity. Interventions aimed at reducing the level of indoor allergens have been found effective in improving asthma outcomes [20]. Environmental interventions focusing on reduction of cockroaches have resulted in a decrease in the level of the

allergens and improved asthma symptoms in urban residents [21, 22]. However, extermination alone may have only minimal or fleeting effects on asthma morbidity unless it is accompanied by patient education and behavior modification that can augment and sustain the effects of environmental interventions. Behavior changes in parents/adolescents to control the pests and to increase treatment adherence in combination with environmental interventions would provide the best chance to achieve enduring optimum asthma control and contain healthcare costs [2].

Conclusion

This study complements the literature by examining a wide range of self-reported allergies simultaneously, which offered the opportunity not only to compare the prevalence of common allergies but also to assess relative implications of each allergy for asthma burden in urban adolescents. Our findings suggest that not all allergies equally predict increased asthma morbidity. For instance, although dust mite or plant allergies are highly prevalent, their implications for adverse asthma outcomes appear minimal. On the other hand, pest allergies involving cockroaches and mice are consistently linked to greater asthma morbidity. To ameliorate the burden of asthma in urban adolescents effectively, addressing widespread allergies is needed through sustainable interventions modifying urban environments along with increasing patient awareness about allergens and their impact on asthma outcomes. Furthermore, our findings call for clinicians' careful assessment of allergy status in urban adolescents with asthma, and proactive management of known or potential allergies to prevent and minimize adverse outcomes of asthma.

Abbreviations
NAEPP: National Asthma Education and Prevention Program; ED: Emergency Department; OR: odds ratio.

Authors' contributions
HR as the principal investigator of the study made substantial contributions to conception and design of the study as well as acquisition, analysis and interpretation of data. HR played a leading role in developing and writing the manuscript. TL made substantial contributions to data analysis and interpretation and drafting the analysis and results sections. DH was involved in data analysis and drafting the result section. AG contributed to data management and drafting and critically reviewing the manuscript for important intellectual content. All authors read and approved the final manuscript.

Author details
[1] University of Rochester School of Nursing, 601 Elmwood Ave. Box SON, Rochester, NY 14642, USA. [2] Department of Biostatistics and Computational Biology, University of Rochester Medical Center, 601 Elmwood Ave., Box 630, Rochester, NY 14642, USA.

Acknowledgements
Not applicable.

Competing interests

The authors declare that they have no competing interests.

Funding

This study was supported by the National Institute of Health/ National Institute for Nursing Research (NIH/NINR R01NR014451) for the implementation of the study protocol including data collection, analysis and interpretation.

References

1. Center for Disease Control and Prevention. Most recent asthma data. http://www.cdc.gov/asthma/most_recent_data.htm. Accessed 10 June 2017.
2. Milligan KL, Matsui E, Sharma H. Asthma in Urban children: epidemiology, environmental risk factors, and the public health domain. Curr Allergy Asthma Rep. 2016;16(4):33.
3. Akinbami LJ, Moorman JE, Liu X. Asthma prevalence, health care use, and mortality: United States, 2005–2009. Natl Health Stat Rep. 2011;32:1–16.
4. Akinbami LJ, Moorman JE, Garbe PL, Sondik EJ. Status of childhood asthma in the United States, 1980–2007. Pediatrics. 2009;123(Supplement 3):S131–45.
5. Akinbami LJ, Moorman JE, Simon AE, Schoendorf KC. Trends in racial disparities for asthma outcomes among children 0–17 years, 2001–2010. J Allergy Clin Immunol. 2014;134(3):547–53. https://doi.org/10.1016/j.jaci.2014.05.037.
6. Busse WW, Mitchell H. Addressing issues of asthma in inner-city children. J Allergy Clin Immunol. 2007;119(1):43–9.
7. Etzel RA. How environmental exposures influence the development and exacerbation of asthma. Pediatrics. 2003;112(1):S233.
8. Genuneit J, Seibold AM, Apfelbacher CJ, et al. Overview of systematic reviews in allergy epidemiology. Allergy. 2017. https://doi.org/10.1111/all.13123.
9. Hill DA, Grundmeier RW, Ram G, Spergel JM. The epidemiologic characteristics of healthcare provider-diagnosed eczema, asthma, allergic rhinitis, and food allergy in children: a retrospective cohort study. BMC Pediatr. 2016. https://doi.org/10.1186/s12887-016-0673-z.
10. Friedlander JL, Sheehan WJ, Baxi SN, et al. Food allergy and increased asthma morbidity in a School-based inner-city asthma study. J Allergy Clin Immunol Pract. 2013;1(5):479–84.
11. Liu AH, Jaramillo R, Sicherer SH, et al. National prevalence and risk factors for food allergy and relationship to asthma: results from the National Health and Nutrition Examination Survey 2005–2006. J Allergy Clin Immunol. 2010;126(4):798–806.
12. National Heart, Lung, and Blood Institute. Expert panel report 3: Guidelines for the diagnosis and management of asthma. 2007.
13. Camacho-Rivera M, Kawachi I, Bennett GG, Subramanian SV. Associations of neighborhood concentrated poverty, neighborhood racial/ethnic composition, and indoor allergen exposures: a cross-sectional analysis of los angeles households, 2006-2008. J Urban Health. 2014;91(4):661–76.
14. Gergen PJ, Togias A. Inner city asthma. Immunol Allergy Clin North Am. 2015;35(1):101–14.
15. Wilson J, Dixon SL, Breysse P, et al. Housing and allergens: a pooled analysis of nine US studies. Environ Res. 2010;110(2):189–98.
16. Stevenson LA, Gergen PJ, Hoover DR, Rosenstreich D, Mannino DM, Matte TD. Sociodemographic correlates of indoor allergen sensitivity among United States children. J Allergy Clin Immunol. 2001;108(5):747–52.
17. Marchetti P, Pesce G, Villani S, et al. Pollen concentrations and prevalence of asthma and allergic rhinitis in Italy: evidence from the GEIRD study. Sci Total Environ. 2017;584:1093–9.
18. Palao-Ocharan P, Dominguez-Ortega J, Barranco P, Diaz-Almiron M, Quirce S. Does the profile of sensitization to grass pollen allergens have clinical relevance? J Investig Allergol Clin Immunol. 2016;26(3):188–9.
19. Gent JF, Belanger K, Triche EW, Bracken MB, Beckett WS, Leaderer BP. Association of pediatric asthma severity with exposure to common household dust allergens. Environ Res. 2009;109(6):768–74.
20. Crocker DD, Kinyota S, Dumitru GG, et al. Effectiveness of home-based, multi-trigger, multicomponent interventions with an environmental focus for reducing asthma morbidity: a community guide systematic review. Am J Prev Med. 2011. https://doi.org/10.1016/j.amepr e.2011.05.012.
21. Morgan WJ, Crain EF, Gruchalla RS, et al. Results of a home-based environmental intervention among urban children with asthma. N Engl J Med. 2004;351(11):1068–80.
22. Gergen PJ, Mortimer KM, Eggleston PA, et al. Results of the national cooperative inner-city asthma study (NCICAS) environmental intervention to reduce cockroach allergen exposure in inner-city homes. J Allergy Clin Immunol. 1999;103:501–6.

13

Expression of intelectin-1 in bronchial epithelial cells of asthma is correlated with T-helper 2 (Type-2) related parameters and its function

Taiji Watanabe[1], Kazuyuki Chibana[1*], Taichi Shiobara[1], Rinna Tei[1], Ryosuke Koike[1], Yusuke Nakamura[1], Ryo Arai[1], Yukiko Horigane[1], Yasuo Shimizu[1], Akihiro Takemasa[1], Takeshi Fukuda[2], Sally E. Wenzel[3] and Yoshiki Ishii[1]

Abstract

Background: Intelectin-1 (ITLN-1) is secreted by intestinal goblet cells and detectable in blood. Its expression is increased in IL-13-overexpressing mouse airways. However, its expression and function in human airways is poorly understood.

Methods: Distal and proximal bronchial epithelial cells (BECs) were isolated from bronchoscopic brushings of disease control (D-CON), COPD, inhaled corticosteroid-treated asthma (ST-Asthma) and inhaled corticosteroid-naïve asthma (SN-Asthma) patients. *ITLN-1* mRNA expression in freshly isolated BECs, primary cultured BECs with or without IL-13 and inhibition effects of mometasone furoate (MF) were investigated by quantitative real-time PCR (qPCR). Correlations between *ITLN-1* mRNA and Type-2 related parameters (e.g. FeNO, IgE, *iNOS, CCL26, periostin* and *DPP4* mRNA) were analyzed. ITLN-1 protein distribution in asthmatic airway tissue was assessed by immunohistochemistry. Bronchial alveolar lavage (BAL) and serum ITLN-1 protein were measured by ELISA. The effect of recombinant human (rh) ITLN-1 on stimulated production of CXCL10 and phospho(p)-STAT1 expression examined in lung fibroblasts.

Results: *ITLN-1* mRNA was expressed in freshly isolated BECs and was correlated with Type-2 related parameters. ITLN-1 protein was increased in goblet cells in SN-Asthmatics and increased in SN-Asthmatic BAL fluid. There were no any differences in serum ITLN-1 concentration between ST and SN-Asthma. IL-13 enhanced ITLN-1 expression and inhibited by MF from BECs in vitro, while rhITLN-1 inhibited CXCL10 production and p-STAT1 expression in HFL-1 cells.

Conclusion: ITLN-1 is induced by IL-13 and expressed mainly in goblet cells in untreated asthma where its levels correlate with known Type-2 related parameters. Further, ITLN-1 inhibits Type-1 chemokine expression.

Keywords: Intelectin-1, Bronchial asthma, Bronchial epithelial cells, IL-13, Type-2 related parameters

Background

Asthma affects nearly 300 million people worldwide but is a heterogeneous disorder comprised of different inflammatory characteristics. Type-2 cytokines (specifically, interleukin (IL)-4, IL-5, and IL-13) are known to play a substantial pathobiological role in many cases.

These cytokines, including IL-13 contribute to a Type-2-high molecular asthma phenotype in about 50% of patients with asthma, and are widely believed to play important roles in asthma pathophysiology [1–7]. Furthermore, IL-13-induced periostin [8] and DPP4 can be measured in peripheral blood and are used as biomarkers to predict the efficacy of anti-IL-13 antibodies in human asthma patients [9–11].

Intelectin-1 (ITLN-1) was cloned in 1998 by Komiya et al. from the murine intestinal tract [12]. Human ITLN-1 is a prophylactic soluble lectin discovered that recognizes

*Correspondence: kchibana@dokkyomed.ac.jp
[1] Department of Pulmonary Medicine and Clinical Immunology, Dokkyo Medical University School of Medicine, Tochigi, Japan
Full list of author information is available at the end of the article

galactofuranose in the bacterial cell wall [13]. The expression of ITLN-1 in the gastrointestinal tract is strongly induced by parasitic infections [14, 15], suggesting that it is associated with prophylaxis in the gastrointestinal tract. ITLN-1 has been primarily studied in the gastrointestinal tract where it is expressed in intestinal goblet cells, primarily from fetal small intestine. It is detected in blood and can be measured intraluminally as well [16]. ITLN-1 is increased in the airways of IL-13-overexpressing mice, where it appears to be a protein component of mucus associated with intense eosinophilic airway inflammation [17, 18]. However, its expression and role in human asthmatic airways is poorly understood. ITLN-1 was also reported as one of the adipocytokine with anti-inflammatory effects [19]. CXCL10 is a chemokine that attracts T-helper (Th)1 cells [20] and strongly induced by IFNγ. When viral infection occurs, viral recognition receptors, such as Toll-like receptor 3 (TLR3) expressed on BECs, are activated to produce inflammatory cytokines and chemokines, including CXCL10 [21]. Autocrine activation of interferon (IFN) receptors further activates Janus kinase-Signal Transducers and Activator of Transcription (JAK-STAT) signaling pathway, promoting an antiviral state. Moreover, fibroblast like cell produce type I IFN and CXCL10 after stimulation with double stranded RNA [22], perhaps contributing to the pathogenesis of viral infections. Little knowledge exists concerning how the fibroblasts respond to ITLN-1 and which signaling pathways might be involved.

We hypothesized that whether ITLN-1 was induced by IL-13 and correlated to type-2 related markers and inhibited Th1 signaling pathway. In this study, we evaluated ITLN-1 mRNA and protein expression in airway cells, tissue and fluid from asthma, COPD, and disease control subjects obtained via bronchoscopy. BAL and serum ITLN-1 levels were also measured. We compared expression of ITLN-1 mRNA with various Type-2 related parameters. Finally, we investigated a possible function of ITLN-1 in the airways.

Methods
Study population
We conducted a retrospective study of 61 patients who visited the Department of Pulmonary Medicine and Clinical Immunology of Dokkyo Medical University

Hospital from June 2009 to March 2014 (Table 1). Bronchial brushings were performed to analyze the expression levels of ITLN-1 mRNA. Transbronchial lung biopsy (TBLB) and endobronchial biopsy (EBB) were performed. All subjects met the American Thoracic Society criteria for asthma and had a pre-bronchodialator FEV1 greater than 80% of predicted with an FEV1/FVC greater than 70%. The ST-Asthma group was regularly treated with inhaled corticosteroids (ICS), while the Steroid Naïve (SN)-Asthma group had symptoms, such as cough with wheezing and night time dyspnea, but had not been treated with ICS or oral corticosteroid (OCS) for at least 6 months. Patients were defined as having COPD if the forced expiratory volume in 1 s (FEV1)/forced vital capacity (FVC) (FEV1/FVC) was <70% with fixed bronchial obstruction after bronchodilator. Disease control subjects (D-CON) were defined as those without asthma/COPD who had undergone bronchoscopy because of abnormal chest X-ray shadows. Lung cancer was found in most of D-CON and COPD patients by bronchoscopy. D-CON (as opposed to healthy control) participants were studied, as research bronchoscopy on healthy individuals is not allowed in Japan. Written informed consent was obtained from all participants to perform the procedure and utilize extra tissue/cells for research purposes. This study was approved by the Ethics Committee of Dokkyo Medical University School of Medicine (hop-m22095).

Bronchoscopy with bronchial epithelial cell brushing
Bronchial brushings were performed with a standard, sterile, single-sheathed nylon cytology brush (Olympus T-260; Olympus, Tokyo, Japan). A total of 4 brushings were performed in the distal and proximal airways. Distal bronchial epithelial cells (BECs) were obtained from airways situated about 1 cm away from the pleura, as identified by X-ray guidance [7]. Proximal BECs were collected by scraping directly from the second carina. TBLB and EBB were available from a small number of participants for ITLN-1 expression by immunohistochemistry. We did not collect bronchial alveolar lavage (BAL) and serum samples at the beginning of this study. Given the results of microarray study [7] that strongly expressed ITLN-1 mRNA in SN-Asthma as well as IL-13 stimulated cells, we decided to accumulate serum and BAL samples

Table 1 Total subjects in this study

	N	Age	M:F	FEV1/FVC (%)	FEV1 (%)	FeNO (ppb)	ICS (µg)	OCS use	Smoker (N:E:C)
D-CON	13	61 ± 5***	11:2	78 ± 2	93 ± 3	27 ± 3	0	0	4:8:1
COPD	17	72 ± 2*	14:3	50 ± 4*	57 ± 6	32 ± 7	0	0	1:7:9
ST-Asthma	13	51 ± 4	10:3	73 ± 5	88 ± 6	45 ± 5	723 ± 86	2	3:8:2
SN-Asthma	18	48 ± 4	13:5	73 ± 3	83 ± 3	129 ± 2*	0	0	6:10:2

*p < 0.0001 vs ST or SN-Asthma, ***p < 0.05 vs other groups

from asthma patients subsequently. Some cases were not able to collect BAL samples because of severe cough or hypoxemia. Finally, total 18 subjects (5 ST-Asthma and 13 SN-Asthma) were able to collect BAL and 16 subjects (6 ST-Asthma and 10 SN-Asthma) serum samples (Tables 2, 3). Table 4 shows 3 subjects who were received bronchoscopy pre and post ICS-treatment.

Quantitative real-time PCR

Expression of *ITLN-1, iNOS, CCL26, periostin* and *DPP4* mRNA in BECs and the expression of *CXCL10* mRNA in HFL-1 cells were following reverse transcription (RT), and then real-time quantitative SYBR Green fluorescent PCR, as described previously [2, 3, 7]. First-strand cDNA was synthesized using the PrimeScript RT reagent Kit (Takara Bio Inc., Shiga, Japan) with both oligo (dT) primers and random hexamers. Reverse transcription was performed with a Takara PCR Thermal Cycler MP (TP3000). The following are the primer sequences used for amplification of *ITLN-1, iNOS, CCL26, periostin, DPP4, CXCL10,* and *GAPDH*: *ITLN-1*: forward primer, TGAGGGTCACCGGATGTAAC, reverse primer, GGACTGGCCTCTGGAAAGTA. *iNOS*: forward primer, GACCAGTACGTTTGGCAATG, reverse primer, TTTCAGCATGAAGAGCGATTT. *CCL26*: forward primer, GCTGCTTCCAATACAGCCACA, reverse primer, TCCTTGGATGGGTACAGACTTTC. *periostin*: forward primer, TGTTGCCCTGGTTATATGAGAA, reverse primer, ACATGGTCAATGGGCAAAAC. *DPP4*: forward primer, GCACGGCAACACATTGAA,

reverse primer, TGAGGTTCTGAAGGCCTAAATC. *CXCL10*: forward primer, GAAAGCAGTTAGCAAGGAAAGGT, reverse primer, GACATATACTCCATGTAGGGAAGTGA. *GAPDH*: forward primer, GCACCGTCAAGGCTGAGAAC, reverse primer, TGGTGAAGACGCCAGTGGA. *B2M*: forward primer, TTCTGGCCTGGAGGCTATC, reverse primer, TCAGGAAATTTGACTTTCCATTC. *RPLP0*: forward primer, TCTACAACCCTGAAGTGCTTGAT, reverse primer, CAATCTGCAGACAGACACTGG.

The 12.5 μL PCR contained 2 μL of cDNA template, 25 μM in 0.5 μL each forward and reverse primers and 6.25 μL of SYBR Premix Ex Taq (Takara). *GAPDH* was evaluated by using the same PCR protocol as for the interest genes-related pathway elements. DNA was amplified for 40 cycles via denaturation for 5 s at 95 °C and annealing for 30 s at 60 °C, using the Takara Thermal Cycler Dice (TP900). PCR assays were performed and analyzed using the Thermal Cycler Dice Real Time System version 4.2 (Takara Bio Inc). The specificity of the reactions was determined by melting curve analysis. The relative expression of each gene of interest and *GAPDH* were calculated using the ΔΔCt method.

Correlations between Type-2 related parameters and ITLN-1 expression

FeNO was measured before bronchoscopy at a flow rate of 50 mL/s using the nitric oxide analyzer (NOA) 280i® (Sievers, CO). Correlations between FeNO, serum IgE (measured in the hospital's clinical lab.) and *ITLN-1*

Table 2 Subjects for analysis of BAL ITLN-1 protein

	N	Age	M:F	FEV1/FVC (%)	%FEV1 (%)	FeNO (ppb)	ICS (μg)
ST-Asthma	5	53 ± 4	4:1	81 ± 3	90 ± 8	53 ± 11	520 ± 120
SN-Asthma	13	51 ± 4	10:3	71 ± 3	82 ± 4	124 ± 23	0

Table 3 Subjects for analysis of serum ILTN-1 protein

	N	Age	M:F	FEV1/FVC (%)	%FEV1 (%)	FeNO (ppb)	ICS (μg)
ST-Asthma	6	53 ± 6	3:3	80 ± 5	96 ± 6	42 ± 31	800 ± 120
SN-Asthma	10	43 ± 5	8:2	77 ± 4	86 ± 5	147 ± 24**	0
Healthy control	8	25 ± 1**	5:3	ND	ND	19 ± 2	0

**p < 0.01 vs other groups

Table 4 Subjects for analysis of ILTN-1 mRNA pre or post ICS treatment

	N (distal: proximal)	Age	M:F	FEV1/FVC (%)	%FEV1 (%)	FeNO (ppb)	ICS (μg)
ST-Asthma (post treatment)	6 (3:3)	65 ± 4	3:0	69 ± 4	84 ± 4	51 ± 4	400
SN-Asthma (pre treatment)	6 (3:3)	65 ± 4	3:0	68 ± 4	89 ± 4	171 ± 49***	0

***p < 0.05 vs ST-Asthma

mRNA expression in distal and proximal BECs from both ST and SN-Asthma subjects were analyzed. We also measured correlations between *ITLN-1* mRNA and *iNOS, CCL26, periostin* and *DPP4* mRNA in distal and proximal BECs from the same subjects.

Immunohistochemistry

Transbronchial lung biopsies (TBLB) and EBB from SN-Asthma, and ST-Asthma subjects were fixed in formalin. Serial 4 μm sections were immunostained using a rabbit polyclonal antibody against ITLN-1 (1:500) (Abcam, MA) with Dako EnVisionTM FLEX Mini Kit High pH detection system including secondary anti-rabbit antibody for detection. Data were collected using an all-in-one fluorescence microscope, BZ-X700 (KEYENCE, Tokyo, Japan).

Quantification of ITLN-1 and CXCL10 protein by ELISA

BAL fluid from 18 asthma subjects, 5 ST-Asthma and 13 SN-Asthma (Table 2) and serum from 6 ST-Asthma, and 10 SN-Asthma subjects (Table 3) was collected. There was a little overlap in three study groups. Cell culture supernatants were performed on ALI cultured BECs and HFL-1 cells. ITLN-1 (Immuno-Biological Laboratories Co., Gunma, Japan) or CXCL10 (R&D Systems, Minneapolis, MN) were measured by commercial sandwich ELISAs. Assay ranges are 0.31–20 ng/mL for ITLN-1 and 7.8–500 pg/mL for CXCL10, respectively.

Culture methods for primary BECs and HFL-1 cells

Freshly isolated BECs were seeded into 60 mm tissue-culture dishes coated with rat-tail type I collagen (BD Discovery Labware, Bedford, MA) in bronchial epithelial growth medium (catalog no. CC-3170, Lonza) in a humidified HEPA-filtered cell culture incubator, supplemented with 5% CO_2. When the BECs reached 80% confluence, cells were passaged and seeded onto collagen-coated polyester 12-well transwell inserts with BEBM/DMEM. When the cell layer reached 100% confluence in the transwells, the culture method was shifted to the air–liquid interface (ALI) condition by removing the apical medium and maintain this condition for 10 days [4, 23]. BECs were stimulated with or without IL-13 (10 ng/mL), purchased from Peprotech (Rocky Hill, NJ) and Mometasone Furoate (MF) at a concentration of 1 μM (Sigma St Louis, MO).

Human fetal lung fibroblasts (HFL-1; lung, diploid, human, passage 3–7) were obtained from the American Type Culture Collection (Manassas, VA). HFL-1 cells were seeded into 24-well tissue culture plates at a density of 4×10^4 cells/well and cultured at 37 °C in a 5% CO_2-humidified incubator in Ham's F12K medium (Sigma, St Louis, MO) containing 10% heat inactivated FBS. Cells were pretreated with recombinant human ITLN-1 (rhITLN-1) (ATGen, Gyeonggi-do, South Korea) at

concentrations up to 500 ng/mL for 30 min and then further stimulated with a combination with TNF, IL-1β, and IFN-γ at 10 ng/mL (PeproTech, Rocky Hill, NJ). Cell-culture supernatants and extracts were harvested 24 h later.

Western blot analysis for phospho-STAT1

Protein samples (10 μg) from HFL-1 were resolved on NuPage Novex 4–12% Bis–Tris gel (Thermo Fisher Scientific, MA) electrophoresis, transferred, and immunoprobed with mouse monoclonal antibody for p-STAT1, total STAT1 (t-STAT1) (1:1000 and 1:500 respectively, Cell Signaling Technologies Inc. MA). Alkaline phosphatase conjugated secondary antibody (Thermo Fisher Scientific) was followed by Chemiluminescent detection (ChemiDoc XRD-J Bio-Rad Laboratories, Inc., CA). Densitometry was performed using the Quantity One (Bio-Rad) and p-STAT1 indexed to t-STAT1.

Statistical analysis

Variables were checked for normality of distribution. As the majority of data were not normally distributed, data were analyzed using nonparametric tests. The Kruskal–Wallis version of the Wilcoxon rank sum test was used to compare overall differences among the groups (the overall p value). When the overall p value was <0.05, intergroup comparisons were done using the Wilcoxon test for multiple comparisons. All other normal distributed data were analyzed using paired t tests compared control and stimulated responses. p values <0.05 were considered significant. Linear regression analysis was used to determine the correlation with Type-2 related parameters and *ITLN-1* mRNA. The statistical software used was the JMP version 10 (SAS Institute, Cary, NC).

Results

Subjects

Thirteen ST-Asthma, 18 SN-Asthma, 13 D-CON and 17 COPD subjects underwent bronchoscopic airway brushing (Table 1). D-CON and COPD were older than ST or SN-Asthma subjects (*p < 0.0001, ***p < 0.05). FEV1/FVC and %FEV1 in COPD were lower than in D-CON, ST and SN-Asthma (*p < 0.0001). FeNO was significantly higher in SN-Asthma than the other groups (*p < 0.0001). Mean ICS dose are represented Beclometasone dipropionate (BDP) equivalent dose. Two subjects were using OCS (predonisolone 5 mg/day). Not all subject's cells were available for every experiments due to the limited numbers of epithelial cells obtained at the time of brushing. Table 2 includes 5 ST and 13 SN-Asthma who underwent BAL. FeNO in SN-Asthma tended to higher than ST-Asthma but this was not significant (p = 0.08). Blood sample was collected from 6 ST-Asthma, 10 SN-Asthma and 8 healthy controls. (Table 3). FeNO in SN-Asthma were significantly higher than SN-Asthma (**p < 0.01).

ITLN-1 mRNA expression in freshly isolated BECs and correlation with Type-2 related parameters in steroid naïve asthma

The mean counts of freshly isolated BECs from all the subjects were $4.4 \pm 0.6 \times 10^5$ from distal, and $4.9 \pm 1.1 \times 10^5$ from proximal (4 brushes each) brushings. They were over 90% pure and 80% viable. *ITLN-1* mRNA expression in freshly isolated BECs was significantly higher in the SN-Asthma group than in the other groups in both distal and proximal airway samples (overall p < 0.0001). There were no differences in *ITLN-1* mRNA levels between distal and proximal samples among the groups (Fig. 1). Positive correlations were seen between *ITLN-1* mRNA expression in the distal BECs and FeNO and IgE in SN-Asthma patients (Fig. 2a: r = 0.84, p < 0.0001, N = 16 and b: r = 0.79 p = 0.0002, N = 16, respectively). *ITLN-1* mRNA was also positively correlated with *iNOS, CCL26, periostin* and *DPP4* mRNA (Fig. 2c–f), respectively. *ITLN-1* mRNA and peripheral blood eosinophil numbers were marginally correlated (r = 0.49 p = 0.0556, N = 16, data not shown). In proximal BECs, *ITLN-1* mRNA was also correlated with FeNO, *iNOS, CCL26* and *periostin* mRNA. In contrast, in ST-Asthma, *ITLN-1* mRNA expression was low and there were no correlations with any Type-2 related parameters (Additional file 1: Table S1).

ITLN-1 appears to be primarily expressed by goblet cells

Immunostaining of a small number of distal airway biopsy sections indicated that ITLN-1 protein was strongly expressed in goblet cells and weakly in brush border. Figure 3a shows representative staining from 3 SN-Asthma subjects stained with ITLN-1 antibody and isotype control IgG (Fig. 3b). Figure 3c (ITLN-1) and d (IgG) were representative staining from 3 ST-Asthma

subjects after ICS (mometasone furoate; MF) treatment. Figure 3c and d was same subject with Fig. 3a, b after ICS treatment. Unfortunately, there were not enough biopsies of sufficient quality to evaluate differences among groups. Figure 3e shows *ITLN-1* mRNA expressions in freshly isolated BECs samples in series of before and after ICS (MF) treatment in 6 samples from 3 subjects. Closed markers represent distal BECs and open diamonds are proximal BECs. *ITLN-1* mRNA in both distal and proximal BECs significantly decreased after ICS treatments.

ITLN-1 protein in BAL and serum

ITLN-1 was detected in BAL and higher in SN-Asthma than ST-Asthma cases, although the concentrations were very low (Fig. 4a). In contrast, ITLN-1 was easily detected in serum in ST and SN-Asthma cases. Unexpectedly, there was no difference between the ST and SN-Asthma groups (p = 0.21) in Fig. 4b. Serum and BALF albumin concentration were determined by ELISA. The ratio of ITLN-1/albumin was significantly higher in SN-Asthma (Additional file 2: Figure S1).

ITLN-1 mRNA and protein is induced by IL-13 in primary cultured BECs

ITLN-1 mRNA expression and protein were measured with or without IL-13 stimulation (10 ng/mL) in primary human BEC derived from both ST and SN-Asthma cultured in ALI. *ITLN-1* mRNA expression and protein were significantly enhanced by IL-13 stimulation (Fig. 5a, b). However, amount of *ITLN-1* mRNA was very low compared with freshly isolated BECs. Interestingly, ITLN-1 protein was detected only in apical supernatant. There were no differences in *ITLN-1* mRNA or protein expression between SN-Asthma and ST-Asthma groups after IL-13 stimulation (Additional file 3: Figure S2a, b). Figure 5c and d show the inhibition effect of MF for induced *ITLN-1* mRNA and protein by IL-13. MF inhibited IL-13 induced *ITLN-1* mRNA significantly, and modest inhibition effect for ITLN-1 protein. *ITLN-1* mRNA expression was significantly enhanced by IL-13 stimulation normalized by other housekeeping genes (*B2M* and *RPLP0*) (Additional file 4: Figure S3)

CXCL10 mRNA and protein expression in HFL-1 cells is inhibited by ITLN-1

To determine whether the Type-2 associated ITLN-1 could functionally inhibit Type-1 associated inflammation, CXCL10 expression was induced by the combination of TNF, IL1β and IFN-γ (Cytomix) in HFL-1 cells and the inhibitory effects of ITLN-1 was evaluated (Fig. 6a, b). ITLN-1 (500 ng/mL) alone did not affect CXCL10 expression or production. However, ITLN-1 pretreatment (30 min) reduced Cytomix-induced *CXCL10* mRNA and protein in a concentration-dependent

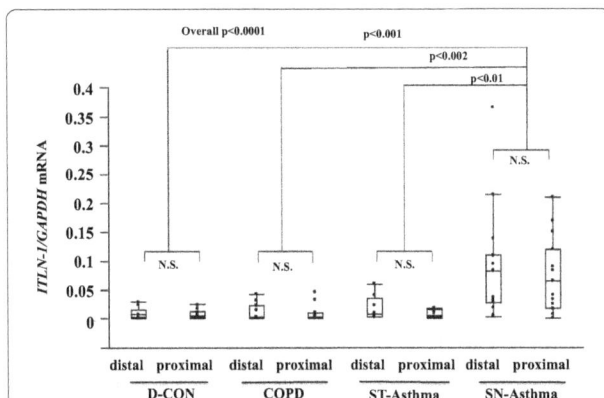

Fig. 1 *ITLN-1* mRNA expression in freshly isolated BECs from each group by qPCR. *ITLN-1* mRNA was significantly enhanced in freshly isolated distal and proximal BECs in SN-Asthma (p < 0.01) compared with other groups. Intergroup comparisons were done using the Wilcoxon test for multiple comparisons

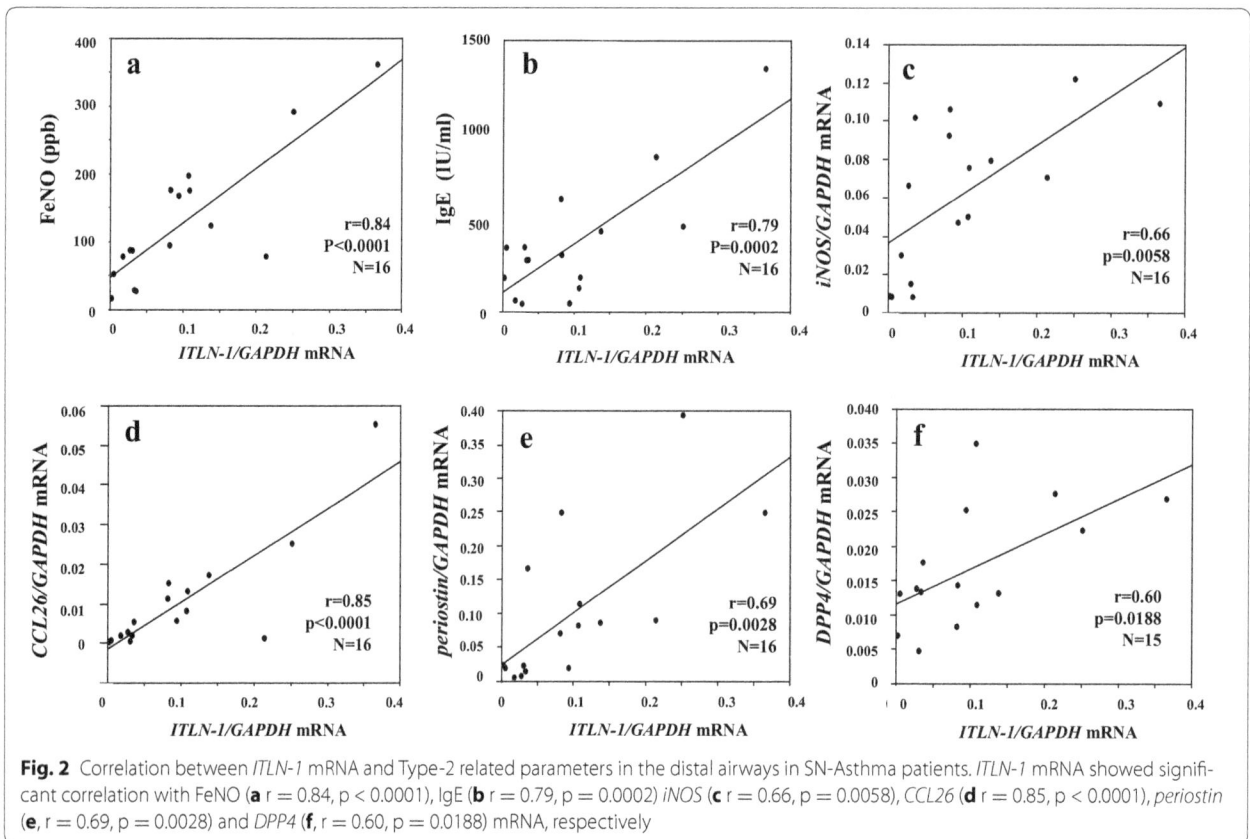

Fig. 2 Correlation between *ITLN-1* mRNA and Type-2 related parameters in the distal airways in SN-Asthma patients. *ITLN-1* mRNA showed significant correlation with FeNO (**a** r = 0.84, p < 0.0001), IgE (**b** r = 0.79, p = 0.0002) *iNOS* (**c** r = 0.66, p = 0.0058), *CCL26* (**d** r = 0.85, p < 0.0001), *periostin* (**e**, r = 0.69, p = 0.0028) and *DPP4* (**f**, r = 0.60, p = 0.0188) mRNA, respectively

manner. To investigate intracellular signal transduction, we examined STAT1 as a signal transduction pathway of IFN-γ. ITLN-1 decreased cytomix induced p-STAT1 at 5 and 15 min (p = 0.0006, p = 0.0063, respectively), supporting an inhibitory effect on this pathway.

Discussion

In this study, ITLN-1 was induced by IL-13 and mainly expressed in goblet cells of the distal and proximal airways in SN-Asthma patients. In the SN-Asthma group, *ITLN-1* mRNA correlated with FeNO, IgE, *iNOS*, *CCL26*, *periostin* and *DPP4* mRNA, all Type-2 related parameters. Finally, our results suggest that ITLN-1 might lead to Type-2-bias by attenuating IFN-γ signaling.

Kupermann et al. reported that ITLN-1 increased in an asthma model and in BECs from asthma subjects [17]. Similar to our data (Fig. 5a, b), Zen et al. showed that ITLN-1 expression increased in NHBE cells stimulated by IL-13 and in the lungs of mice after intranasal IL-13 administration and found ITLN-1 among the induced genes [24]. Gu et al. reported that ITLN-1 is required for expression of IL-13-induced monocyte chemotactic protein (MCP)-1 and -3 in lung epithelial cells and promotes

allergic airway inflammation [25]. Thus, ITLN-1 appears to be strongly related to Type-2 inflammation in vitro and in vivo. However, no reports have compared ITLN-1 with other asthma biomarkers or revealed its function in human asthma.

In this study, *ITLN-1* mRNA significantly correlated with FeNO and serum IgE, as well as *iNOS*, *CCL26*, *periostin* and *DPP4* mRNA in SN-Asthma, as these genes are known to be induced in BECs stimulated with IL-13. Kerr et al. showed that ITLN-1 in sputum is significantly higher in eosinophil-high groups, supporting an association of ITLN-1 with Type-2-high asthma [18]. Immunostaining showed that ITLN-1 protein was expressed in BECs, and suggested it was particularly expressed in goblet cells. The expression levels closely resembled those in intestinal epithelial cells published in previous reports [15, 18].

As Fig. 1 shows, *ITLN-1* mRNA expression was significantly higher in freshly isolated BECs from the SN-Asthma group than in the other groups, we hypothesized that ITLN-1 in BAL or more importantly in serum, could be a useful asthma biomarker. Comparing SN-Asthma and ST-Asthma groups only, BAL-ITLN-1 was detected

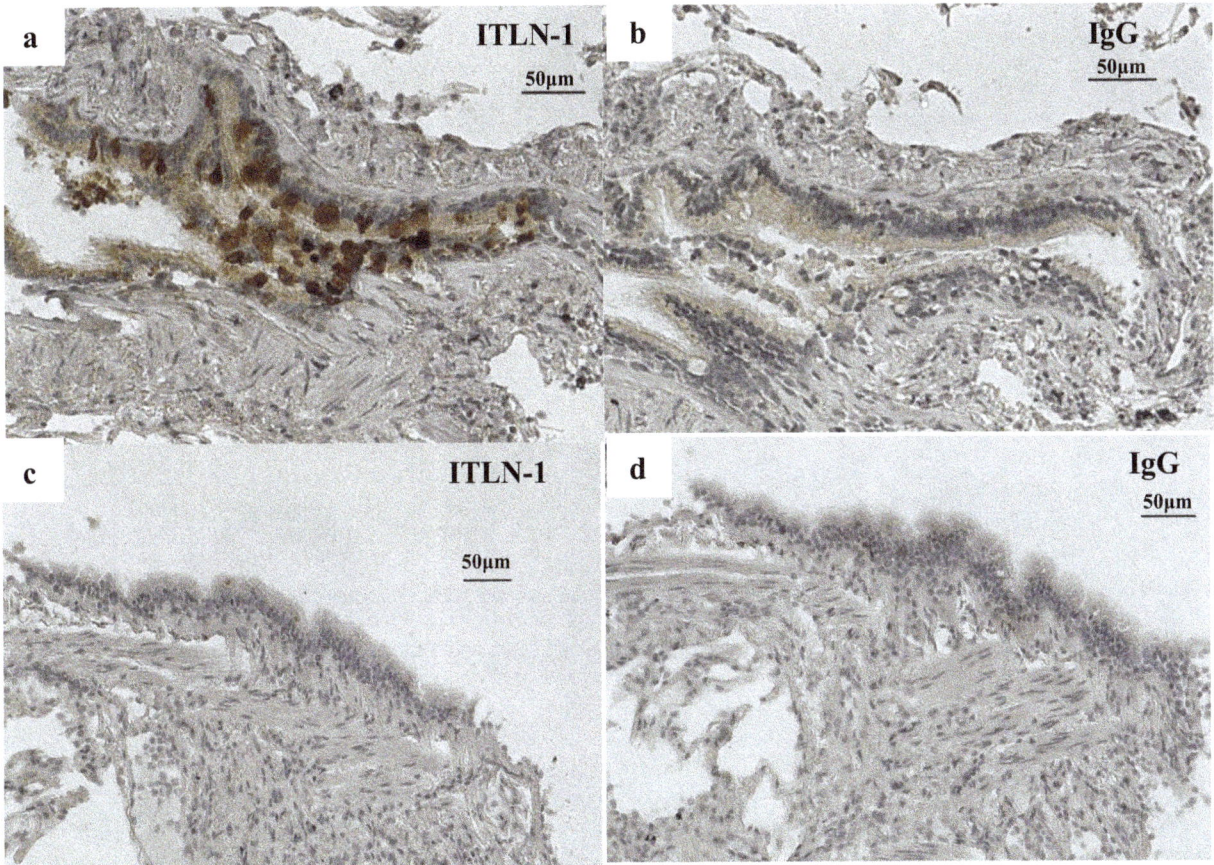

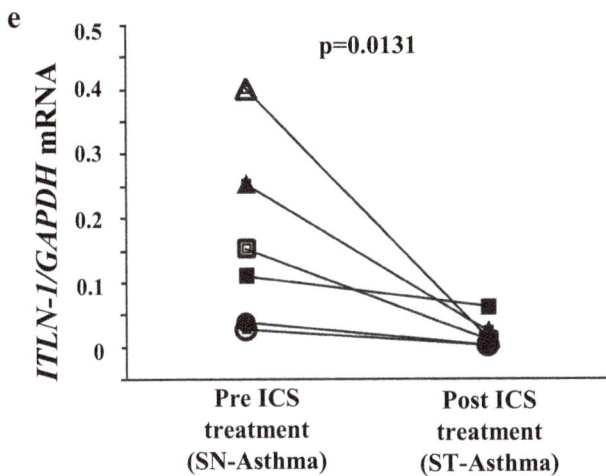

Fig. 3 Immunohistochemistry of ITLN-1 expression in airway tissue. Representative distal BECs of SN-Asthma (**a**, **b**), and ST-Asthma (**c**, **d**) samples were stained with anti-ITLN-1 antibody (**a**, **c**) and IgG isotype control (**b**, **d**). The fields are 200 magnificent and antibodies are 1:500 diluted, respectively. ITLN-1 staining is mainly in the goblet cells in SN-Asthma. **e** *ITLN-1* mRNA expressions before and after ICS (MF) treatment from 3 patients with 6 samples. *Closed markers* represent distal BECs and *open markers* are proximal BECs. *Circles*, *triangles* and *squares* are represented subjects individually. *Additional small tables* shows *ITLN-1* mRNA values pre and post ICS treatments. Comparisons were done using the Wilcoxon test

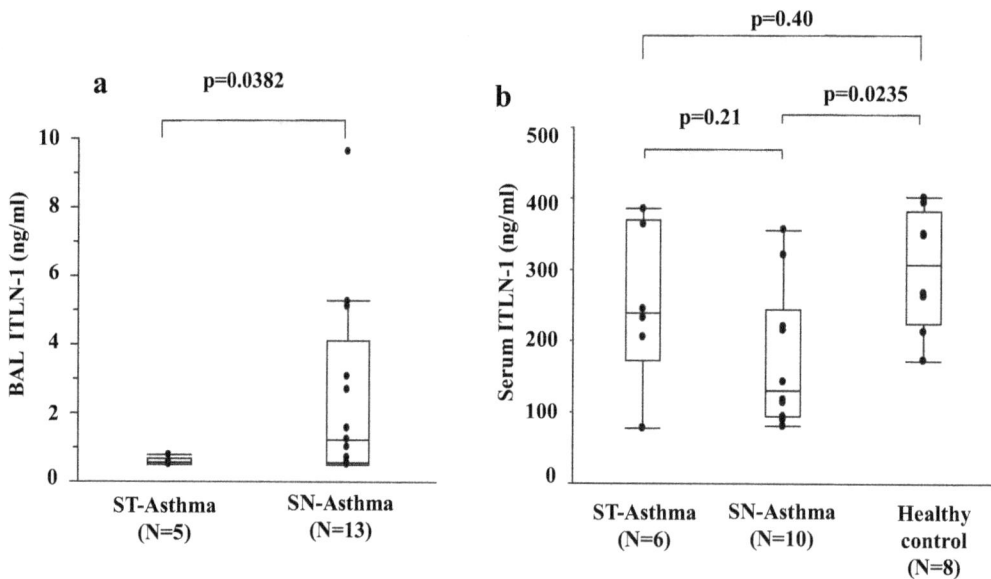

Fig. 4 ITLN-1 concentration in BAL and serum. **a** ITLN-1 concentration from BAL samples. ITLN-1 concentration was low (0.5–11.3, mean 2.4 ng/mL) but detectable by ELISA. ITLN-1 is higher in SN-Asthma (n = 13) than in ST-Asthma (n = 5) subjects (p = 0.0382, Wilcoxon test). **b** Serum ITLN-1 concentration is abundant (77.3 to 402 ng/mL, mean 236.5 ng/mL). Serum ITLN-1 is no difference between ST and SN-Asthma subjects (p = 0.21) and ST-Asthma and healthy controls (p = 0.40). However, IT LN-1 is significantly higher than SN-Asthma (p = 0.0235). These comparisons were done using the Wilcoxon test

at low levels (range 0.5–9.6 ng/mL), and was significantly higher than in SN-Asthma as compared to ST-Asthma (Fig. 4a). However, BAL fluid collection is invasive, therefore we evaluated serum for ITLN-1. ITLN-1 was abundant in serum (range 77.3–385 ng/mL); but serum ITLN-1 was indistinguishable between ST-Asthma and SN-Asthma patients. This could be because systemic ITLN-1 may originate primarily from the intestinal tract or other organs as opposed to the airways. Moreover, ITLN-1 is expressed in goblet cells and mainly released into the lumens of the airways, such that the amount derived from the airways is not likely to reflect the serum ITLN-1. Thus, it does not appear that serum ITLN-1 will be a valid asthma biomarker.

As described earlier, ITLN-1 is a protective lectin against parasites and microorganisms. Suzuki et al. reported that ITLN-1 is a receptor of lactoferrin which helps to protect against infections [26]. It has been reported that ITLN-1 is expressed in the brush border of intestinal cells and binding of lactoferrin results in activation of signal transduction pathways that control infections. However, data on lactoferrin expression are controversial, with Kerr et al. also reporting increases in lactoferrin asthmatic sputum, while a

recent gene array data suggested lower mRNA expression in asthma, particularly Type-2/severe asthma [18, 27]. Thus, further studies are needed to better understand the interactions between ITLN-1 and lactoferrin in asthma.

We also wished to examine the potential functions of ITLN-1 in the airway particularly in relation to Type-1 inflammation. Previously, it was reported that ITLN-1 was one of an adipokine with anti-inflammatory effect [19]. CXCL10 (IP-10) is strongly induced by IFN-γ and is a biomarker of Th1/Type-1 inflammation [28]. We hypothesized that ITLN-1 might skew cellular responses away from Type-1 pathways. Thus, we investigated whether rhITLN-1 could inhibit CXCL10 expression after stimulation with cytomix. ITLN-1 significantly inhibited cytomix induced CXCL10 in HFL-1 cells in a concentration-dependent manner, accompanied by a decrease in phosphorylation of STAT1. These results suggest that ITLN-1 could contribute to a Type-2-high bias in asthmatic airways.

The study limitations include the clinical/observational nature of the study which did not include specific bronchodilator responsiveness testing or methacholine challenge to confirm the asthma diagnosis, particularly

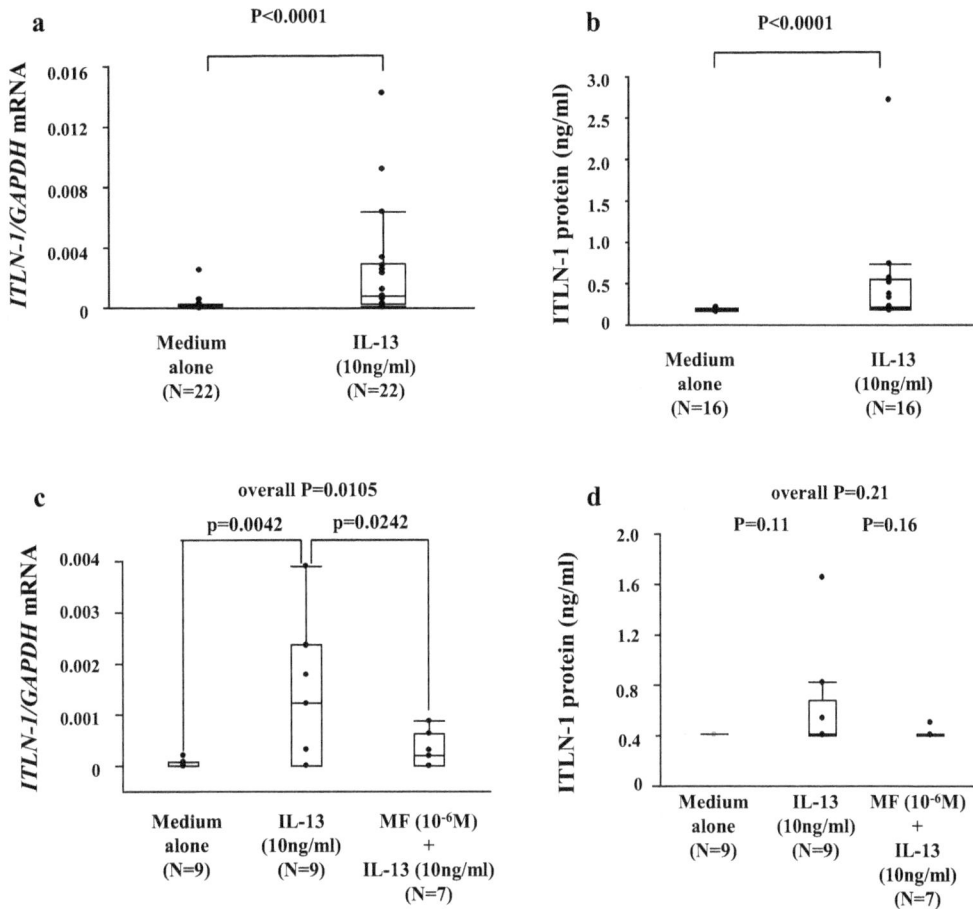

Fig. 5 *ITLN-1* mRNA expression and protein production induced by IL-13 in primary cultured BECs in vitro. **a** *ITLN-1* mRNA expression with or without IL-13 stimulation, in BECs from-asthma patients (p < 0.0001). **b** ITLN-1 protein production enhanced with or without IL-13 stimulation, in BECs from asthma patients (p < 0.0001). **c** Inhibitory effect of MF (1 μM) induced *ITLN-1* mRNA expression by IL-13 stimulation asthma subjects. MF significantly decreased *ITLN-1* mRNA expression (p = 0.0242). **d** MF inhibited modestly induced ITLN-1 protein production from BECs from asthma subjects. Comparisons were done using the Wilcoxon test

in the mild steroid naïve patients. However, despite this lack of objective data, differences in epithelial ITLN-1 expression were apparent on the basis of steroid treatment and in relation to known Type-2 related parameters. We also lacked a true healthy control group. However, it is difficult to perform bronchoscopies in healthy individuals in Japan. Finally, these studies were done as add-on research studies to clinically indicated bronchoscopies in all patients. Therefore, the availability of BAL and tissue samples was limited to a small number of patients.

Conclusions

ITLN-1 is expressed in untreated asthmatic bronchial epithelial cells, particularly in goblet cells, in association with Type-2 related parameters. However, it appears to be suppressed by corticosteroids in vivo, and epithelial ITLN-1 does not appear to contribute substantially to serum

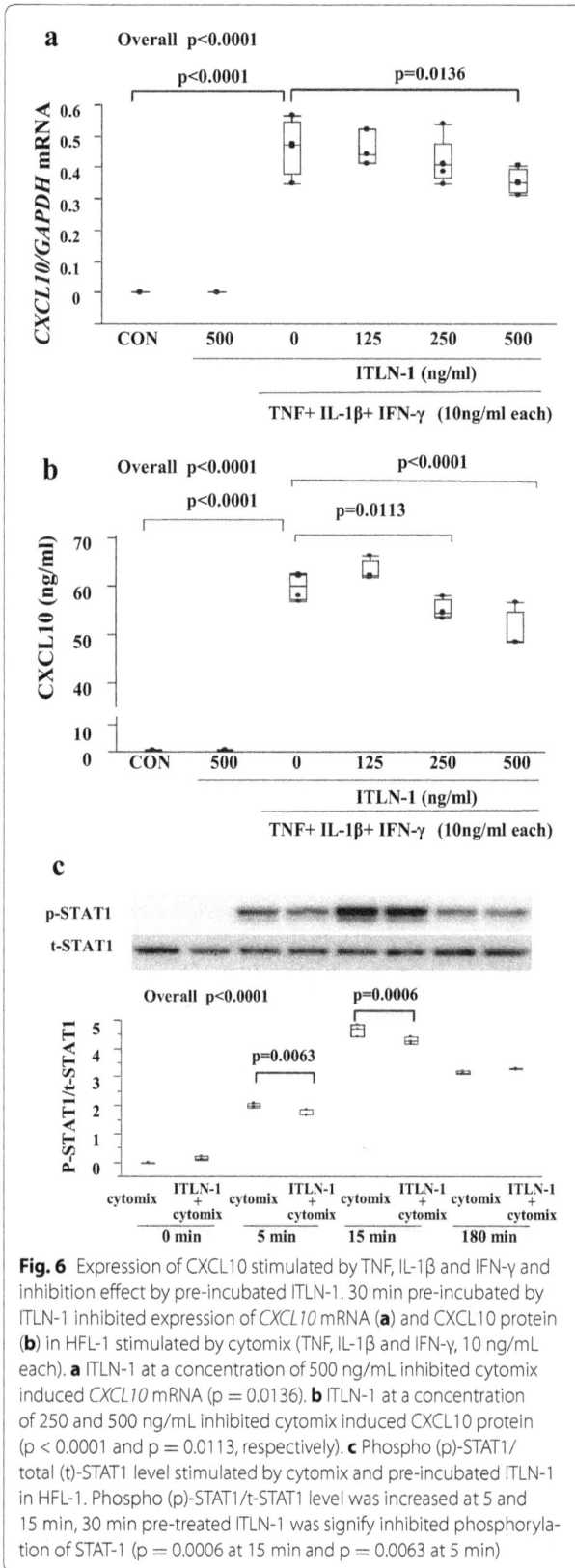

Fig. 6 Expression of CXCL10 stimulated by TNF, IL-1β and IFN-γ and inhibition effect by pre-incubated ITLN-1. 30 min pre-incubated by ITLN-1 inhibited expression of *CXCL10* mRNA (**a**) and CXCL10 protein (**b**) in HFL-1 stimulated by cytomix (TNF, IL-1β and IFN-γ, 10 ng/mL each). **a** ITLN-1 at a concentration of 500 ng/mL inhibited cytomix induced *CXCL10* mRNA (p = 0.0136). **b** ITLN-1 at a concentration of 250 and 500 ng/mL inhibited cytomix induced CXCL10 protein (p < 0.0001 and p = 0.0113, respectively). **c** Phospho (p)-STAT1/ total (t)-STAT1 level stimulated by cytomix and pre-incubated ITLN-1 in HFL-1. Phospho (p)-STAT1/t-STAT1 level was increased at 5 and 15 min, 30 min pre-treated ITLN-1 was signify inhibited phosphorylation of STAT-1 (p = 0.0006 at 15 min and p = 0.0063 at 5 min)

levels, making it unsuitable as a Type-2 asthma biomarker. Its true role in asthma requires further study, perhaps in association with lactoferrin, but it has the potential to further skew inflammation away from Type-1 and towards a Type-2 process.

Abbreviations
ITLN-1: intelectin-1; rhITLN-1: recombinant human ITLN-1; BECs: bronchial epithelial cells; FeNO: fractional exhaled nitric oxide; DPP4: dipeptidyl peptidase-4; iNOS: inducible nitric oxide synthase; CCL26: chemokine ligand 26; D-CON: disease control; ICS: inhaled corticosteroid; OCS: oral corticosteroid; SN-Asthma: ICS-naïve bronchial asthma; ST-Asthma: ICS-treated bronchial asthma; TBLB: transbronchial lung biopsy; EBB: endobronchial biopsy; BAL: bronchial alveolar lavage; ALI: air–liquid interface; HFL-1: human fetal fibroblasts; CXCL10: C-X-C motif chemokine 10; STAT1: signal transducer and activator of transcription 1.

Authors' contributions
TW, KC, TS, TR, RK, YN, RA, YH, and AT carried out sampling BECs and PCR studies, and drafted the manuscript. TW, KC, YH and TS carried out the immunoassays. TW, KC, YS, SW and YI participated in the design of the study and performed the statistical analysis. TW, KC, TF, SW and YI conceived of the study, and participated in its design and coordination and helped to draft the manuscript. All authors read and approved the final manuscript.

Author details
[1] Department of Pulmonary Medicine and Clinical Immunology, Dokkyo Medical University School of Medicine, Tochigi, Japan. [2] Dokkyo Medical University School of Medicine, 880 Kitakobayashi Mibumachi, Shimotsuga-gun, Tochigi 321-0293, Japan. [3] Pulmonary Allergy and Critical Care Medicine, Department of Medicine, University of Pittsburgh, 3459 Fifth Ave., Pittsburgh, PA 15213, USA.

Acknowledgements
We thank Reiko Komura and Kazumi Okazaki, who measured FeNO.

Competing interests
The authors declare that they have no competing interests.

Funding
This study was by a Dokkyo Medical University, Young Investigator Award (No. 2013-16).

References

1. Wenzel S, Castro M, Corren J, Maspero J, Wang L, Zhang B, Pirozzi G, Sutherland ER, Evans RR, Joish VN, et al. Dupilumab efficacy and safety in adults with uncontrolled persistent asthma despite use of medium-to-high-dose inhaled corticosteroids plus a long-acting β2 agonist: a randomised double-blind placebo-controlled pivotal phase 2b dose-ranging trial. Lancet. 2016;388:31–44.

2. Asakura T, Ishii Y, Chibana K, Fukuda T. Leukotriene D4 stimulates collagen production from myofibroblasts transformed by TGF-beta. J Allergy Clin Immunol. 2004;114:310–5.

3. Chibana K, Ishii Y, Asakura T, Fukuda T. Up-regulation of cysteinyl leukotriene 1 receptor by IL-13 enables human lung fibroblasts to respond to leukotriene C4 and produce eotaxin. J Immunol. 2003;170:4290–5.

4. Chibana K, Trudeau JB, Mustovich AT, Hu H, Zhao J, Balzar S, Chu HW, Wenzel SE. IL-13 induced increases in nitrite levels are primarily driven by increases in inducible nitric oxide synthase as compared with effects on arginases in human primary bronchial epithelial cells. Clin Exp Allergy. 2008;38:936–46.

5. Yamamoto M, Tochino Y, Chibana K, Trudeau JB, Holguin F, Wenzel SE. Nitric oxide and related enzymes in asthma: relation to severity, enzyme function and inflammation. Clin Exp Allergy. 2012;42:760–8.

6. Zhao J, Maskrey B, Balzar S, Chibana K, Mustovich A, Hu H, Trudeau JB, O'Donnell V, Wenzel SE. Interleukin-13-induced MUC5AC is regulated by 15-lipoxygenase 1 pathway in human bronchial epithelial cells. Am J Respir Crit Care Med. 2009;179:782–90.

7. Shiobara T, Chibana K, Watanabe T, Arai R, Horigane Y, Nakamura Y, Hayashi Y, Shimizu Y, Takemasa A, Ishii Y. Dipeptidyl peptidase-4 is highly expressed in bronchial epithelial cells of untreated asthma and it increases cell proliferation along with fibronectin production in airway constitutive cells. Respir Res. 2016;17:28.

8. Takayama G, Arima K, Kanaji T, Toda S, Tanaka H, Shoji S, McKenzie AN, Nagai H, Hotokebuchi T, Izuhara K. Periostin: a novel component of subepithelial fibrosis of bronchial asthma downstream of IL-4 and IL-13 signals. J Allergy Clin Immunol. 2006;118:98–104.

9. Corren J, Lemanske RF, Hanania NA, Korenblat PE, Parsey MV, Arron JR, Harris JM, Scheerens H, Wu LC, Su Z, et al. Lebrikizumab treatment in adults with asthma. New Engl J Med. 2011;365:1088–98.

10. Izuhara K, Conway SJ, Moore BB, Matsumoto H, Holweg CT, Matthews JG, Arron JR. Roles of periostin in respiratory disorders. Am J Respir Crit Care Med. 2016;193:949–56.

11. Brightling CE, Chanez P, Leigh R, O'Byrne PM, Korn S, She D, May RD, Streicher K, Ranade K, Piper E. Efficacy and safety of tralokinumab in patients with severe uncontrolled asthma: a randomised, double-blind, placebo-controlled, phase 2b trial. Lancet Respir Med. 2015;3:692–701.

12. Komiya T, Tanigawa Y, Hirohashi S. Cloning of the novel gene intelectin, which is expressed in intestinal paneth cells in mice. Biochem Biophys Res Commun. 1998;251:759–62.

13. Tsuji S, Uehori J, Matsumoto M, Suzuki Y, Matsuhisa A, Toyoshima K, Seya T. Human intelectin is a novel soluble lectin that recognizes galacto-furanose in carbohydrate chains of bacterial cell wall. J Biol Chem. 2001;276:23456–63.

14. Pemberton AD, Knight PA, Gamble J, Colledge WH, Lee JK, Pierce M, Miller HR. Innate BALB/c enteric epithelial responses to Trichinella spiralis: inducible expression of a novel goblet cell lectin, intelectin-2, and its natural deletion in C57BL/10 mice. J Immunol. 2004;173:1894–901.

15. French AT, Knight PA, Smith WD, Pate JA, Miller HR, Pemberton AD. Expression of three intelectins in sheep and response to a Th2 environment. Vet Res. 2009;40:53.

16. Tsuji S, Tsuura Y, Morohoshi T, Shinohara T, Oshita F, Yamada K, Kameda Y, Ohtsu T, Nakamura Y, Miyagi Y. Secretion of intelectin-1 from malignant pleural mesothelioma into pleural effusion. Br J Cancer. 2010;103:517–23.

17. Kuperman DA, Lewis CC, Woodruff PG, Rodriguez MW, Yang YH, Dolganov GM, Fahy JV, Erle DJ. Dissecting asthma using focused transgenic modeling and functional genomics. J Allergy Clin Immunol. 2005;116:305–11.

18. Kerr SC, Carrington SD, Oscarson S, Gallagher ME, Solon M, Yuan S, Ahn JN, Dougherty RH, Finkbeiner WE, Peters MC, Fahy JV. Intelectin-1 is a prominent protein constituent of pathologic mucus associated with eosinophilic airway inflammation in asthma. Am J Respir Crit Care Med. 2014;189:1005–7.

19. Zhong X, Li X, Liu F, Tan H, Shang D. Omentin inhibits TNF-alpha-induced expression of adhesion molecules in endothelial cells via ERK/NF-kappaB pathway. Biochem Biophys Res Commun. 2012;425:401–6.

20. Bhushan B, Homma T, Norton JE, Sha Q, Siebert J, Gupta DS, Schroeder JW Jr, Schleimer RP. Suppression of epithelial signal transducer and activator of transcription 1 activation by extracts of Aspergillus fumigatus. Am J Respir Cell Mol Biol. 2015;53:87–95.

21. Matsukura S, Kokubu F, Kurokawa M, Kawaguchi M, Ieki K, Kuga H, Odaka M, Suzuki S, Watanabe S, Takeuchi H, et al. Synthetic double-stranded RNA induces multiple genes related to inflammation through Toll-like receptor 3 depending on NF-kappaB and/or IRF-3 in airway epithelial cells. Clin Exp Allergy. 2006;36:1049–62.

22. Yoshizawa T, Hammaker D, Sweeney SE, Boyle DL, Firestein GS. Synoviocyte innate immune responses: I. Differential regulation of interferon responses and the JNK pathway by MAPK kinases. J Immunol. 2008;181:3252–8.

23. Chu HW, Balzar S, Seedorf GJ, Westcott JY, Trudeau JB, Silkoff P, Wenzel SE. Transforming growth factor-β2 induces bronchial epithelial mucin expression in asthma. Am J Pathol. 2004;165:1097–106.

24. Zhen G, Park SW, Nguyenvu LT, Rodriguez MW, Barbeau R, Paquet AC, Erle DJ. IL-13 and epidermal growth factor receptor have critical but distinct roles in epithelial cell mucin production. Am J Respir Cell Mol Biol. 2007;36:244–53.

25. Gu N, Kang G, Jin C, Xu Y, Zhang Z, Erle DJ, Zhen G. Intelectin is required for IL-13-induced monocyte chemotactic protein-1 and -3 expression in lung epithelial cells and promotes allergic airway inflammation. Am J Physiol Lung Cell Mol Physiol. 2010;298:L290–6.

26. Suzuki YA, Shin K, Lonnerdal B. Molecular cloning and functional expression of a human intestinal lactoferrin receptor. Biochemistry. 2001;40:15771–9.

27. Modena BD, Tedrow JR, Milosevic J, Bleecker ER, Meyers DA, Wu W, Bar-Joseph Z, Erzurum SC, Gaston BM, Busse WW, et al. Gene expression in relation to exhaled nitric oxide identifies novel asthma phenotypes with unique biomolecular pathways. Am J Respir Crit Care Med. 2014;190:1363–72.

28. Yoshikawa M, Wada K, Yoshimura T, Asaka D, Okada N, Matsumoto K, Moriyama H. Increased CXCL10 expression in nasal fibroblasts from patients with refractory chronic rhinosinusitis and asthma. Allergol Int. 2013;62:495–502.

14

Visual analogue scale (VAS) as a monitoring tool for daily changes in asthma symptoms in adolescents

Hyekyun Rhee[1]*⊙, Michael Belyea[2] and Jennifer Mammen[1]

Abstract

Background: Success in asthma management hinges on patients' competency to detect and respond to ever-changing symptom severity. Thus, it is crucial to have reliable, simple, and sustainable methods of symptom monitoring that can be readily incorporated into daily life. Although visual analogue scale (VAS) has been considered as a simple symptom assessment method, its utility as a daily symptom monitoring tool in adolescents is unknown. This study was to determine the concurrent validity of VAS in capturing diurnal changes in symptoms and to examine the relationships between VAS and asthma control and pulmonary function.

Methods: Forty-two adolescents (12–17 years old) with asthma completed daily assessment of symptoms twice per day, morning and bedtime, for a week using VAS and 6-item symptom diary concurrently. Asthma control was measured at enrollment and 6 month later, and spirometry was conducted at enrollment. Pearson correlations, multilevel modeling and regression were conducted to assess the relationships between VAS and symptom diary, asthma control and FEV1.

Results: Morning and evening VAS was positively associated with symptom diary items of each corresponding time frame of the day ($r = 0.41$–0.58, $p < 0.0001$). Morning VAS was significantly predicted by morning diary data reflecting nocturnal wakening ($\beta = 2.13$, $p = 0.033$) and morning symptoms ($\beta = 4.09$, $p = 0.002$), accounting for 57% of the total variance of morning VAS. Similarly, changes in four evening diary items, particularly shortness of breath ($\beta = 2.60$, $p = 0.028$), significantly predicted changes in evening VAS, accounting for 55% of the total variance. Average VAS scores correlated with asthma control ($r = 0.65$, $p < 0.001$) and FEV1 ($r = -0.38$, $p = 0.029$), and were predictive of asthma control 6 months later ($\beta = 0.085$, $p = 0.006$).

Conclusions: VAS is a valid tool capturing diurnal changes in symptoms reflected in a multi-item symptom diary. Moreover, VAS is a valid measure predicting concurrent and future asthma control. The findings suggest VAS can be a simple alternative to daily dairies for daily symptom monitoring, which can provide invaluable information about current and future asthma control without substantially increasing self-monitoring burdens for adolescent patients.

Clinical Trial Registration NCT01696357. Registered 18 September 2012

Keywords: Visual analogue scale, Asthma symptom monitoring, Adolescents, Symptom diary, Asthma control

Background

Asthma symptom monitoring incorporated in daily routines is essential to successful asthma self-management [1–3]. Symptom monitoring is linked to fewer cases of asthma exacerbation and acute care visits, as well as better functional outcomes and higher quality of life in children and adolescents [4]. Recognition of symptoms through monitoring allows patients to take necessary management actions (e.g., adjusting medication, altering activity level, avoiding or minimizing triggers, or seeking assistance). Moreover, patients' symptom monitoring

*Correspondence: Hyekyun_rhee@urmc.rochester.edu
[1] University of Rochester, School of Nursing, 601 Elmwood Avenue, Box SON, Rochester, NY 14642, USA
Full list of author information is available at the end of the article

is an essential source of information in implementing guideline based treatment.

Expert Panel Report 3 (EPR-3) by the National Heart, Lung and Blood Institute [3] recommends that each patient be taught to recognize symptom patterns indicating inadequate asthma control. The need for a patient completed monitoring tool that can capture the variability and changing nature of asthma between office visits has been recognized [5, 6]. To address the need, symptom diaries have been suggested especially for those with uncontrolled or persistent asthma, as it can aid in the identification of asthma of higher severity [3, 7]. Asthma diaries completed on a daily basis minimize recollection errors [8], and are a better means for identifying patients with persistent asthma compared to retrospective reports of usually previous 4 weeks, as in a periodic self-assessment form completed at the time of an office visit (e.g., asthma control test) [7].

Structured daily diaries often consist of multiple items assessing various symptoms and asthma related impairments, which can be burdensome to children and adolescents, resulting in poor adherence. This calls for an alternative symptom monitoring strategy that is simple and conducive to daily use by young patients. A visual analogue scale (VAS) can be the alternative to multiple item diaries for daily symptom monitoring. VAS has been found useful in assessing patient's subjective experience or perception of a variety of clinical phenomena [9]. VAS scores have been shown to be associated with varying levels of asthma control [10–12] and pulmonary function [11, 12]. A simple VAS performed better in capturing asthma severity compared to other structured assessment methods of multiple categories measuring the same construct [13]. For being a single item with minimal wording, VAS requires little time or literacy to complete. These advantages render VAS suitable for daily use for symptom monitoring, particularly in pediatric patients.

The extent to which the VAS performs as an alternative to multiple item diaries for a daily symptom assessment tool for adolescents remains to be explored. In particular, demonstrating its capacity to capture diurnal and day-to-day variations in symptoms would be critical to be considered as a symptom monitoring tool. The purpose of this study was to determine the concurrent validity of VAS in capturing diurnal changes in symptoms and to examine the relationships between VAS and asthma control and pulmonary function.

Methods
Study sample and setting
This study was the secondary analysis of data originally collected for a study that examined the validity of a newly developed automated device monitoring asthma symptoms [14]. Eligibility criteria included age 13 through 17, having physician-diagnosed asthma at least 1 year, and ability to understand spoken and written English. Those with other diagnoses producing asthma-like symptoms (e.g., cardiac disease and cystic fibrosis) were excluded. Subjects were recruited from the pediatric emergency department (ED) and outpatient clinics (primary practice and pediatric pulmonary specialty clinic) in a major university medical center located in the Northeastern U.S. Of a total of 42 participants, the majority (69%) were recruited from the emergency department, and the remaining were from the study flyers (24%) and clinician referrals (8%).

Study measures
Visual analogue scale (VAS)
The VAS was 100 mm long with 3 anchors dividing 3 zones (green, yellow, and red). For each symptom, the green zone (0–20 mm) labeled "no symptoms", the yellow zone (21–50 mm) "mild symptoms" and the red zone (50–100 mm) "very bad symptoms" [13, 15]. Teens marked any point on the zone according to their perception of symptoms. The distance between the 0 mm mark and the placement of the "X" was measured to provide a numeric interpretation of their symptom perception. VAS was used twice, morning (VAS-am) and bedtime (VAS-pm).

Asthma Control Diary (ACD)
This 6-item diary measures the levels of symptoms on a 7-point scale from zero (no symptom) to 6 for consistent symptoms [16]. The diary data were collected electronically using an iPod to increase participants' adherence and convenience. By sending automatic reminders and restricting the time of entry, the electronic diaries were useful in ascertaining adherence and reinforcing proper entry time, thereby reducing the recollection bias and risk of fabrication. Morning questions (2 items) pertained to nocturnal wakening and morning symptoms, and bedtime questions (4-items) assessed the degree of activity limitation, shortness of breath, and wheeze they experienced during the day and use of short-acting beta agonist (SABA) in previous 24 h. Each item was evaluated separately in the analysis.

Forced expiratory volume in one second (FEV1)
Spirometry test (KoKo®: Pulmonary Data Service; Louisville, CO, USA) was conducted on the first day of the 7-day trial to obtain FEV1 in accordance with the American Thoracic Society standards [17].

Asthma control questions consisting of 4 questions were devised for the study based on four impairment based asthma control criteria provided by EPR3. The criteria including the frequency of the limitation of daily activity, nocturnal wakening, asthma symptoms and use of SABA in the past 4 weeks were measured on a 5-point scale. Asthma control questions were administered at enrollment and at the 6-months follow-up. A total score was computed; higher scores indicating poor asthma control.

Demographic and asthma-related information was collected, including gender, age, race, annual family income, years with asthma diagnosis and current medications.

Data collection procedure

Institutional Review Board within the academic institution affiliated with the principal investigator (HR) reviewed and approved the study for human subject protection. Informed consent was obtained from parents and assent from adolescents prior to data collection. At enrollment, a demographic form, asthma control questions and spirometry were administered. Adolescents completed a paper form VAS twice a day, morning and bedtime, for 7 days. Simultaneously, electronic asthma diaries were completed using an iPod programed to push morning and evening questions at the designated timeframes each day for 7 days. Automatic reminders were sent until the completion of scheduled diary questions within the timeframe. Asthma control questions were repeated at the 6-month follow up.

Data analysis

Pearson correlations were computed to assess the relationships between VAS and ACD, asthma control and FEV1. A multilevel regression model for longitudinal data was used to assess the relationships between VAS and daily asthma symptoms reported in ACD measured twice a day for seven consecutive days. Morning and evening VAS measures were analyzed using two hierarchical models: (1) a model with time varying covariates, and (2) a final model with the addition of the demographic covariates. Diary symptoms were grand mean centered, where 0 represented the average level of the measure, and entered simultaneously into the model.

In the first model, asthma symptoms as time-varying predictors of VAS were entered into the model. In these models, VAS was modeled with an intercept, linear slope, and with the time-varying covariates entered simultaneously (nocturnal wakening and morning symptoms for morning VAS and activity limitation, shortness of breath, wheezing, and SABA use for evening VAS). Using daily asthma symptoms as time-varying covariates tests whether they can explain changes in the overall trajectory of VAS. Such tests would examine whether VAS and asthma symptoms measured at the within-person level changed together.

In the second model, age, sex, and race were entered as time fixed demographic variables. The introduction of time fixed covariates tests whether the association between VAS and asthma symptoms persists after controlling for the demographic variables. Multilevel regression analysis, using all available data from each participant, was conducted using the Mixed procedure in SAS. Ordinary least squares regression analysis was conducted to examine the extent to which VAS predicted asthma control after 6 months. All statistical analyses were conducted in SAS (v.9.3). The level of significance was set at p < 0.05 for all tests.

Results

Forty-two adolescents (mean age 15.2 years; SD = 1.5) participated: 60% (n = 25) females, 57% (n = 24) minority and 52% (n = 22) with annual household income less than $30,000. Based on the EPR-3 classification criteria, 36% (n = 15) and 33% (n = 14) of the sample reported not well controlled and very poorly controlled asthma, respectively.

Correlations between VAS and Asthma Control Diary Questions

The relationships between average VAS for morning and evening and each time-corresponding diary data obtained for 7 days were examined in 41 persons. One participant's electronic diary data were lost due to unknown technical glitches. Table 1 displays the summary of correlation coefficients between VAS and each of items of ACD. Significant correlations were found between VAS and ACD, ranging from r = 0.41 to 0.58.

Morning VAS and morning diary variables

Table 2 displays the descriptive statistics of morning VAS (VAS-am) data over 7 days.

Multilevel regression models for the 7 measurement points were conducted. Model 1 (Table 3) was computed to examine the relationship between VAS-am and two morning diary items, nocturnal wakening and bad morning symptoms, as time varying covariates.

Table 1 Correlations between VAS and asthma diary items

	VAS-am	VAS-pm
Morning diary items		
Nocturnal wakening	0.45***	
Morning symptoms	0.55***	
Evening diary items		
Activity limitation		0.41***
Shortness of breath		0.52***
Wheezing		0.58***
Short acting beta agonist use		0.42***

*** p = <.0001

Table 2 Descriptive statistics for morning VAS

Time point	N	Mean	SD	Skewness	Kurtosis	Range
VAS Day 1	34	19.18	19.85	1.69	2.95	0–82
VAS Day 2	41	18.41	16.77	1.20	0.91	0–63
VAS Day 3	41	18.95	19.82	1.79	3.25	0–84
VAS Day 4	41	16.98	15.50	1.09	0.84	0–65
VAS Day 5	41	15.93	17.24	1.87	3.86	0–75
VAS Day 6	41	17.05	17.50	1.17	0.48	0–64
VAS Day 7	41	15.59	15.21	0.70	−0.96	0–50
Average	41	17.33	14.58	0.79	−0.49	0–50.71

Table 3 Morning VAS predicted by the morning diary items as time varying covariates

	Model 1			Model 2		
	Standard			Standard		
	Estimate	SE	p	Estimate	SE	p
Effect						
Intercept	18.13	2.17	≤.001	−0.70	−0.70	0.974
Time	−0.24	0.33	0.479	−0.32	0.34	0.360
Nocturnal wakening	2.21	0.98	0.024	2.13	0.99	0.033
Morning symptoms	3.79	1.20	0.002	4.09	1.29	0.002
Age				0.81	1.34	0.557
Sex (1 = female)				5.18	4.25	0.224
Race (1 = non-white)				5.77	4.26	0.177

The average starting or initial level of morning VAS was 18.13 (t = 8.35, p = 0.001). The linear slope (time) was not significant indicating that the level of reported VAS-am was relatively stable for each individual for 7 days as a whole. However, tests of the random effects indicated significant individual differences in the intercepts or starting values for VAS-am (z = 3.73, p < 0.0001) and individual differences in its slopes or linear change over time approached significance (z = 1.46, p < 0.07). Changes in nocturnal wakening (β = 2.21, p = 0.024) and morning symptoms (β = 3.79, p = 0.002) were significantly related to changes in morning VAS. Including age, gender and race as covariates (Model 2, Table 3) did not substantially change these relationships. Approximately 57% of the total variance of VAS-am scores was accounted for by Model 2.

Evening VAS and evening diary variables
Table 4 displays the means and distributions for evening VAS (VAS-pm) over 7 days.

Model 1 examined the relationship between VAS-pm and the evening diary variables of limited activity, shortness of breath, wheeze, and SABA use as time varying covariates. Model 1 (Table 5), indicates that on average,

the starting or initial level of VAS-pm for participants was 18.58. The linear trend for the group as a whole was not significant indicating that the overall average VAS-pm was relatively stable.

Shortness of breath had a significant effect on VAS-pm (β = 2.27, p = 0.04) after controlling for other items, such that changes in shortness of breath predicted changes in VAS-pm scores above and beyond other evening diary items. Wheezing approached significance. Including age, gender, and race as covariates (Model 2) further reduced the effect of wheezing, but did not change the relationship between shortness of breath and VAS-pm. Females reported higher VAS-pm. The total variance accounted for in VAS-pm scores by Model 2 was approximately 55%.

VAS and asthma control and FEV1
Adjusting for age, gender and race, average VAS scores from 7 days correlated with asthma control questions (r = 0.65, p < 0.001) and FEV1 (r = −0.38, p = 0.029). Average VAS was predictive of asthma control at 6 months (β = 0.085, p = 0.006) after controlling for age, gender and race. VAS along with demographic variables accounted for 33% of variance of asthma control at 6-months.

Table 4 **Descriptive statistics for evening VAS**

Time point	N	Mean	Std D	Skewness	Kurtosis	Range
VAS Day 1	41	18.80	19.82	1.77	3.30	0–87
VAS Day 2	40	19.83	21.13	1.84	4.12	0–100
VAS Day 3	41	20.95	20.36	1.24	0.95	0–77
VAS Day 4	40	17.98	17.20	1.49	2.45	0–75
VAS Day 5	40	15.10	15.13	1.31	1.33	0–63
VAS Day 6	41	18.05	17.84	1.18	0.89	0–74
VAS Day 7	41	18.37	17.37	1.08	0.65	0–70
Average	41	18.44	15.83	1.00	0.27	0–62.86

Table 5 **Evening VAS predicted by the evening diary items as time varying covariates**

	Model 1 Standard			Model 2 Standard		
	Estimate	SE	p	Estimate	SE	p
Effect						
Intercept	18.58	2.83	<0.001	−19.62	19.10	0.311
Time	−0.13	0.49	0.795	−0.08	0.52	0.874
Activity limitation	0.11	0.89	0.904	0.21	0.93	0.821
Shortness of breath	2.27	1.11	0.042	2.60	1.18	0.028
Wheezing	2.27	1.20	0.060	2.11	1.24	0.089
SABA use	−0.45	1.67	0.786	−0.95	1.67	0.571
Age				1.97	1.21	0.104
Sex (1 = female)				9.00	3.81	0.019
Race (1 = non-white)				3.41	3.83	0.375

Discussion

This study demonstrates that VAS can be a reasonable alternative to symptom diaries for daily symptom monitoring in adolescents with asthma. To our knowledge, this is the first study to provide evidence for VAS' capacity to reflect diurnal and daily variation in asthma symptoms. In an earlier cross-sectional study, VAS appropriately differentiated between good, usual and bad breathing days in children with asthma [18]. A prospective study also supported VAS as an instrument that could reasonably detect symptom variations between two discrete observation points with 2 weeks apart in adult patients with allergic rhinitis [19]. Our findings provide more specific evidence that VAS can capture symptom fluctuations occurring not only day-to-day but also within each day.

Consistent with earlier studies [11, 20, 21], we found moderate correlation between VAS and pulmonary function, supporting VAS as a tool for measuring airway obstruction. Validity and clinical usefulness of VAS has often been evaluated in comparison to an objective assessment of airway obstruction such as FEV1. Studies have shown correlations between the degrees of symptoms indicated on VAS and FEV1 in adults [12, 22] and children with asthma [11, 23]. The relationships between VAS and pulmonary function do not appear to be affected by age and gender of children [11]. In fact, symptom perception measured on VAS reliably correlated with pulmonary function in children with asthma across a broad age ranging from 5 to 15 years [24]. Furthermore, in an earlier study [21], VAS was able to discriminate children with bronchial obstruction (FEV1 <80% predicted) from those with normal lung function through the demonstration of significant group differences in VAS scores at a single point. Also, changes in symptom perceptions after use of bronchodilator in children with asthma were also adequately captured by VAS, which was suggestive of bronchial reversibility [21]. Based on the evidence, the authors advocated for the potential application of VAS in establishing an asthma diagnosis in the absence of spirometer in some office settings [21]. Overall, accumulated evidence including ours is overwhelmingly in favor of VAS of symptom perception as a proxy measure of airway obstruction.

As in a previous study [25], we found a moderate to strong correlation between VAS and symptom control. It is important to recognize that traditional measures of symptom control often fail to capture the full extent of symptoms, particularly in adolescent populations, resulting in underestimation of symptoms [26, 27]. Therefore, the lack of decisive correlation between VAS and a conventional measure of asthma control should not be interpreted as an indication of inadequacy of the VAS. On the contrary, it is equally likely that unexplained variance between the VAS and the conventional asthma control measure may have been due to the conventional measure' limited capacity to fully represent the construct of symptom control. Nonetheless, demonstrated correlations between VAS and symptom diary items were close to or well above 0.5, indicating large effect size [28]. Similar to our findings, a large cross-sectional epidemiological study of nearly 30,000 adult patients demonstrated that VAS measured symptom severity accurately and predicted asthma control as defined by Global Initiative for Asthma [10]. This earlier study also showed no differences in VAS scores between patient-rated versus physician-rated, supporting the reproducibility of the measure across different raters. Furthermore, we found that VAS was predictive of asthma control 6 months later. To our knowledge, this is the first study providing the evidence of predictive validity of VAS longitudinally. The possibility of gauging future asthma morbidity using simple VAS has important clinical implications as it could help patients and clinicians determine plans for long-term treatment.

Taken all together, VAS scores could be a simple, reliable indicator of asthma control in adolescents, when used daily. VAS is easily understood and can be a useful tool in improving children's perceptual ability [29]. However, there are mixed reports regarding when VAS would be useful and valid in asthma monitoring. Some reported that VAS more adequately measured symptom control when severity is low [20, 30]. Given that accuracy of symptom perception in children and adolescents shows a marked decrease when symptom severity elevates [27, 31], perhaps VAS may be more appropriate for those with intermittent to mild severity. Conversely, others provided evidence demonstrating VAS to be more useful in those with moderate to severe asthma [12] or airway obstruction (FEV1 <80%) [11]. Similarly, in another study [32] VAS scores reflected peak exploratory flow rates more adequately when children experienced actual symptoms compared to symptom-free times, hence supporting use of VAS only for moderate to severe cases of asthma. In order for VAS to be considered as a daily symptom monitoring tool, however, it is essential that it be sufficiently sensitive to wide range of symptom severity from low

to high. Although this study offers a glimpse of the possibility that VAS could capture the broader spectrum of symptom severity, further research is required to provide more conclusive evidence in a large sample of adolescents with differing levels of symptom control.

VAS is a simple and straightforward method to assess daily variations of asthma symptoms and the degrees of asthma control and airway obstruction. The simplicity makes the measure less dependent on users' literacy or attention capability and requires very little time to complete. Nonetheless, by allowing responses to vary along the line of continuum, VAS could adequately assess and quantify subtle changes in an individual's perception about a subjective attribute such as symptoms over time [9, 33]. Evidence that VAS effectively captured positive changes in asthma condition responding to bronchodilation [21] provides further support for the tool's usefulness in assessing treatment effects and preventing overestimation of asthma control through improved symptom perception [34]. These benefits render VAS a practical daily symptom assessment tool that can potentially maximize users' long-term compliance, through which symptom perception can be improved and asthma morbidity can be prevented or detected at an earlier stage.

This study is subject to several limitations germane to the study design. First, a small convenient sample of adolescents with asthma limits the generalizability of the findings. It is also worth mentioning that despite a large portion of our sample having been recruited from the emergency department, average VAS scores were generally low indicating mild symptoms albeit with wide variations. In USA, low income families tend to use the ED for usual asthma care or management that could have been handled at primary care practices [35, 36]. Hence, ED visits do not always suggest higher symptom severity in such populations. A large-scale study using a sample representing a broad spectrum of symptom severity is warranted to assure the replicability of our findings prior to broad clinical implementation of VAS as a symptom monitoring tool. Second, our relatively brief observation period (7 days) prevented us from establishing the validity of VAS for an extended period during which symptom variations may become more pronounced. Third, we were unable to assess changes in VAS scores responding to treatment (e.g., short-term vs. long-term medication) during the observation period. Strategically timed administration of VAS before and after specific medication is needed to assess the usefulness of VAS as a tool capturing treatment effect. In addition, it is unclear whether and how VAS could be used to discriminate different levels of asthma control corresponding to the EPR3 guidelines. Such information might have provided further compelling evidence supporting the clinical utility of VAS. Lastly, this study relied primarily on a symptom diary against which changes in VAS scores were compared. Given adolescents' poor perception of asthma symptoms [27, 37, 38], the sole reliance on the symptom diary may raise a question of validity. To date existing daily symptom monitoring is predominantly self-report in nature. Therefore, comparing one measure of self-report (symptom diary) to another (VAS) is justified to make a case for comparability between two monitoring methods. Nonetheless, further research, such as comparison with daily peak flow, is needed to augment the adequacy of VAS as a daily monitoring tool. Use of VAS in conjunction with peak flow monitoring has been reported to increase symptom perception and medication adherence [39]. Moreover, research establishing the criterion validity of VAS by examining its correlations with airway inflammation (e.g., nitric oxide) and disease burden (e.g., asthma exacerbation, acute healthcare utilization or school absenteeism) is warranted.

Despite the identified limitations, this study has important clinical implications. Demonstrated correlations between the VAS and a daily symptom assessment and an asthma control measure suggest that the single-item VAS be a viable alternative to multiple-question, multiple-choice methods. Inability to identify day to day variations in symptoms often presents challenges for appropriate clinical decision-making. Current retrospective recall methods or multi-item symptom diaries have been found inadequate, due to recall bias or poor patient compliance. In contrast, VAS is a simple, one-step solution to current practice of symptom monitoring, and has the potential to aid tracking daily symptoms in real time without substantially increasing burdens for patients.

Conclusions

Success in asthma management hinges on patients' competency to detect and respond to ever-changing symptom severity. Thus, it is crucial to have valid and simple methods of symptom assessment that can be readily incorporated into daily life with minimal patient or provider burden. This study supports VAS as the simplest possible symptom tracking tool for adolescents in ambulatory settings. Future research is warranted to determine the effectiveness and long-term sustainability of VAS and to explore the extent to which daily VAS would facilitate patients' self-management and providers' clinical decision making (e.g. medication management). To enhance daily accessibility and adherence, VAS digital versions downloaded onto smart phones can be considered. This will not only facilitate real time, long-term symptom tracking and increase its appeal to adolescent patients but also holds potential for integration with electronic medical records, enhancing clinical usefulness of VAS data.

Abbreviations

ACD: Asthma Control Diary; EPR3: Expert Panel Report 3; FEV1: forced expiratory volume in one second; SABA: short acting beta agonist; VAS: visual analogue scale; VAS-am: morning VAS; VAS-pm: evening VAS.

Authors' contributions

HR as the principal investigator of the study made substantial contributions to conception and design of the study as well as acquisition, analysis and interpretation of data. HR played a leading role in developing and writing the manuscript. MB made substantial contributions to data analysis and interpretation and drafting the analysis and results sections. JM was involved in data collection and contributed to drafting and critically reviewing the manuscript for important intellectual content. All authors read and approved the final manuscript.

Author details

[1] University of Rochester, School of Nursing, 601 Elmwood Avenue, Box SON, Rochester, NY 14642, USA. [2] Arizona State University, College of Nursing and Health Innovation, 500 N. 3rd Street, Phoenix, AZ 85004, USA.

Acknowledgements

The authors would like to acknowledge Ms. Eileen Fairbanks for coordinating the study including participant recruitment, data collection and database management.

Competing interests

The authors declare that they have no competing interests.

Funding

This study was supported by the National Institute of Health/National Institute for Nursing Research (NIH/NINR R01NR011169) for the implementation of the study protocol including data collection, analysis and interpretation.

References

1. Bruzzese JM, Bonner S, Vincent EJ, Sheares BJ, Mellins RB, Levison MJ, Wiesemann S, Du Y, Zimmerman BJ, Evans D. Asthma education: the adolescent experience. Patient Educ Couns. 2004;55(3):396–406.
2. Davis KJ, DiSantostefano R, Peden DB. Is Johnny wheezing? Parent-child agreement in the childhood asthma in America survey. Pediatr Allergy Immunol. 2011;22(1-Part-I):31–5.
3. National Heart, Lung, and Blood Institute. Expert Panel Report 3: guidelines for the diagnosis and management of asthma; 2007.
4. Bhogal S, Zemek R, Ducharme FM. Written action plans for asthma in children. Cochrane Database Syst Rev. 2006. doi:10.1002/14651858.CD005306.pub2.
5. Yawn BP, Brenneman SK, Allen-Ramey F, Cabana MD, Markson LE. Assessment of asthma severity and asthma control in children. Pediatrics. 2006;118(1):322–9.
6. Rhee H, Fairbanks E, Butz A. Symptoms, feelings, activities and medication use in adolescents with uncontrolled asthma: lessons learned from asthma diaries. J Pediatr Nurs. 2014;29(1):39–46.

7. Reznik M, Sharif I, Ozuah PO. Classifying asthma severity: prospective symptom diary or retrospective symptom recall? J Adolesc Health. 2005;36(6):537–8.

8. Hensley MJ, Chalmers A, Clover K, Gibson PG, Toneguzzi R, Lewis PR. Symptoms of asthma: comparison of a parent-completed retrospective questionnaire with a prospective daily symptom diary. Pediatr Pulmonol. 2003;36(6):509–13.

9. Wewers ME, Lowe NK. A critical review of visual analogue scales in the measurement of clinical phenomena. Res Nurs Health. 1990;13(4):227–36.

10. Ohta K, Jean Bousquet P, Akiyama K, Adachi M, Ichinose M, Ebisawa M, Tamura G, Nagai A, Nishima S, Fukuda T, Morikawa A, Okamoto Y, Kohno Y, Saito H, Takenaka H, Grouse L, Bousquet J. Visual analog scale as a predictor of GINA-defined asthma control. The SACRA study in Japan. J Asthma. 2013;50(5):514–21.

11. Tosca MA, Silvestri M, Olcese R, Pistorio A, Rossi GA, Ciprandi G. Breathlessness perception assessed by visual analogue scale and lung function in children with asthma: a real-life study. Pediatr Allergy Immunol. 2012;23(6):537–42.

12. Gupta D, Aggarwal AN, Subalaxmi MV, Jindal SK. Assessing severity of asthma: spirometric correlates with visual analogue scale (VAS). Indian J Chest Dis Allied Sci. 2000;42(2):95–100.

13. Halterman JS, Yoos HL, Kitzman H, Anson E, Sidora-Arcoleo K, McMullen A. Symptom reporting in childhood asthma: a comparison of assessment methods. Arch Dis Child. 2006;91(9):766–70.

14. Rhee H, Belyea MJ, Sterling M, Bocko MF. Evaluating the validity of an automated device for asthma monitoring for adolescents: correlational design. J Med Internet Res. 2015;17(10):e234.

15. Yoos HL, Kitzman H, McMullen A, Henderson C, Sidora K. Symptom monitoring in childhood asthma: a randomized clinical trial comparing peak expiratory flow rate with symptom monitoring. Ann Allergy Asthma Immunol. 2002;88(3):283–91.

16. Juniper EF, O'Byrne PM, Ferrie PJ, King DR, Roberts JN. Measuring asthma control. Clinic questionnaire or daily diary? Am J Respir Crit Care Med. 2000;162(4):1330–4.

17. American Thoracic Society. Standardization of spirometry. Am J Respir Crit Care Med. 1995;152:1107–36.

18. Carrieri VK, Kieckhefer G, Janson-Bjerklie S, Souza J. The sensation of pulmonary dyspnea in school-age children. Nurs Res. 1991;40(2):81–5.

19. Demoly P, Bousquet PJ, Mesbah K, Bousquet J, Devillier P. Visual analogue scale in patients treated for allergic rhinitis: an observational prospective study in primary care. Clin Exp Allergy. 2013;43(8):881–8.

20. Bijl-Hofland ID, Cloosterman SGM, Folgering HTM, Akkermans RP, van Schayck CP. Relation of the perception of airway obstruction to the severity of asthma. Thorax. 1999;54(1):15–9.

21. Tosca MA, Silvestri M, Rossi GA, Ciprandi G. Perception of bronchodilation assessed by visual analogue scale in children with asthma. Allergol Immunopathol (Madr). 2013;41(6):359–63.

22. Ciprandi G, Schiavetti I, Sorbello V, Ricciardolo FL. Perception of asthma symptoms as assessed on the visual analog scale in subjects with asthma: a real-life study. Respir Care. 2016;61(1):23–9.

23. Horak E, Grässl G, Skladal D, Ulmer H. Lung function and symptom perception in children with asthma and their parents. Pediatr Pulmonol. 2003;35(1):23–8.

24. Chen E, Oliver-Welker T, Rodgers D, Strunk RC. Developing measures of symptom perception for children with asthma. J Allergy Clin Immunol. 2007;119(1):248–50.

25. Yoos HL, McMullen A. Symptom perception and evaluation in childhood asthma. Nurs Res. 1999;48(1):2–8.

26. Mammen JR, Rhee H, Norton SA, Butz AM. Perceptions and experiences underlying self-management and reporting of symptoms in teens with asthma. J Asthma. 2017;54(2):143–52.

27. Rhee H, Belyea MJ, Elward KS. Patterns of asthma control perception in adolescents: associations with psychosocial functioning. J Asthma. 2008;45:600–6.

28. Cohen J. Statistical power analysis for the behavioral sciences. 2nd ed. New Jersey: Lawrence Erlbaum Associates; 1988.

29. Fritz GK, McQuaid EL, Spirito A, Klein RB. Symptom perception in pediatric asthma: relationship to functional morbidity and psychological factors. J Am Acad Child Adolesc Psychiatry. 1996;35(8):1033–41.

30. Mittal V, Khanna P, Panjabi C, Shah A. Subjective symptom perceptual accuracy in asthmatic children and their parents in India. Ann Allergy Asthma Immunol. 2006;97(4):484–9.

31. Yoos HL, Kitzman H, McMullen A, Sidora K. Symptom perception in childhood asthma: how accurate are children and their parents? J Asthma. 2003;40(1):27–39.

32. Yoos HL, McMullen A. Symptom monitoring in childhood asthma: how to use a peak flow meter. Pediatr Ann. 1999;28:31–9.

33. Patrician PA. Single-item graphic representational scales. Nurs Res. 2004;53(5):347–52.

34. Sanchez-Solis M. Could a visual analogue scale be useful, in real life, to manage children with asthma? Allergol Immunopathol (Madr). 2013;41(6):357–8.

35. Rand CS, Butz AM, Kolodner K, Huss K, Eggleston P, Malveaux F. Emergency department visits by urban African American children with asthma. J Allergy Clin Immunol. 2000;105(1 Pt 1):83–90.

36. Keet CA, Matsui EC, McCormack MC, Peng RD. Urban residence, neighborhood poverty, race/ethnicity, and asthma morbidity among children on Medicaid. J Allergy Clin Immunol. 2017. doi:10.1016/j.jaci.2017.01.036.

37. Britto MT, Byczkowski TL, Hesse EA, Munafo JK, Vockell AB, Yi MS. Overestimation of impairment-related asthma control by adolescents. J Pediatr. 2011;158(6):1028–30.

38. Fuhlbrigge AL, Guilbert T, Spahn J, Peden D, Davis K. The influence of variation in type and pattern of symptoms on assessment in pediatric asthma. Pediatrics. 2006;118(2):619–25.

39. Bheekie A, Syce JA, Weinberg EG. Peak expiratory flow rate and symptom self-monitoring of asthma initiated from community pharmacies. J Clin Pharm Ther. 2001;26(4):287–96.

15

The course of asthma during pregnancy in a recent, multicase–control study on respiratory health

A. Grosso[1]*[iD], F. Locatelli[2], E. Gini[1], F. Albicini[1], C. Tirelli[1], I. Cerveri[1] and A. G. Corsico[1]

Abstract

Background: Over the years it has been widely stated that approximately one-third of asthmatic women experience worsening of the disease during pregnancy. However, the literature has not been reviewed systematically and the meta-analytic reviews include old studies. This study aimed to examine whether the prevalence of worsening asthma during pregnancy is still consistent with prior estimate or it has been reduced.

Methods: A detailed Clinical Questionnaire on respiratory symptoms, medical history, medication, use of services, occupation, social status, home environment and lifestyle was administered to random samples of the Italian population in the frame of the Gene Environment Interactions in Respiratory Diseases (GEIRD) study. Only clinical data belong to 2.606 subjects that completed the clinical stage of the GEIRD study, were used for the present study.

Results: Out of 1.351 women, 284 self-reported asthma and 92 of them had at least one pregnancy. When we considered the asthma course during pregnancy, we found that 16 women worsened, 31 remained unchanged, 25 improved. Seven women had not the same course in the different pregnancies and 13 did not know. The starting age of ICS use almost overlaps with that of asthma onset in women with worsening asthma during pregnancy (19 years ± 1.4), unlike the other women who started to use ICS much later (30.3 years ± 12). In addition, the worsening of asthma was more frequent in women with an older age of onset of asthma (18 years ± 9 vs 13 years ± 10). Among women who completed the ACT during the clinical interview, the 50% of women who experienced worsening asthma during pregnancy (6/12) had an ACT score below 20.

Conclusion: Asthma was observed to worsen during pregnancy in a percentage much lower to that generally reported in all the previous studies. There is still room in clinical practice to further reduce worsening of asthma during pregnancy by improving asthma control, with a more structured approach to asthma education and management prepregnancy.

Keywords: Asthma control, Pregnancy, Inhaled corticosteroids

Background

Asthma is the most common respiratory disorder complicating pregnancy and it is associated with a range of adverse maternal and perinatal outcomes. Its prevalence among pregnant women varies among studies from 4 to 8% and appears to have increased over recent decades. Several studies have demonstrated that the use of inhaled corticosteroid (ICS) for the treatment of asthma does not affect fetal growth, and that maternal uncontrolled asthma has a greater impact on the fetus and placenta [1–3]. Even though asthma is a potentially serious medical condition and despite known risks of poorly controlled asthma during pregnancy, a large proportion of women still have a sub-optimal asthma control, principally due to concerns about surrounding risks of pharmacological agents, particularly ICS, and uncertainties regarding the effectiveness and the safety of different management strategies.

*Correspondence: amelia.grosso@gmail.com
[1] Division of Respiratory Diseases, IRCCS "San Matteo" Hospital Foundation, University of Pavia, Vaile C. Golgi 19, 27100 Pavia, Italy
Full list of author information is available at the end of the article

The course of asthma during pregnancy, evaluated in numerous retrospective and prospective studies over the years, has resulted to be variable. It has been stated that about one-third of asthmatic women experience worsening of the disease during pregnancy [4–7]. However, the literature has not been reviewed systematically and the meta-analytic reviews include old studies that vary in population characteristics such as asthma severity and treatment received. Many of these old studies have several methodologic inadequacy, such as low power or lack of control for confounders.

While a number of factors that may worsen asthma have been proposed in the literature, the mechanisms involved are largely undefined, and thus a woman's asthma course during pregnancy is often unpredictable [8].

The aim of our study was to examine whether the prevalence of worsening asthma during pregnancy is still consistent with prior estimates or it has been reduced. For this purpose, we used data of our population-based Gene-Environment Interactions in Respiratory Disease (GEIRD) study.

Methods

Study design

GEIRD is a multicase–control study on respiratory health, involving seven Italian centres. Cases and controls were identified through a two-stage screening process in pre-existing cohorts and in new random samples from the Italian general population.

In the first stage (2007–2010), eligible subjects were administered a screening questionnaire on respiratory symptoms. In the second stage (2008–2016) all the responders with symptoms suggestive of asthma, chronic obstructive pulmonary disease (COPD) or chronic bronchitis (CB) and a random sample of subjects without respiratory symptoms or with symptoms suggestive of rhinitis, were referred to clinical centres to undergo the "phenotypization" protocol. Protocol and descriptive characteristics of the GEIRD study are available on the web site http://www.geird.org [9].

Study population and procedures

For the present study we used clinical data belonging to 2606 subjects, who completed the stage 2 of the GEIRD study. Clinical data were obtained by means of a structured medical interview through the Clinical Questionnaire, a modification of the European Community Respiratory Health Survey (ECRHS) questionnaire (http://www.ecrhs.org) including detailed questions on respiratory symptoms, medical history, medication, use of services, occupation, social status, home environment and lifestyle. For the evaluation of regular ICS use and patient adherence to anti-asthmatic treatment the questions: *"Since the last survey have you used inhaled corticosteroids?"*, *"How old were you when you first started to use inhaled corticosteroids?"*, *"Have you used inhaled corticosteroids every year since the last survey?"*, *"If you are prescribed medicines for your breathing, do you normally take: A) all of the medicines? B) most of the medicines? C) some of the medicines? D) none of the medicines"* were used [10].

On the basis of the answers to the Clinical Questionnaire, a woman was considered to have asthma if she answered affirmatively to both questions: *"Have you ever had asthma?"* and *"Was this confirmed by a doctor?"*.

The asthma course during pregnancy was evaluated with the specific question: *"What happened to your asthma during your pregnancies? A) got better B) got worse C) stayed the same D) not the same for all pregnancies E) don't know"*.

Participants were considered to have allergic rhinitis if they answered positively to this question: *"Do you have any nasal allergies including hay fever?"*.

Atopy was assessed by skin prick tests (SPT). Individuals with at least one positive SPT were considered to be atopic. The allergens selected in all centres were *Cupressus arizonica, Graminacee mix Dermatophagoides pteronyssinus, Artemisia vulgaris, Dermatophagoides farina, Ambrosia artemisifolia, Alternaria tenuis, Parietaria Judaica, Dog dander, Corylus avellana, Cat hair, Olea europea, Betula verrucosa, Cladosporium herbarum* (ALK diagnostics, Denmark) (Mailing 1993).

In a subsample of 50 asthmatic women, we also evaluated the asthma control by means of the Asthma Control Test (ACT™). Patients assigned scores of 1–5 to each item, resulting in the following grading system: uncontrolled/partly controlled asthma with score ≤ 20; well controlled asthma with score > 20 [11]. These data refer to the time of the clinical interview and they cannot be used as an indicator of asthma control before pregnancy.

No clinical data before pregnancy are available.

Statistical analysis

Women who answered *"D) not the same (asthma) for all pregnancies"* were excluded from the statistical analyses. The sample who answered *"E) don't know"* was included in the group of those unchanged/improved asthma. The relationship of the main determinants of unchanged/improved asthma during pregnancy and worsened asthma during pregnancy was evaluated by Fisher's exact test for categorical variables and by Wilcoxon–Mann–Whitney non-parametric test for continuous variables. The statistical analyses were performed using Stata 14.0 (StataCorp, College Station, TX, USA).

Results

Out of 1351 women, 284 (mean age 44.4 ± 9) self-reported asthma and 92 of them had at least one pregnancy.

When we considered the asthma course during pregnancy, we found that 16 women worsened, 31 remained unchanged, 25 improved. Seven women had not the same course in the different pregnancies and 13 did not know.

Table 1 reports the results of the associations between considered factors and outcomes in the univariate analysis. Women who reported that the asthma was different from pregnancy to pregnancy were removed from the statistical analysis, because it was not possible to include it in either group, as there is no information on the number of pregnancies and on the course of asthma during each pregnancy. Instead, the sample who answered "don't know" was included in the group of those "improved" or

Table 1 **Characteristics of women with worsened asthma and women with not worsened asthma during pregnancy**

Characteristics	"Not worsened" asthmatics (n = 69)	"Worsened" asthmatics (n = 16)	p
Smoking status, n (%)			
Current smoker	13 (18.8)	3 (18.8)	1.0
Former/never smoker	56 (81.2)	13 (81.2)	
BMI category (kg/m²), n (%)			
< 18.5	3 (4.5)	0 (0.0)	0.710
18.5–24	44 (65.7)	12 (75.0)	
25–29	14 (2.9)	4 (25.0)	
> 30	6 (8.9)	0 (0.0)	
Asthmatic treatment adherence category, n (%)			
Null/poor	7 (19.0)	1 (7.7)	0.662
High/moderate	30 (81.4)	12 (92.3)	
Age of asthma onset (year), mean ± SD			
	13.3 ± 10.2	18.2 ± 9.5	0.09
Allergic rhinitis, n (%)			
No	14 (21.5)	3 (20.0)	0.602
Yes	51 (78.5)	12 (80.0)	
Atopy, n (%)			
No	10 (15.4)	2 (13.0)	0.602
Yes	55 (84.6)	13 (87.0)	
Starting age of anti-asthmatic drug use (year), mean ± SD			
	22.3 ± 15	19.3 ± 10.0	0.553
Starting age of ICS use (year), mean ± SD			
	30.3 ± 12	19 ± 1.4	0.2465
Regular ICS use, n (%)			
No	49 (71.0)	7 (44.0)	*0.046*
Yes	20 (29.0)	9 (56.0)	

Significant p value is highlighted in italic (p < 0.05)

ICS, inhaled corticosteroid; BMI, body mass index; p, values compared between groups

"unchanged" (N = 69). The reason is related to the fact that those who have no memory for a negative condition, most likely did not experience it. The worsening of asthma during pregnancy was significantly associated with a more regular use of ICS (p < 0.05). The starting age of ICS use almost overlaps with that of asthma onset in women with worsening asthma during pregnancy (19 years ± 1.4), unlike the other women who started to use ICS much later (30.3 years ± 12). In addition, the worsening of asthma was more frequent in women with an older age of onset of asthma (18 years ± 9 vs 13 years ± 10). Among 50 women who completed the ACT during the clinical interview, 16 (32%) showed uncontrolled/partially controlled asthma (score < 20). In particular, 50% of women who experienced worsening asthma during pregnancy (6/12) had ACT score below 20, versus 26% of those with no worsening asthma during pregnancy ("unchanged"/"improved"/"don't know" group). The percentage of women with a good treatment adherence was found to be higher in those with worsening asthma during pregnancy than in the other group, even if the difference was not statistically significant (respectively 92 and 81%).

When we considered smoking habits, BMI, presence of atopy and rhinitis, no statistically significant difference between the two groups was found in the univariate analysis.

Discussion

The main finding in the present analysis is that asthma was observed to worsen during pregnancy in a percentage much lower that the one generally reported in all the previous studies, 18.8% (16/85) versus 30%. A meta-analytic review of 14 studies, conducted before 1990, assessing changes in the course of asthma throughout pregnancy suggested that approximately one-third of pregnant asthmatic women experience a symptomatic improvement, one-third experience a worsening, and one-third remain the same [12]. In our knowledge, at present, there are only few published data recently collected and the use of heterogeneous methods, such as the subjective nature and different definitions of asthma symptoms and control, makes the comparison with the older studies difficult.

The worsening of asthma during pregnancy represented an important problem in the management of the disease, taking into account the increased risk for preterm delivery, low birth weight preeclampsia and Cesarean delivery. Some studies indicated that over one-third of women may discontinue their asthma medications during pregnancy, many without consulting their doctors and that only half of the pregnant women with asthma used their controller drugs regularly during pregnancy

[13, 14]. The undermedication of pregnant women with asthma may contribute to worsening of asthma symptoms in some women during pregnancy [15].

Over the past 20 years, there was an evolving understanding of heterogeneous airways disease, a broader evidence base, increasing interest in targeted treatment, and evidence about effective implementation approaches. Substantial advances have been made in knowledge about a wide range of new effective therapies and understanding of many important aspects of asthma care. In the past medication would not have included inhaled corticosteroids, which are a mainstay of treatment today. Inhaled corticosteroids are the treatment of choice for all levels of persistent asthma and asthma guidelines around the world strongly recommend that women continue their asthma medications during pregnancy to maintain adequate control [13].

It has been well documented that the course of asthma during pregnancy may be influenced by the various physiologic changes during pregnancy, as well as the severity of the pre-existing disease and that in general after delivery, asthma returns to the severity that was present before pregnancy [6, 7, 16, 17]. Our results indirectly confirm the influence of the severity of the disease in the asthma worsening that was present despite a more frequent regular use of ICS and a higher treatment adherence. A further confirmation comes from the result of a low ACT score in the subsample of 50 women.

Also, the age of asthma onset was higher in this group than in the other and it is well known that adult-onset asthma has a low remission rate, a worse prognosis and a poorer response to standard asthma treatment [18]; in general, asthma in adult-onset usually relates with severe types of the disease. The concomitant presence of rhinitis worsens the asthma control in these subjects, as shown by the Rhinasthma's score. The score was on average higher in asthmatics who reported worsening of the disease (31.36 ± 25.92), although the difference with the comparison group was not significant, probably because of the small number of cases. Differently from Grzeskowiak et al. no influence of smoking habits and BMI on worsening asthma during pregnancy was found in our sample.

Strengths and limits of the study

Strengths of our study include the use of data recently collected from more than 1300 women randomly drawn from the general population rather than from clinically selected groups, the collection of high quality data, the standardized questionnaires and protocol procedures. Nonetheless, our study has several limitations. The first weakness is the relatively limited number of cases, which also precludes the multivariate analysis on the factors

associated with the worsening of asthma during pregnancy. Another important limitation is that we fully rely on self-reported data. In addition, we have only data on asthma control and on use of ICS referred to the time of the clinical interview and not those before pregnancy.

Conclusion

The most interesting findings of this study are that: (1) the prevalence of asthma worsening during pregnancy is actually reduced compared to the past and (2) the worsening is significantly related to the severity of the disease, as indicated by the more regular use of ICS and by the presence of an ACT score below 20. There is still room in clinical practice to further reduce worsening of asthma during pregnancy by improving asthma control, with a more structured approach to asthma education and management pre-pregnancy.

Authors' contributions
AG and IC conceived and designed the study. AG and IC prepared a preliminary draft of the manuscript. FA, EG, CT and AG contributed to the data collection. FL performed statistical analysis. AGC contributed to the interpretation of data, revised the paper critically for important intellectual content. All authors read and approved the final manuscript.

Author details
[1] Division of Respiratory Diseases, IRCCS "San Matteo" Hospital Foundation, University of Pavia, Vaile C. Golgi 19, 27100 Pavia, Italy. [2] Unit of Epidemiology and Medical Statistics, Department of Diagnostics and Public Health, University of Verona, Verona, Italy.

Acknowledgements
Not applicable.

Competing interests
The authors declare that they have no competing interests.

Funding
The GEIRD project was funded by the Cariverona Foundation (Bando 2006), the Italian Ministry of Health (RF-2009-1471235), Chiesi Farmaceutici and the Italian Medicines Agency (AIFA). The funders had no role in study design, data collection and analysis, decision to publish, or preparation of the manuscript.

References
1. NAEPP expert panel report. Managing asthma during pregnancy: recommendations for pharmacologic treatment-2004 update. National Heart, Lung, and Blood Institute; National Asthma Education and Prevention Program Asthma and Pregnancy Working Group. J Allergy Clin Immunol. 2005;115:34–46.
2. Louik C, Schatz M, Hernández-Díaz S, Werler MM, Mitchell AA. Asthma in pregnancy and its pharmacologic treatment. Ann Allergy Asthma Immunol. 2010;105:110–7.
3. Grzeskowiak LE, Smith B, Roy A, Dekker GA, Clifton VL. Patterns, predictors

and outcomes of asthma control and exacerbations during pregnancy: a prospective cohort study. ERJ Open Res. 2016;2:00054–2015.

4. Charlton RA, Hutchison A, Davis KJ, de Vries CS. Asthma management in pregnancy. PLoS ONE. 2013;8(4):e60247.

5. Bain E, Pierides KL, Clifton VL, Hodyl NA, Stark MJ, Crowther CA, Middleton P. Interventions for managing asthma in pregnancy. Cochrane Database Syst Rev. 2014. https://doi.org/10.1002/14651858.CD010660.pub2.

6. Katz O, Sheiner E. Asthma and pregnancy: a review of two decades. Expert Rev Respir Med. 2008;2:97–107.

7. Gluck JC. The change of asthma course during pregnancy. Clin Rev Allergy Immunol. 2004;26:171.

8. Schatz M. Interrelationships between asthma and pregnancy: a literature review. J Allergy Clin Immunol. 1999;103(2 Pt 2):S330–6.

9. de Marco R, Accordini S, Antonicelli L, Bellia V, Bettin MD, Bombieri C, Bonifazi F, Bugiani M, Carosso A, Casali L, Cazzoletti L, Cerveri I, Corsico AG, Ferrari M, Fois AG, Lo Cascio V, Marcon A, Marinoni A, Olivieri M, Perbellini L, Pignatti P, Pirina P, Poli A, Rolla G, Trabetti E, Verlato G, Villani S, Zanolin ME, GEIRD Study Group. The gene-environment interactions in respiratory diseases (GEIRD) project. Int Arch Allergy Immunol. 2010;152(3):255–63.

10. Corsico AG, Cazzoletti L, de Marco R, Janson C, Jarvis D, Zoia MC, Bugiani M, Accordini S, Villani S, Marinoni A, Gislason D, Gulsvik A, Pin I, Vermeire P, Cerveri I. Factors affecting adherence to asthma treatment in an international cohort of young and middle-aged adults. Respir Med. 2007;101(6):1363–7 **Epub 2006 Dec 26**.

11. Braido F, Baiardini I, Menoni S, Gani F, Senna GE, Ridolo E, Schoepf V, Rogkakou A, Canonica GW. Patients with asthma and comorbid allergic rhinitis: is optimal quality of life achievable in real life? PLoS ONE. 2012;7(2):e31178.

12. Juniper EF, Newhouse MT. Effect of pregnancy on asthma: systematic review and meta-analysis. In: Schatz M, Zeiger RS, Claman HN, editors. Asthma and immunological diseases in pregnancy and early infancy. New York: Marcel Dekker; 1993. p. 223–50.

13. Lim A, Stewart K, Abramson MJ, Walker SP, George J. Multidisciplinary approach to management of maternal asthma (MAMMA [copyright]): the PROTOCOL for a randomized controlled trial. BMC Public Health. 2012;12:1094.

14. Yilmaz I, Erkekol FO, Celen S, Karaca MZ, Aydin O, Celik G, Misirligil Z, Mungan D. Does drug adherence change in asthmatic patients during pregnancy? Multidiscip Respir Med. 2013;8:38.

15. Kwon HL, Belanger K, Bracken MB. Effect of pregnancy and stage of pregnancy on asthma severity: a systematic review. Am J Obstet Gynecol. 2004;190:1201e10.

16. Schatz M, Dombrowski MP, Wise R, Thom EA, Landon M, Mabie W, Newman RB, Hauth JC, Lindheimer M, Caritis SN, Leveno KJ, Meis P, Miodovnik M, Wapner RJ, Paul RH, Varner MW, O'sullivan MJ, Thurnau GR, Conway D, McNellis D. Asthma morbidity during pregnancy can be predicted by severity classification. J Allergy Clin Immunol. 2003;112:283–8.

17. Mirzakhani H, O'Connor G, Bacharier LB, Zeiger RS, Schatz MX, Weiss ST, Litonjua AA. Asthma control status in pregnancy, body mass index, and maternal vitamin D levels. J Allergy Clin Immunol. 2017;140:1453–6.

18. de Nijs SB, Venekamp LN, Bel EH. Adult-onset asthma: is it really different? Eur Respir Rev. 2013;22(127):44–52.

16

A case series evaluating the serological response of adult asthma patients to the 23-valent pneumococcal polysaccharide vaccine

C. R. Laratta[1], K. Williams[2], D. Vethanayagam[1], M. Ulanova[2] and H. Vliagoftis[1,3*]

Abstract

Background: Asthma is an independent risk factor for invasive pneumococcal disease; however, the immune response of adult asthma patients to pneumococcal vaccination is unknown. We explore the serologic response of patients with moderate to severe asthma to the 23-valent pneumococcal polysaccharide vaccine (PPSV23).

Methods: Seventeen moderate to severe adult asthma patients that had not been vaccinated against pneumococcus over the 5 previous years were prospectively recruited from a tertiary care asthma clinic. Serum was analyzed for the presence of antibodies to five capsular polysaccharide (CP) antigens (6B, 9V, 19A, 19F, 23F) before and 4 weeks after PPSV23 vaccination.

Results: There was a wide variability in baseline anti-CP antibody concentrations. Other than for serotype 19A, our patients frequently have baseline anti-CP antibody concentrations below 1 µg/mL (35% for serotype 19F, 41% for serotypes 9V and 23F, and 59% for serotype 6B). All post-vaccination geometric mean antibody concentrations were significantly higher than baseline. In the 31 tests where the baseline antibody concentration was <1 µg/mL, 77.4% had at least a twofold increase post-vaccination. Despite this, a large proportion of post-vaccination anti-CP antibody concentrations remained <1 µg/mL (51.6% of tests). Nine patients had at least one anti-CP antibody concentration <1 µg/mL post-vaccination. There was no difference between these patients and the remaining eight patients in demographic or clinical variables.

Conclusions: Patients with moderate to severe asthma have variable baseline and low post-vaccination antibody concentrations to common CP antigens included in the PPSV23 vaccine. The clinical relevance of these observations remains to be determined since the threshold concentration in adults required for clinical protection from invasive pneumococcal disease is uncertain.

Keywords: Invasive pneumococcal disease, Vaccination, Pneumococcal polysaccharide vaccine, Serology, Antibodies, Asthma, Obstructive airways disease, Prevention, Capsular polysaccharide serotypes, Pneumococcal vaccine, PPSV23, Vaccine responsiveness, Corticosteroids

Background

Invasive pneumococcal disease (IPD) is a common cause of morbidity in adults, occurring at a rate of 9.1 and 9.7 cases per 100,000 people in the North America according to the Centers for Disease Control and Prevention ABCs report [1], and the Public Health Agency of Canada [2], respectively. Vaccinations with pneumococcal capsular polysaccharides (CP) reduce morbidity from IPD [3]. Bigham and colleagues reviewed cases of IPD in British Columbia in 2000, and identified that 89% of the serotypes causing IPD are included into the 23-valent pneumococcal polysaccharide vaccine (PPSV23) [4].

Adults with asthma are at higher risk of developing IPD than the general population [5]. Asthma is a chronic condition affecting as many as 15–20% of the population

*Correspondence: hari@ualberta.ca
[3] Division of Pulmonary Medicine, Department of Medicine, University of Alberta, Room 3-105 Clinical Sciences Building, 11350 83 Avenue, Edmonton, AB T6G 2G3, Canada
Full list of author information is available at the end of the article

in developed countries [6]; a population in whom reduction of morbidity and healthcare utilization through preventative measures is an important objective. The Public Health Agency of Canada recognizes asthma "as a high-risk condition warranting vaccination to prevent IPD" and recommends that "adults requiring medical attention for asthma in the last 12 months" should receive one dose of PPSV23 to prevent IPD [7]. These recommendations are similar to other North American guidelines regarding pneumococcal vaccination [8]; however, there remains uncertainty regarding the efficacy of pneumococcal immunization in this population.

Literature on the clinical or serological effect of vaccination in patients with asthma, or on the effects of asthma treatments on vaccination response is limited [9, 10]. In a recent Canadian study, the estimated number of patients with asthma that would need to be vaccinated to prevent one case of IPD may be as low as 246 in low-risk adults and 135 in high-risk adults [11]; however, a number of assumptions had to be used for this analysis as there are limited data specific to this population. Pneumococcal vaccination has been shown to decrease documented pneumococcal pneumonia-related hospitalizations in asthma patients, but have little difference on the risk of pneumonia [12]. Lee et al. [13] demonstrated that children and adolescents with asthma had lower baseline antibody concentrations prior to pneumococcal immunization than healthy children, but post-vaccination geometric mean concentrations (GMC) and the ability to achieve a twofold response were comparable to healthy children. Ohshima and colleagues [14] analyzed serological response to PPSV23 of 40 patients with chronic lung disease including 7 patients with asthma, but did not separately report the results of patients with asthma. Lahood et al. [15] studied pre- and post-vaccination antibody levels for serotypes 3, 7F, 9N, and 14, in a small group of steroid-dependent or non-steroid dependent asthma patients. They found that both groups were able to increase their antibody levels in response to PPSV23; no significant differences between the two groups were noted [15]. Clinical and serological markers of vaccine efficacy in patients with asthma have not yet been established for other respiratory vaccines, such as the influenza vaccine [16]. Limited studies have assessed the impact of high dose inhaled corticosteroid (ICS) therapy or oral corticosteroid therapy on vaccine response in other patient populations [17–19], and there is no data on any vaccine effectiveness with concomitant omalizumab treatment.

As the literature contains very little data on the immunogenicity of vaccination in asthma patients, we have examined baseline antibody concentrations to common pneumococcal serotypes in 17 adult asthma patients, and

studied the ability of PPSV23 to increase post-vaccination antibody concentrations. Importantly, we included moderate to severe asthma patients taking high-dose ICS therapy, oral corticosteroid therapy, or biologic therapy, as these patients are at the highest risk of IPD.

Methods

Patients and vaccination procedure

We prospectively evaluated the serological response to PPSV23 in a case series of patients with moderate to severe asthma. The study protocol was approved by the University of Alberta Health Research Ethics Board. All patients provided written informed consent. Nineteen patients attending the University of Alberta asthma clinics were enrolled between November 2011 and June 2014. For two enrolled patients, the attending physician questioned the diagnosis of asthma in follow-up visits, and these patients were subsequently excluded from analysis. Fourteen of the 17 patients met criteria for severe asthma as defined per the European Respiratory Society/American Thoracic Society guidelines for severe asthma [20]. Three patients were not using high dose inhaled corticosteroids when recruited and did not meet criteria for severe asthma. However, all these patients were on omalizumab and therefore had a prior diagnosis of moderate to severe asthma, since this is a requirement for treatment with omalizumab in Alberta. Therefore we report all the subjects as having moderate to severe asthma. Six patients had a smoking history. Co-morbid COPD was diagnosed in two of these six patients prior to recruitment. The other four were all under the age of forty, three had a smoking history of only 3–4 pack years and all 4 had no evidence of COPD on pulmonary function testing. One 27 year old non-smoker had a reduced diffusing capacity, but had a normal chest radiograph and no other respiratory diagnosis except from asthma. None of the patients had received the pneumococcal vaccine within the last 5 years. At the time of enrolment, serum was collected for determination of antibodies against pneumococcal CP antigens, and was stored at −70 °C until analysis. Following blood collection, the patient received the PPSV23 vaccine (Pneumovax 23, Merck Sharp & Dohme Corporation, USA) through an intramuscular injection. Three to six weeks later, the serum collection was repeated to follow the antibody response and the sera stored at −70 °C until analysis. Clinical data were obtained through chart review. Pulmonary function testing was performed according to previously published standards [21–23].

Determination of pneumococcal antibodies

Pre-vaccination and post-vaccination sera were analyzed for antibodies against the following serotype-specific CP antigens: 6B, 9V, 19A, 19F, 23F. Enzyme-linked immuno-sorbent assay (ELISA) was used to quantify antibodies as per previously published protocols [24]. The lower limit of detection was 0.01 µg/mL. Since there is no consensus with regards to immunological correlates of protection, the following sets of criteria were used to evaluate vaccine response: (a) a significant increase in GMC post-vaccination [25–29]; a twofold increase in antibody concentration [30–36], specifically for ≥ 2 serotype-specific antigens [30]; or (b) achieving a threshold of 0.35, 1, or 5 µg/mL [25–27, 30, 32, 37, 38].

Statistical analyses

Data for each patient were coded with a unique identifier. Continuous variables are shown as mean ± standard error of the mean for normally distributed data, and median ±interquartile range (IQR) or 95% confidence interval (CI) for data not normally distributed. The time interval between baseline and post-vaccination serological testing was missing for a single patient, and was included in the analysis as the maximum interval required by any other patient, which was 44 days. Serological measurements are shown as GMC or geometric mean fold rise with two-sided 95% CI. Log-transformed serological data were compared using paired t test after normality was confirmed using the Shapiro–Wilk normality test. Continuous variables were compared using the Mann–Whitney U test for unpaired data and Wilcoxon signed rank test for paired data. Categorical variables were compared using the Chi square test or Fisher's exact test. Pre-vaccination and post-vaccination sera GMCs were compared using a two-sample paired t-test after logarithmic transformation. Statistical analyses were performed using GraphPad Prism (GraphPad Prism version 5.00 for Windows, GraphPad Software, San Diego California USA, http://www.graphpad.com).

Results

Seventeen patients were included in the analysis, 53% males, mean age 47.4 ± 3.4 years (median 51 years, IQR 33–60 years), with a mean body mass index (BMI) 30.8 ± 1.8 kg/m². Patient demographics are outlined in Table 1. Thirteen patients were on high dose ICS therapy. Of the remaining 4 patients, all were on low to moderate dose ICS therapy with the addition of daily oral corticosteroid therapy (1 patient), or omalizumab (3 patients). No patient was smoking at the time of inclusion; however,

Table 1 Patient demographics

	Case series (n = 17)
Age in years	51 (IQR 33–60)
Male gender	9 (53%)
Body mass index (kg/m²)	30.8 ± 1.8
History of smoking	6 (35%)
Co-morbid chronic obstructive pulmonary disease	2 (12%)
FEV1[†] (% predicted)	67.3 ± 4.6
FVC[††] (% predicted)	90.8 ± 3.4
FEV1/FVC	60.9 ± 2.3
Taking high dose inhaled corticosteroid therapy	13 (76%)
Taking an additional controller agent	16 (94%)
Taking omalizumab therapy	3 (18%)
Taking daily systemic corticosteroid therapy	4 (24%)

[†] *FEV1* forced expiratory volume in one second

[††] *FVC* forced vital capacity

35% of patients had a history of smoking. Two patients had significant non-respiratory co-morbidities, i.e. type II diabetes mellitus and neuromuscular disease. Among 14 patients that had quantitative serum immunoglobulin evaluation, 13 had levels within normal limits, and one had IgA deficiency (0.58 g/L; normal range 0.70–4.00 g/L).

The mean time between vaccination and follow-up serological testing was 31.7 ± 2.3 days (minimum and maximum time was 16 and 44 days, respectively). Ten patients had at least one baseline serotype-specific antibody concentration <1 µg/mL (Table 2). For capsular antigens 6B and 23F, the anti-CP antibody concentrations were ≤ 0.35 µg/mL in 41 and 29% of the patients, respectively (Table 2). After vaccination with PPSV23, there was a significant increase in antibody GMCs against all CP antigens, and all post-vaccination antibody GMCs were >1 µg/mL (Table 3). Among all the serotype-specific antibodies, the lowest geometric mean fold rise was found for the serotype 19A; however, the baseline

Table 2 Number (%) of patients with baseline antibody levels below predefined thresholds of 0.35, 1.00, and 5.00 µg/mL

Pneumococcal serotype	Number of patients with baseline anti-CP antibody concentrations failing to achieve specified threshold concentration		
	≤0.35 µg/mL	<1.00 µg/mL	<5.00 µg/mL
6B	7 (41%)	10 (59%)	16 (94%)
9V	2 (12%)	7 (41%)	16 (94%)
19A	0 (0%)	1 (6%)	7 (41%)
19F	3 (18%)	6 (35%)	13 (76%)
23F	5 (29%)	7 (41%)	16 (94%)

Table 3 Response to pneumococcal vaccination in the overall cohort

Pneumococcal serotype	Serum samples	Anti-CP GMC[†] (95% CI) (µg/mL)	Mean fold rise (95% CI)
6B	Baseline	0.54 (0.21–1.38)	–
	Post-vaccination	2.13 (0.72–6.28)**	3.96 (1.70–9.22)
9V	Baseline	1.19 (0.64–2.22)	–
	Post-vaccination	4.25 (2.19–8.24)***	3.57 (1.84–6.93)
19A	Baseline	7.78 (4.2–14.4)	–
	Post-vaccination	15.34 (8.39–28.05)**	1.97 (1.26–3.09)
19F	Baseline	1.70 (0.64–4.56)	–
	Post-vaccination	7.76 (3.26–18.46)***	4.56 (2.26–9.21)
23F	Baseline	0.94 (0.43–2.08)	–
	Post-vaccination	3.81 (1.56–9.30)****	4.03 (2.35–6.92)

[†] *Anti-CP GMC* anti-capsular polysaccharide geometric mean concentration

** $p < 0.01$, *** $p < 0.001$, **** $p < 0.0001$

anti-19A antibody levels were the highest in comparison to other serotypes (i.e. 7.78 µg/mL, 95% CI 4.2–14.4 µg/mL).

The overall substantial increase in GMC was a result of a highly variable individual response to vaccination. Individual changes in anti-CP antibody concentrations post-vaccination for each patient are outlined in Fig. 1, organized by the baseline antibody levels of <1.00, 1.00–4.99, or ≥5.00 µg/mL. As can be seen in Fig. 1, the post-vaccination anti-CP antibody concentrations increased in some patients and decreased in others, and these changes were not consistent between serotypes. Fold change in serotype-specific antibody concentrations for each patient is shown in Fig. 2.

Although we tried to collect post vaccination serum 3–6 weeks after vaccination, we had some 6 subjects that came back outside this interval. In order to ensure that our findings are not accounted for by either a short or long interval between the vaccination and follow-up serology, we analyzed the data separately for those with follow-up blood collection less than 3 weeks or more than 6 weeks after vaccination. Notably, the three patients who had blood for determination of antibody concentrations collected less than 3 weeks (3 patients) or more that 6 weeks (3 patients) after vaccination all achieved a twofold increase to at least two antigens, and only one had antibody concentrations <1.00 µg/mL in the post-vaccination serum collection (capsular antigens 6B and 23F). The data for these three patients is shown in Additional file 1 under patient identifiers 9, 10, 12, 13, 16 and 17. Excluding these patients from the analyses did not change the results (data not shown).

The serological response of asthma patients to the PPSV23 was variable among patients as well as among serotype-specific antibodies within individual patients.

When a twofold rise in concentration was used as a marker of response, the majority of the patients responded to the vaccination, i.e. 13 out of the 17 patients (76.5%) mounted a twofold response to ≥2 antigens. Very high baseline antibody concentrations may have contributed to the inability of some patients to achieve a twofold rise in post-vaccination antibody concentrations. For example, in one patient, the anti-19A CP antibody level increased from 82.55 to 119.55 µg/mL, which is a 1.45-fold rise. Four patients mounted a twofold antibody increase to 0–1 antigens, 4 had a twofold response to 4 antigens, and 4 patients had a twofold response to all 5 antigens.

When achievement of a certain threshold concentration was used to determine the response to vaccination, the results were again highly variable. In Table 4, we summarize the antibody responses of patients who had a baseline antibody concentration below 1 µg/mL. Ten patients had at least one baseline anti-CP antibody concentration <1 µg/mL. After vaccination, nine patients had at least one anti-CP antibody concentration <1 µg/mL. Eight of the 9 patients in this group had a baseline antibody concentration <1 µg/mL, but the ninth patient had an anti-CP antibody concentration <1 µg/mL post-vaccination only (1.23 µg/mL at baseline and 0.30 µg/mL post-vaccination for the capsular antigen 6B). In these 9 patients, post-vaccination levels <1 µg/mL were detected against serotype 6B (7 patients), 9V (2 patients), 19F (3 patients), and 23F (4 patients). In the individuals with a baseline antibody concentration <1 µg/mL, only 19% of the serotype-specific antibodies increased to ≥5 µg/mL post-vaccination indicating that PPSV23 was able to induce a robust vaccine response in a minority of these patients.

Contingency analysis and logistical regression were used to determine whether any patient-related factors

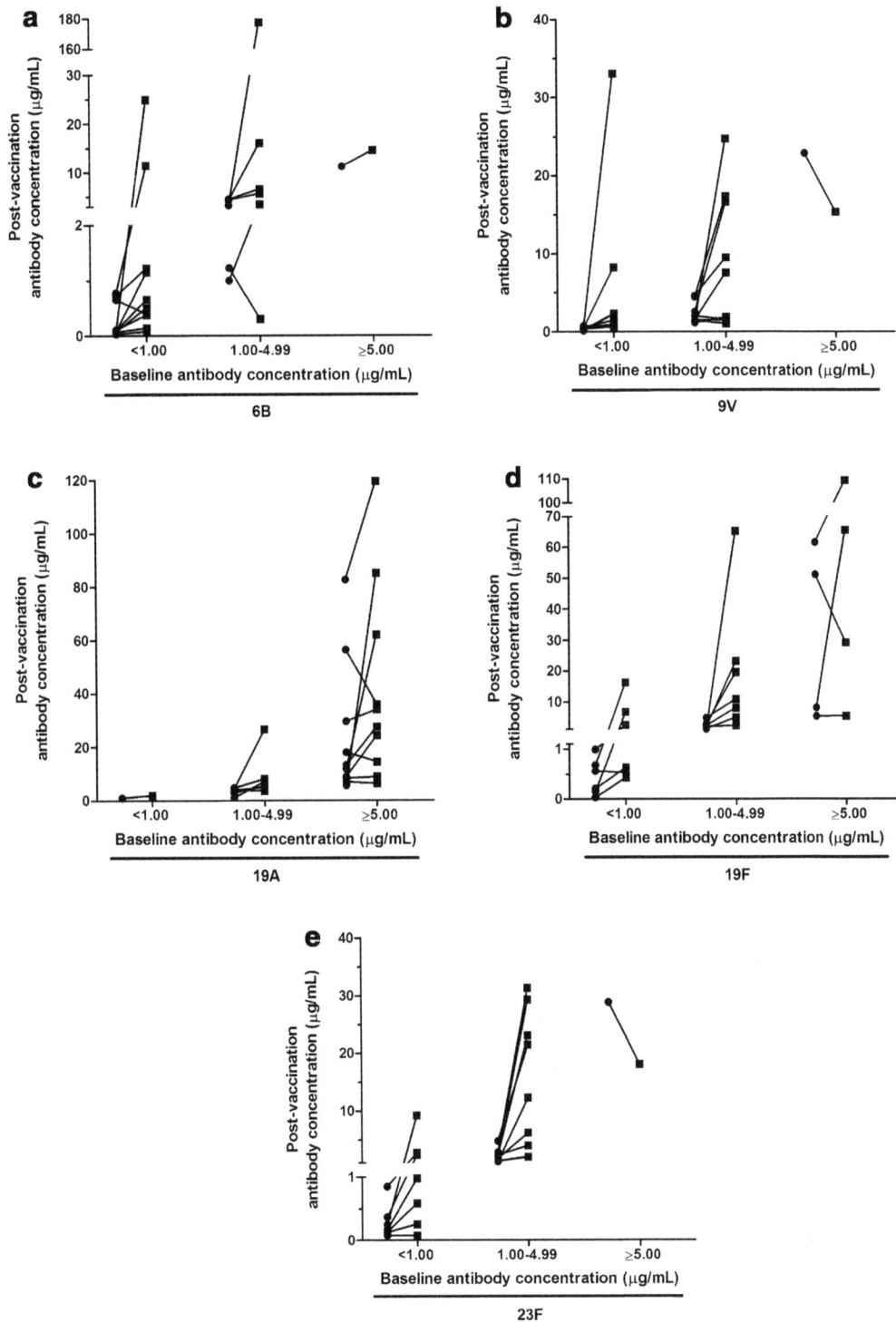

Fig. 1 Individual antibody responses to vaccination for capsular antigens **a** 6B, **b** 9V, **c** 19A, **d** 19F, **e** 23F. The patients are displayed in three categories: those who started with a baseline concentration <1 µg/mL, between 1 and 4.99 µg/mL, and ≥5 µg/mL

were associated with response to vaccination. There was no predilection for gender or age to affect response to immunization with PPSV23 within our case series; however, all patients included were younger than 65 years. The phenotype of asthma including timing of onset, or atopy as documented on skin prick testing,

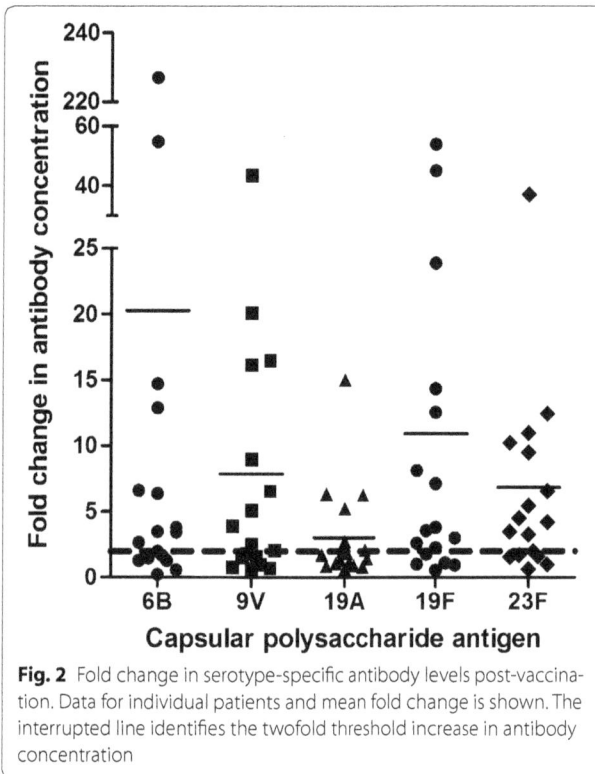

Fig. 2 Fold change in serotype-specific antibody levels post-vaccination. Data for individual patients and mean fold change is shown. The interrupted line identifies the twofold threshold increase in antibody concentration

peripheral eosinophil count, or IgE concentration was not associated with a response to vaccination. Obesity was not associated with vaccine response either. Treatment with biologics, high dose inhaled corticosteroid therapy, or systemic steroids, was not associated with the ability to mount a response to vaccination (data not shown). Similarly, there was no significant association between the presence of daily corticosteroid use or steroid burst in the last year with either the inability to mount a ≥twofold response in antibody concentrations to at least two capsular antigens [relative risk (RR) 0.70, 95% CI 0.13–3.85; p = 1.0], or to increase in the post-vaccination anti-CP antibody concentration to ≥1 μg/mL (RR 0.42, 95% CI 0.15–1.21; p = 0.15).

Discussion

Preventative strategies to reduce the impact of IPD in patients with asthma may have substantial impact on patient morbidity, with secondary gains in the form of reduced health care utilization and a decreased need for health care resources. This study presents pre- and post-vaccination antibody concentrations of adult patients with moderate to severe asthma immunized with PPSV23. In this population, baseline anti-CP GMCs are highly variable among both individuals and serotypes, consistent with previous findings in the general population, the elderly, and adults with chronic or immunosuppressive medical conditions [14, 26, 27, 31, 32, 34–36, 38–42]. Comparable baseline serologic data are limited to one study by Lahood et al. [15], that also reports highly variable baseline antibody concentrations in asthma patients. Of the serotype-specific antibodies included in our analysis, the highest baseline concentrations were found against serotype 19A, raising the possibility that asthma patients in our population may be exposed to this serotype in the community. Serotype 19A has been implicated as a cause of "replacement disease" following the introduction of 7-valent pneumococcal protein-conjugate vaccine (PCV) [43, 44].

A response to vaccination has been defined with a variety of methods in the literature, such as the ability to achieve a significant rise in GMC, fold rise in antibody concentration, or an antibody concentration threshold that is considered protective; however, interpretation of these data is complicated in that immunological correlates of protection have not been established for adults [45]. Antibody thresholds conferring clinical protection are likely to be serotype specific, as suggested from studies in children [46]. Published data on adult immunization with PPSV23 are of limited comparative value as the subjects are often populations with high prevalence of IPD, such as subjects with asplenia [36, 37]. The knowledge on serologic responses to PPSV23 in patients with asthma is very limited, with only two small studies available [13, 15]. Lee et al. [13] report a twofold rise in

Table 4 Response to vaccination of patients with baseline antibody concentrations of <1 μg/mL

Pneumococcal serotype	Twofold response to vaccination	Post-vaccination anti-CP[†] antibody concentration		
		≥0.35 μg/mL	≥1.00 μg/mL	≥5.00 μg/mL
6B (n = 10)	8	7	3	1
9V (n = 7)	5	7	5	2
19A (n = 1)	0	1	1	0
19F (n = 6)	5	5	3	2
23F (n = 7)	6	6	3	1

[†] *CP* capsular polysaccharide

antibodies in 41.6–87.5% of their 24 pediatric asthma patients after vaccination with PPSV23, which is comparable to our data. Absolute antibody concentrations from this study cannot be compared to our results because they were expressed as % of reference serum [13]. Lahood et al. [15] performed a study comparing 14 adult asthma patients on prednisone to 14 adult asthma patients not taking prednisone, and reported increases in antibody concentrations 4 weeks after vaccination with PPSV23 [15]. As they report post-vaccination antibody concentrations measured by a different immunoassay, their data cannot be directly compared to our results.

Our study suggests that patients with asthma may remain at risk of developing IPD after receiving vaccination with PPSV23, as they may not achieve an adequate antibody concentration threshold that confers clinical protection. Indeed, although the majority of our patients (13 out of 17) responded to immunization with a twofold increase in antibody concentrations to at least 2 antigens out of 5, 9 patients had at least one post-vaccination antibody concentration <1 μg/mL. In comparison, in an earlier study, 4–6 weeks post-PPSV23 immunization, most of healthy adults had the concentrations of serotype-specific pneumococcal antibody >1 μg/mL, i.e. 73 and 82% against the serotype 6B, 88 and 83% against 19F, and 85 and 85% against 23F, for subjects of 20–69 and ≥70 years of age, respectively [47].

Although interpretation of these findings is complicated by the fact that immunologic correlates of protection against IPD in adults are not well described, it has been demonstrated that non-immunocompromised 50–85 year old subjects who developed culture-verified pneumococcal pneumonia post PPSV immunization, failed to achieve a >1 μg/mL antibody concentration threshold for the infecting serotype [48]. These data support our suggestion that 9 out of 17 asthma patients in our study may remain at risk of pneumococcal infection.

Although this is a pilot study with a small number of participants, our report intends to draw attention to an urgent need to improve pneumococcal immunity in adults with moderate to severe asthma who are highly susceptible to IPD. In this category of patients, immunization with the pneumococcal polysaccharide vaccine may be insufficient for inducing protective immunity against S. pneumoniae. As an option, immunization with the conjugate protein pneumococcal vaccine (PCV13) should be considered because it may confer better immune response to the capsular polysaccharide antigens in certain categories of immunocompromised adults [49–51]. In Canada, PCV13 has recently been approved for immunization of immunocompromised adults, including subjects with primary immunodeficiency, malignant neoplasms, hematopoietic stem cell, solid organ, or

islet transplantation, treatment with immunosuppressive therapy, and HIV-infection (Canadian Immunization Guide). However, with regards to using PCV13 for immunization of adults it is important to consider that it contains only 13 capsular polysaccharides as compared to 23 in PPSV23, and was designed to primarily target the most important pediatric S. pneumoniae serotypes. More research is needed to develop optimal immunization strategy for asthma patients, in particular, to determine the prevalence of various S. pneumoniae serotypes in IPD and pneumococcal pneumonia in this group of patients and to address the impact of various asthma treatments on immune response to pneumococcal immunization.

There are several limitations to this study, including a small number of asthma patients, and a risk of selection bias, given that we did not enrol consecutive patients from our asthma clinic. In addition, an interval between pre- and post-immunization samples varied among the participants although this unlikely affected our results, considering that the half-life of IgG is approximately 4 weeks [52], and the majority of studies of the response to PPSV23 vaccination in various populations report serologic testing between 25 and 46 days post-immunization [25, 30, 38, 51, 53, 54]. In addition, exclusion of participants with short or long intervals between pre- and post-vaccination evaluation of antibody concentrations did not change the results of our analysis. In our study, we did not address the functional antibody activity, which would require an opsonophagocytic assay. Finally, the lack of a healthy control group for direct comparison of immune responses to immunization is a limitation of this study. However, the response of healthy adults to PPSV23 has been previously reported by several other studies [55]. One of the advantages of our study is that it is prospective in nature. This study is also important in that it explores vaccination in a population that may derive significant benefit from optimized protection against IPD, and in whom optimization of preventative therapy may result in large gains in terms of health-care utilization and resource allocation.

Conclusions

While many adult patients with asthma are able to generate at least a twofold increase in antibody concentrations in response to immunization, the majority of patients had at least one post-vaccination anti-CP antibody concentration <1 μg/mL, and may not be achieving a threshold associated with clinical protection against IPD. The clinical relevance of these observations remains to be determined since the threshold concentration in adults required for clinical protection from IPD is unknown. Further research is required to determine if PPSV23 or other pneumococcal vaccines are capable of inducing adequate post-vaccination anti-CP antibody concentrations that confer clinical protection. The timing of vaccination in this patient population should also be studied, as high baseline antibody concentrations to serotype 19A in our population may indicate frequent exposure to this serotype. Further research into these questions is required in order to optimize recommendations to prevent IPD in this at-risk population.

Abbreviations

IPD: invasive pneumococcal disease; CP: capsular polysaccharide; PPSV23: 23-valent pneumococcal polysaccharide vaccine; GMC: geometric mean concentration; IQR: interquartile range; CI: confidence interval; BMI: body mass index; FEV1: forced expiratory volume in one second; FVC: forced vital capacity; PCV: pneumococcal protein-conjugate vaccine.

Authors' contributions

CL contributed to data collection, analysis and drafting the manuscript. KW and MU contributed to data collection, data analysis and manuscript preparation. DV contributed to data collection and manuscript preparation. HV contributed to data collection, analysis and manuscript preparation. All authors read and approved the final manuscript.

Author details

[1] Pulmonary Research Group, Department of Medicine, University of Alberta, Edmonton, AB, Canada. [2] Medical Sciences Division, Northern Ontario School of Medicine, Lakehead University Campus, Thunder Bay, ON, Canada. [3] Division of Pulmonary Medicine, Department of Medicine, University of Alberta, Room 3-105 Clinical Sciences Building, 11350 83 Avenue, Edmonton, AB T6G 2G3, Canada.

Acknowledgements

We thank Dr. Maria Ospina, Ph.D., for reviewing the methods used for data analysis.

Competing interests

C. Laratta, K. Williams, D. Vethanayagam, and H. Vliagoftis have no competing interests related to the content of this manuscript. M. Ulanova has received an investigator-initiated research grant from Pfizer, but this funding was not used for this project.

Funding

The study was funded by grants from the National Sanitarium Association and Canadian Institutes of Health Research to H. Vliagoftis.

References

1. Centers for Disease Control and Prevention Active Bacterial Core Surveillances. ABCs report: *Streptococcus pneumoniae*, 2014. 2016. Available at http://www.cdc.gov/abcs/reports-findings/survreports/spneu14.html. Accessed 19 June 2016.

2. Public Health Agency of Canada. Immunization and vaccines. Invasive pneumococcal disease. 2016. Available at http://www.phac-aspc.gc.ca/im/vpd-mev/pneumococcal-pneumococcie/professionals-professionnels-eng.php. Accessed 19 June 2016.

3. Davis SM, Deloria-Knoll M, Kassa HT, O'Brien KL. Impact of pneumococcal conjugate vaccines on nasopharyngeal carriage and invasive disease among unvaccinated people: review of evidence on indirect effects. Vaccine. 2013;32(1):133–45.

4. Bigham M, Patrick DM, Bryce E, Champagne S, Shaw C, Wu W, et al. Epidemiology, antibiotic susceptibility, and serotype distribution of Streptococcus pneumoniae associated with invasive pneumococcal disease in British Columbia- a call to strengthen public health pneumococcal immunization programs. Can J Infec Dis Med Microbiol. 2003;14(5):261–6.

5. Boikos C, Quach C. Risk of invasive pneumococcal disease in children and adults with asthma: a systematic review. Vaccine. 2013;31(42):4820–6.

6. Subbarao P, Mandhane PJ, Sears MR. Asthma: epidemiology, etiology and risk factors. Can Med Assoc J. 2009;181(9):E181–90.

7. Public Health Agency of Canada: Infectious Diseases. National Advisory Committee on Immunization. Update on the use of pneumococcal vaccines: addition of asthma as a high-risk condition. 2014. Available at http://www.phac-aspc.gc.ca/naci-ccni/acs-dcc/2014/pvaa-vaaa_0414-eng.php. Accessed 19 June 2016.

8. Nuorti J, Whitney C. Updated recommendations for prevention of invasive pneumococcal disease among adults using the 23-valent pneumococcal polysaccharide vaccine (PPSV23). MMWR Recomm Rep. 2010;59(34):1102–6.

9. Pesek R, Lockey R. Vaccination of adults with asthma and COPD. Allergy. 2011;66(1):25–31.

10. Ochoa-Gondar O, Vila-Corcoles A, Ansa X, Rodriguez-Blanco T, Salsench E, de Diego C, et al. Effectiveness of pneumococcal vaccination in older adults with chronic respiratory diseases: results of the EVAN-65 study. Vaccine. 2008;26(16):1955–62.

11. Okapuu JM, Chétrit E, Lefebvre B, Quach C. How many individuals with asthma need to be vaccinated to prevent one case of invasive pneumococcal disease? Can J Infect Dis Med Microbiol. 2014;25(3):147–50.

12. Lee TA, Weaver FM, Weiss KB. Impact of pneumococcal vaccination on pneumonia rates in patients with COPD and asthma. J Gen Intern Med. 2007;22(1):62–7.

13. Lee H-J, Kang J-H, Henrichsen J, Konradsen HB, Jang S-H, Shin H-Y, et al. Immunogenicity and safety of a 23-valent pneumococcal polysaccharide vaccine in healthy children and in children at increased risk of pneumococcal infection. Vaccine. 1995;13(16):1533–8.

14. Ohshima N, Nagai H, Matsui H, Akashi S, Makino T, Akeda Y, et al. Sustained functional serotype-specific antibody after primary and secondary vaccinations with a pneumococcal polysaccharide vaccine in elderly patients with chronic lung disease. Vaccine. 2014;32(10):1181–6.

15. Lahood N, Emerson SS, Kumar P, Sorensen RU. Antibody levels and response to pneumococcal vaccine in steroid-dependent asthma. Ann Allergy. 1993;70(4):289–94.

16. Cates CJ, Rowe BH. Vaccines for preventing influenza in people with asthma. Cochrane Database Syst Rev. 2013;2:CD000364.

17. Hanania NA, Sockrider M, Castro M, Holbrook JT, Tonascia J, Wise R, et al. Immune response to influenza vaccination in children and adults with asthma: effect of corticosteroid therapy. J Allergy Clin Immunol. 2004;113(4):717–24.

18. de Roux A, Marx A, Burkhardt O, Schweiger B, Borkowski A, Banzhoff A, et al. Impact of corticosteroids on the immune response to a MF59-adjuvanted influenza vaccine in elderly COPD-patients. Vaccine. 2006;24(10):1537–42.

19. Russell AF, Parrino J, Fisher CL Jr, Spieler W, Stek JE, Coll KE, et al. Safety, tolerability, and immunogenicity of zoster vaccine in subjects on chronic/maintenance corticosteroids. Vaccine. 2015;33(27):3129–34.

20. Chung KF, Wenzel SE, Brozek JL, Bush A, Castro M, Sterk PJ, et al. International ERS/ATS guidelines on definition, evaluation and treatment of severe asthma. Eur Resp J. 2014;43:343–73.

21. Miller MR, Hankinson J, Brusasco V, Burgos F, Casaburi R, Coates A, et al. Standardisation of spirometry. Eur Respir J. 2005;26(2):319–38.

22. MacIntyre N, Crapo RO, Viegi G, Johnson DC, van der Grinten CPM, Brusasco V, et al. Standardisation of the single-breath determination of carbon monoxide uptake in the lung. Eur Respir J. 2005;26(4):720–35.

23. Wanger J, Clausen JL, Coates A, Pedersen OF, Brusasco V, Burgos F, et al. Standardisation of the measurement of lung volumes. Eur Respir J. 2005;26(3):511–22.

24. Wernette CM, Frasch CE, Madore D, Carlone G, Goldblatt D, Plikaytis B, et al. Enzyme-linked immunosorbent assay for quantitation of human antibodies to pneumococcal polysaccharides. Clin Diagn Lab Immunol. 2003;10(4):514–9.

25. Hammitt LL, Bulkow LR, Singleton RJ, Nuorti JP, Hummel KB, Miernyk KM, et al. Repeat revaccination with 23-valent pneumococcal polysaccharide vaccine among adults aged 55–74 years living in Alaska: no evidence of hyporesponsiveness. Vaccine. 2011;29(1):2287–95.

26. Manoff SB, Liss C, Caulfield MJ, Marchese RD, Silber J, Boslego J, et al. Revaccination with a 23-valent pneumococcal polysaccharide vaccine induces elevated and persistent functional antibody responses in adults aged 65≥ years. J Infect Dis. 2010;201(4):525–33.

27. Musher DM, Manoff SB, Liss CL, Marchese RD, Raab J, et al. Antibody persistence ten years after first and second doses of 23-valent pneumococcal polysaccharide vaccine, and immunogenicity and safety of second and third doses in older adults. Hum Vaccin. 2011;7(9):919–28.

28. Forstner C, Plefka S, Tobudic S, Winkler HM, Burgmann K, Burgmann H. Effectiveness and immunogenicity of pneumococcal vaccination in splenectomized and functionally asplenic patients. Vaccine. 2012;30(37):5449–52.

29. Schenkein JG, Park S, Nahm MH. Pneumococcal vaccination in older adults induces antibodies with low opsonic capacity and reduced antibody potency. Vaccine. 2008;26(43):5521–6.

30. Brandão AP, de Oliveira TC, de Cunto Brandileone MC, Gonçalves JE, Yara TI, Simonsen V. Persistence of antibody response to pneumococcal capsular polysaccharides in vaccinated long term-care residents in Brazil. Vaccine. 2004;23(6):762–8.

31. Musher DM, Manof SB, Liss C, McFetridge RD, Marchese RD, Bushnell B, et al. Safety and antibody response, including antibody persistence for 5 years, after primary vaccination or revaccination with pneumococcal polysaccharide vaccine in middle-aged and older adults. J Infect Dis. 2010;201(4):516–24.

32. Tobudic S, Plunger V, Sunder-Plassmann G, Riegersperger M, Burgmann H. Randomized, single blind, controlled trial to evaluate the prime-boost strategy for pneumococcal vaccination in renal transplant recipients. PLoS ONE. 2012;7(9):e46133.

33. Waites KB, Canupp KC, Chen YY, DeVivo MJ, Nahm MH. Revaccination of adults with spinal cord injury using the 23-valent pneumococcal polysaccharide vaccine. J Spinal Cord Med. 2008;31(1):53–9.

34. Jackson LA, Neuzil KM, Nahm MH, Whitney CG, Yu O, Nelson JC, et al. Immunogenicity of varying dosages of 7-valent pneumococcal polysaccharide-protein conjugate vaccine in seniors previously vaccinated with 23-valent pneumococcal polysaccharide vaccine. Vaccine. 2007;25(20):4029–37.

35. Ridda I, MacIntyre CR, Lindley R, Gao Z, Sullivan JS, Yuan FF, et al. Immunological responses to pneumococcal vaccine in frail older people. Vaccine. 2009;27(10):1628–36.

36. Stanford E, Print F, Falconer M, Lamden K, Ghebrehewet S, Phin N, et al. Immune response to pneumococcal conjugate vaccination in asplenic individuals. Human Vaccines. 2009;5(2):85–91.

37. Meerveld-Eggink A, de Weerdt O, van Velzen-Blad H, Biesma DH, Rijkers GT. Response to conjugate pneumococcal and Haemophilus influenzae type b vaccines in asplenic patients. Vaccine. 2011;29(4):675–80.

38. Ho Y-L, Brandão AP, de Cunto Brandileone MC, Lopes MH. Immunogenicity and safety of pneumococcal conjugate polysaccharide and free polysaccharide vaccines alone or combined in HIV-infected adults in Brazil. Vaccine. 2013;31(37):4047–53.

39. Malley R, Lipsitch M, Bogaert D, Thompson CM, Hermans P, Watkins AC, et al. Serum antipneumococcal antibodies and pneumococcal colonization in adults with chronic obstructive pulmonary disease. J Infect Dis. 2007;196(6):928–35.

40. Serpa JA, Valayam J, Musher DM, Rossen RD. Pirofski L-a, Rodriguez-Barradas MC. VH3 antibody response to immunization with pneumococcal polysaccharide vaccine in middle-aged and elderly persons. Clin Vaccine Immunol. 2011;18(3):362–6.

41. Elberse KEM, de Greeff SC, Wattimena N, Chew W, Schot CS, van de Pol JE, et al. Seroprevalence of IgG antibodies against 13 vaccine Streptococcus pneumoniae serotypes in the Netherlands. Vaccine. 2011;29(5):1029–35.

42. Macintyre CR, Ridda I, Gao Z, Moa AM, McIntyre PB, Sullivan JS, et al. A randomized clinical trial of the immunogenicity of 7-valent pneumococcal conjugate vaccine compared to 23-valent polysaccharide vaccine in frail, hospitalized elderly. PLoS ONE. 2014;9(4):e94578.

43. Esposito S, Principi N. Pneumococcal vaccines and the prevention of community-acquired pneumonia. Pulm Pharmacol Ther. 2015;32:124–9.

44. Lynch JPI, Zhanel GG. Streptococcus pneumoniae: epidemiology and risk factors, evolution of antimicrobial resistance, and impact of vaccines. Curr Opin Pulm Med. 2010;16(3):217–25.

45. Balmer P, Cant AJ, Borrow R. Anti-pneumococcal antibody titre measurement: what useful information does it yield? J Clin Pathol. 2007;60(4):345–50.

46. Andrews NJ, Waight PA, Burbidge P, Pearce E, Roalfe L, Zancolli M, et al. Serotype-specific effectiveness and correlates of protection for the 13-valent pneumococcal conjugate vaccine: a postlicensure indirect cohort study. Lancet Infect Dis. 2014;14(9):839–46.

47. Musher DM, Sampath R, Rodriguez-Barradas MC. The potential role for protein-conjugate pneumococcal vaccine in adults: what is the supporting evidence? Clin Infect Dis. 2011;52(5):633–40.

48. Ortqvist A, Henckaerts I, Hedlund J, Poolman J. Non-response to specific serotypes likely cause for failure to 23-valent pneumococcal polysaccharide vaccine in the elderly. Vaccine. 2007;25:2445–50.

49. Musher DM, Groover JE, Graviss EA, Baughn RE. The lack of association between aging and postvaccination levels of IgG antibody to capsular polysaccharides of Streptococcus pneumoniae. Clin Infect Dis. 1996;22:165–7.

50. de Roux A, Schmöele-Thoma B, Siber GR, Hackell JG, Kuhnke A, Ahlers N, et al. Comparison of pneumococcal conjugate polysaccharide and free polysaccharide vaccines in elderly adults: conjugate vaccine elicits improved antibacterial immune responses and immunological memory. Clin Infect Dis. 2008;46(7):1015–23.

51. Dransfield MT, Nahm MH, Han MK, Harnden S, Criner GJ, Martinez FJ, et al. Superior immune response to protein-conjugate versus free pneumococcal polysaccharide vaccine in chronic obstructive pulmonary disease. Am J Respir Crit Care Med. 2009;180(6):499–505.

52. Mankarious S, Lee M, Fischer S, Pyun KH, Ochs HD, Oxelius VA, et al. The half-lives of IgG subclasses and specific antibodies in patients with primary immunodeficiency who are receiving intravenously administered immunoglobulin. J Lab Clin Med. 1988;112(5):634–40.

53. Abzug MJ, Song LY, Levin MJ, Nachman SA, Borkowsky W, Pelton SI. Antibody persistence and immunologic memory after sequential pneumococcal conjugate and polysaccharide vaccination in HIV-infected children on highly active antiretroviral therapy. Vaccine. 2013;31(42):4782–90.

54. Cherif H, Landgren O, Konradsen HB, Kalin M, Björkholm M. Poor antibody response to pneumococcal polysaccharide vaccination suggests increased susceptibility to pneumococcal infection in splenectomized patients with hematological diseases. Vaccine. 2006;24(1):75–81.

55. Goldblatt D, Southern J, Andrews N, Ashton L, Burbidge P, Woodgate S, et al. The immunogenicity of 7-valent pneumococcal conjugate vaccine versus 23-valent polysaccharide vaccine in adults aged 50-80 years. Clin Infect Dis. 2009;49:1318–25.

17

A multi-stakeholder perspective on asthma care in Canada: findings from a mixed methods needs assessment in the treatment and management of asthma in adults

Suzanne Murray[1], Sara Labbé[1*] ⓘ, Alan Kaplan[2], Kristine Petrasko[3] and Susan Waserman[4]

Abstract

Background: Although several aspects of asthma care have been identified as being sub-optimal in Canada, such as patient education, practice guideline adoption, and access to care, there remains a need to determine the extent to which these gaps remain, so as to investigate their underlying causes, and potential solutions.

Methods: An ethics-approved mixed methods educational needs assessment was conducted in four Canadian provinces (Alberta, British Columbia, Ontario, and Quebec), combining a qualitative phase (45-min semi-structured interviews with community-based healthcare providers and key stakeholders) and a quantitative phase (15-min survey, healthcare providers only).

Results: A total of 234 participants were included in the study, 44 in semi-structured interviews and 190 in the online survey. Five clinical areas were reported to be suboptimal by multiple categories of participants, and specific causes were identified for each. These areas included: Integration of guidelines into clinical practice, use of spirometry, individualisation of asthma devices to patient needs, emphasis on patient adherence and self-management, and clarity regarding roles and responsibilities of different members of the asthma healthcare team. Common causes for gaps in all these areas included suboptimal knowledge amongst healthcare providers, differing perceptions on the importance of certain interventions, and inadequate communication between healthcare providers.

Conclusions: This study provides a better understanding of the specific causes underlying common gaps and challenges in asthma care in Canada. This information can inform future continuing medical education, and help providers in community settings obtain access to adequate materials, resources, and training to support optimal care of adult patients with asthma.

Keywords: Needs assessment, Asthma, Continuing medical education, Mixed-methods, Clinical challenges, Clinical practice, Guidelines

*Correspondence: labbes@axdevgroup.com
[1] AXDEV Group Inc., 210-8, Place du Commerce, Brossard, QC J4W 3H2, Canada
Full list of author information is available at the end of the article

Background

The prevalence of asthma in Canadian adults has more than tripled over the last three decades, but remains stable since 2004 with a current prevalence of 8.1%, affecting an estimated 2.4 million Canadians [1]. Several aspects of asthma care and management in Canada have previously been identified to be sub-optimal, specifically in relation to patient education, adoption of practice guidelines by healthcare providers, and issues specific to the structure and regulations of the different provincial healthcare systems [2–4]. A 2006 Canadian survey of patients and physicians demonstrated a lack of patient understanding of controlled vs. uncontrolled asthma, and inadequate use of Canadian asthma guidelines by physicians [4]. Poor inhaler technique had also been identified as an important contributor to decreased patient adherence, and sub-optimal asthma control [3]. More recently, a questionnaire was developed to assess family physicians' integration of the Canadian asthma guidelines into practice, and revealed that, despite guideline recommendations, there was a significant lack of education provided to patients [2]. From a systems perspective, lack of access to spirometry testing has been reported as an important barrier to accurate diagnosis and monitoring of asthma [5, 6].

Direct and indirect impacts of asthma have been well documented in the literature for the past two decades, and include significantly reduced patient quality of life, work absenteeism, and substantial healthcare and productivity costs [7–9]. In addition, uncontrolled asthma is responsible for the death of over 200 adults Canadians each year (228 in 2009 [10]), highlighting the importance of investigating potential contributors to sub-optimal care in asthma.

Although multiple barriers have been identified in Canada in the last 20 years, it is not known to what extent these barriers currently remain. In addition, the precise causes of these barriers are often not investigated, limiting the effectiveness of potentially corrective interventions. A previous international study, conducted by a group of researchers that included co-authors SM and SW, compared the state of asthma care in 4 countries (Canada, France, Germany and the United Kingdom) [11] and identified four main challenges: (1) awareness and understanding of asthma including severe asthma, (2) diagnosis of severe asthma, (3) new treatments and personalized medicine, (4) referral process and collaboration between primary care and specialty care.

Study rationale and objectives

To determine the extent to which previously identified gaps and barriers in adult asthma care still exist, as well as their underlying causes and potentially new challenges,

an in-depth mixed methods educational needs assessment was conducted. An educational needs assessment consists of a systematic investigation of how "what is" differs from "what should be", in order to identify the educational needs of a defined population [12]. This study collected the perspectives of community-based (i.e. non-academic) healthcare providers and other key stakeholders from the four largest provinces of Canada (Alberta, British Columbia, Ontario, and Quebec). The objectives of this study were to identify the challenges faced within the Canadian healthcare system, their causes, and to recommend interventions that could bridge these care gaps and ultimately improve patients' asthma care.

Methods

Overview of the mixed methods approach

This Canadian needs assessment used a mixed methods approach which consisted of collecting data through two consecutive phases; a qualitative phase followed by a quantitative phase. The qualitative phase consisted of semi-structured interviews. The qualitative findings were used to design the quantitative online survey. Triangulation of data sources (different categories of participants) and data collection methods (interviews, survey) were used to increase validity of findings [13]. A mixed methods study design allows the benefit of two types of data collection: the depth, breadth and exploratory nature of qualitative methodology, and the precision and analytic power of quantitative methodology [14].

Recruitment

Potential participants were identified mainly through professional listings purchased from independent (not pharmaceutical industry-related) organization in compliance with the ESOMAR/ICC International Code on Market, Opinion and Social Research and Data Analytics [15]. Other recruitment methods included snowball sampling, which consists of asking initial participants to refer potential participants from their own social network [16]. Invitations to participate in the telephone interviews (phase 1) were sent via email, which included a link to a secure website that provided study details, screening questions, and an informed consent agreement. Eligible individuals who consented to participate were then redirected to an availability form to schedule their interviews. Recruitment for telephone interviews closed once targeted numbers of participants were reached. Invitations to participate in the online survey (phase 2) were then sent with the same process, and eligible individuals were redirected to the survey.

Eligibility criteria for healthcare providers included (1) in active practice for a minimum of 3 years, (2) a primary role as a clinician (not research or teaching) from an eligible profession/specialty (see below) in a community setting (non-academic), (3) in either Alberta, British Columbia, Ontario or Quebec, and (4) a minimum caseload of 20 adults patients with asthma per month. Eligible professions were: (1) allergists/clinical immunologists, respirologists, pneumologists (grouped together as "specialists"); (2) general practitioners, family physicians (GP/FP); (3) Community Pharmacists; (4) Nurses; (5) Certified Respiratory Educators (CRE). Nurses and pharmacists who self-reported having a Respiratory Educator certification were classified as CRE. Sample size for each of these groups were determined based on their population size and professional involvement in asthma care in the community setting. Therefore, the target sample for pharmacists and family physicians are higher than for other professionals such as specialists, nurses with asthma patients and CRE.

Administrators were required to have at least 2 years experience in the administration or management of a community clinical institution. Patient advocates were required to be involved with a recognized patient advocacy group at the national or provincial level. Payers were required to be involved or to have been recently involved with a private or public insurer. For the purpose of this study, "policy influencers" were defined as individuals who have expertise in, and influence on health policy, and/or are experts in the field of asthma in Canada.

Data collection

A review of the literature on existing gaps, barriers and challenges in adult asthma care was initially conducted to identify the main areas to be discussed with interview participants in the qualitative phase of the study. These areas of exploration were discussed with clinical experts (co-authors AK, KP and SW) and researchers in the field of medical education (including co-authors SM, SL). The final areas were used to design the interview guide. For each area, open-ended, non-directive questions were designed to collect in-depth data about challenges and barriers to optimal asthma care from participants. The 45-min telephone interviews were conducted by trained interviewers in educational research (including co-authors SM and SL) and conducted in the two official languages of Canada (English and French). Interviews were audio-recorded (with each participant's consent) and transcribed for analysis.

The online survey questions were designed based on the themes that emerged from the qualitative analysis. Survey was completed by healthcare providers only, as they were the primary target for the continuing medical/health education this study aimed to inform. The 15 min survey consisted of six sections: (1) self-assessment of level of knowledge in relation to specific components of asthma guidelines; (2) self-assessment of confidence; (3) skills in relation to specific tasks that should be performed in the treatment and management of asthma patients; (4) perceived importance of these specific tasks in the delivery of optimal asthma care; (5) agreement level with statements related to asthma care; and (6) ranking or perceived importance of significant barriers to the provision of optimal asthma care. Response formats of survey questions included multiple nominal choices, Likert-type scales and visual-analogue scales, all of which were used in previous needs assessments [17].

The 15-min online survey was designed in English and translated into French. To increase validity of data, the survey questions were adapted to the specific roles and responsibilities of the participants; for example, some questions were asked only to nurses, to pharmacists, or to healthcare providers licensed to prescribe. For Sections 1, 2 and 3, participants were asked to self-report their knowledge, confidence and skills in relation to their professional role.

Analysis plan

Transcribed interviews (qualitative phase) were analysed using a four-step approach derived from thematic analysis [18] and directed content analysis [19] using NVivo qualitative data analysis software (QSR International Pty Ltd, Version 7, 2006). These steps consisted of (1) developing the coding tree with pre-determined codes based on the initial areas of investigation and study objectives; (2) coding the transcripts according to the pre-determined codes; (3) refining the coding tree based on data that could not be coded with the predetermined codes; and (4) identification of themes that emerged the most frequently across and within different sources.

Data from the online survey (quantitative phase) was analysed using IBM SPSS 22.0 software (IBM Corporation, Armonk, NY). Data was analysed using frequencies, cross tabulations, means and Chi square. Post-hoc tests were performed when Chi square was significant ($p < 0.05$). To identify potential educational gaps, knowledge and skill answers were recoded from 5-point Likert-type scale into dichotomous variables, either as a 1–3 response ("low" to "acceptable"), or a 4–5 response ("optimal").

Main gaps, barriers and challenges to optimal asthma care as well as their causes such as sub-optimal knowledge, skills, or confidence were identified using the triangulation of data sources (professions) and methodologies (qualitative and quantitative). Data was interpreted by clinical experts (co-authors AK, KP, SW) and educational experts in the field of health care (co-authors SM and SL).

Results

Sample characteristics

The study sample included a total of 233 participants. Semi-structured telephone interviews were conducted with 43 participants (37 health-care providers and 6 non-healthcare providers) and the online survey was completed by 190 health-care providers. Table 1 presents the sample, grouped by professions for each phase. The majority of participants (84%) had more than 10 years of practice and nearly half of healthcare providers (46%) had 50 or more adult asthma patients a month.

The following sections present challenges in adult asthma care, and their underlying causes, as reported by participants in the qualitative and quantitative phases. This manuscript will focus on five clinical areas that were

substantively reported to be problematic by multiple categories of participants: (1) integration of guidelines into clinical practice; (2) use of spirometry; (3) individualisation of asthma devices to patient needs; (4) promotion of patient adherence and self-management; and (5) definition and sharing of roles and responsibilities by asthma healthcare professionals.

Challenges with integration of asthma guidelines into clinical practice

An inadequate level of knowledge was reported by participants regarding the Canadian Thoracic Society (CTS) and the Global Initiative for Asthma (GINA) guidelines for adult asthma care (see Table 2). Overall, knowledge was reported to be lower for the GINA guidelines with

Table 1 Description of the study sample

Profession	Phase I: qualitative (interview)	Phase II: quantitative (online survey)	Total
General practitioners/family physicians	8	79	87
Specialists[a]	8	18	26
Nurses	8	18	26
Pharmacists	5	54	59
Certified Respiratory Educators (CRE)[b]	8	21	29
Non-healthcare providers (sources of triangulation)			
Admins/payers/policy influencers	4	–	4
Patient advocates	2	–	2
Total	*43*	*190*	*233*

[a] Including allergists/clinical immunologists, respirologists and internal medicine specialists

[b] Including nurses and pharmacists who have obtained a Respiratory Educator certification

Table 2 Sub-optimal knowledge reported by healthcare providers

Knowledge area	% (n) of participants who reported sub-optimal knowledge in relation to what it should be, given their professional role[a]						
	GP/FPs. (n = 79)	SPE. (n = 18)	CRE. (n = 21)	Nurses (n = 18)	Pharm. (n = 54)	Total (n = 190)	Significant differences[b]
Canadian Thoracic Society (CTS) guidelines	52%[c] (n = 41)	28%[c] (n = 5)	67% (n = 14)	83% (n = 15)	87%[c] (n = 47)	64% (n = 122)	p < 0.001
Global Initiative for Asthma (GINA) guidelines	77% (n = 61)	33% (n = 6)	57% (n = 12)	94% (n = 17)	93% (n = 50)	77% (n = 146)	NV
Indicators to request or conduct a spirometry test	33%[c] (n = 26)	22% (n = 4)	38% (n = 8)	44% (n = 8)	89%[c] (n = 48)	50% (n = 94)	p < 0.001
Respective responsibilities of healthcare team members regarding patient education, in my practice setting	27% (n = 21)	22% (n = 4)	24% (n = 5)	44% (n = 8)	41% (n = 22)	32% (n = 60)	NS

GP general practitioner, *FP* family physician, *SPE* specialist, *CRE* Certified Respiratory Educator, *Pharm* community pharmacist, *NS* not significant, *NV* Chi square not valid due to distribution

[a] Self-reported 1–3 on a 5-pt scale, where 1 = low, given my professional role 3 = acceptable, but could be improved, given my professional role and 5 = optimal, given my professional role

[b] Significant differences between professions using Chi square (p < 0.05)

[c] Post hoc test indicated for statistical difference

a total of 77% participants reporting sub-optimal knowledge as compared to 64% for the CTS guidelines. Nurses were the professional sub-group reporting the highest gaps in knowledge for these two guidelines, *in relation to what it should be, given their professional role*: 83% for the CTS guidelines (significant differences between professions, p < 0.001) and 94% for the GINA guidelines. More than half of CREs and GP/FPs also reported knowledge gaps in these two guidelines: with CREs reporting less knowledge of the CTS guidelines (67% CTS, vs. 57% for GINA) whereas a higher proportion of GP/FP reported less knowledge of GINA (77% GINA vs. 52% CTS). From one-third to one quarter of specialists reported a gap for each of the guidelines (28% for CTS; 33% for GINA). Interviewed participants explicitly expressed the need to improve overall knowledge of guidelines for the asthma care community, and to enhance implementation in practice:

"I would say that I've worked in six offices in the last ten years, same thing, no-one actually has a consistent evidence-based way of assessing. And yet the checklist is there. (...) The question is, who does this?"

-FP/GP

Discrepancies between these two guidelines were reported by participants of this study. Half of participants (49%) agreed with the statement that "there are discrepancies between the Canadian guidelines and the international guidelines which create confusion on what to do in practice" (see Table 3). This proportion of agreement reached 72% among nurses and SPE compared to 43% of CRE and 41% of GP/FPs (p = 0.035). Discrepancies between guidelines, especially for criteria determining asthma control, were also explicitly reported by interviewed participants, and participants reported a preference for the GINA guidelines over the CTS:

"I find that the Canadian guidelines are not, I guess, tight enough, or they're too relaxed in determining control. So unlike the GINA guidelines where they say zero symptoms not using your beta-2 at all. The Canadian guidelines, I mean they're allowing up to four doses of your beta-2 in a week. And I just find that just that, that will mix up our doctors."

-CRE

"The GINA guidelines, the Global Initiative for Asthma is [sic] up to date, 2016, but our Canadian

Table 3 Participants' level of agreement with statements on asthma care

Level of agreement with...	% (n) of participants who reported agreement with the statement[a]						
	GP/FPs. (n = 79)	SPE. (n = 18)	CRE. (n = 21)	Nurses (n = 18)	Pharm. (n = 54)	Total (n = 190)	Significant differences[b]
I believe there are discrepancies between the Canadian guidelines and the international guidelines which creates confusion of what to do in practice	41% (n = 32)	72% (n = 13)	43% (n = 9)	72% (n = 13)	50% (n = 27)	49% (n = 94)	p = 0.035
Asthma spirometry test is not necessary to diagnose asthma	43%[c] (n = 34)	44% (n = 8)	14% (n = 3)	17% (n = 3)	17% (n = 9)	30% (n = 57)	p = 0.002
Asthma can be diagnosed based on patient history, and response to a medication trial	75% (n = 59)	72% (n = 13)	71% (n = 15)	50% (n = 9)	63% (n = 34)	68% (n = 130)	NS
Most patients with asthma do not proactively help themselves	56% (n = 44)	67% (n = 12)	48% (n = 10)	33% (n = 6)	61% (n = 33)	55% (n = 105)	NS
Managing adult patients with asthma is time-consuming and frustrating	35% (n = 28)	72% (n = 13)	33% (n = 7)	39% (n = 7)	39% (n = 21)	40% (n = 76)	NS
I suspect there is more I should be doing in the care of patients with asthma	72% (n = 57)	67% (n = 12)	81% (n = 17)	89% (n = 16)	87% (n = 47)	78% (n = 149)	NV

GP general practitioner, *FP* family physician, *SPE* specialist, *CRE* Certified Respiratory Educator, *Pharm* community pharmacist, *NS* not significant, *NV* Chi square not valid due to distribution

[a] Participants were asked to indicate their level of agreement with the following statements. Data are the % of participants that selected 3 or 4 on a 4-pt scale (1 = completely disagree, 2 = slightly disagree, 3 = slightly agree, 4 = completely agree)

[b] Significant differences between professions using Chi square (p < 0.05)

[c] Post hoc test indicated for statistical difference

guidelines are not, 2012. And they're not consistent therefore. So, there's contradiction sometimes or there's gaps in what the CTS guidelines talk about. So, it's another confusing picture. I think the GINA guidelines ... should be exercised, they're very complete and they're easier to use."

-FP/GP

Challenges with the use of spirometry for diagnosis and management

When asked about their knowledge of when to request spirometry, an insufficient level of knowledge was reported by nurses (44%), CRE (38%), and GP/FPs (33%).

Almost half of GP/FPs (43%) and specialists (44%) agreed with the statement that "Spirometry test is not necessary to diagnose asthma" as compared to 17% of nurses and 14% of CRE (p = 0.002, see Table 3). In addition, three-quarters of CRE, GP/FPs and SPE (71, 75 and 72% respectively) agreed that asthma can be diagnosed based on patient history and response to a trial of medication. Confirming an asthma diagnosis was also found

not to be necessary at all, or necessary only in specific cases by nearly half of GP/FPs (46%) (see Table 4).

This perception of spirometry not being necessary to diagnose asthma was also an important theme that emerged from the semi-structured interviews:

*"I only diagnose by history and physical. If I think there's some COPD or some other chronic respiratory illness then they may go for spirometry **but I tend to think of spirometry more for COPD** than asthma and so for **asthma patients most of them are just diagnosed by history and physical and I only use the spirometry if I want to rule something else out** and that's it, and then **I give them a trial of medication and see if they're better with the medication."***

-FP/GP

Spirometry was also reported to be underused to monitor asthma control. As summarized in Table 5, over three quarters of CREs (76%) and half of GP/FPs (56%) and nurses (50%) reported using spirometry for monitoring asthma control either never or only at the first consultation, compared to 17% of specialists. CREs were also the

Table 4 Participants' perceived importance of doing specific tasks in their current clinical practice

Perceived importance of...	% (n) of participants who reported the task as necessary						
	GP/FPs. (n = 79)	SPE. (n = 18)	CRE. (n = 21)	Nurses (n = 18)	Pharm. (n = 54)	Total (n = 190)	Significant differences[b]
Confirm diagnosis prior to initiating treatment	54% (n = 43)	94% (n = 17)	Not asked	Not asked	Not asked	62% (n = 60)	NV
Select the type of device based on my patient's preferences	73% (n = 58)	94% (n = 17)	67% (n = 14)	61% (n = 11)	83% (n = 45)	76% (n = 145)	NV
Assess proper use of device with a demonstration	76% (n = 60)	78% (n = 14)	81% (n = 17)	61% (n = 11)	93% (n = 50)	80% (n = 152)	NV

GP general practitioner, *FP* family physician, *SPE* specialist, *CRE* Certified Respiratory Educator, *Pharm* community pharmacist, *NV* Chi square not valid due to distribution

[a] Selected 4 or 5 on a 5-pt scale (1 = Not necessary at all, 3 = necessary only in specific cases, and 5 = always necessary)

[b] Significant differences between professions using Chi square (p < 0.05)

Table 5 Participants reporting of the frequency they are doing specific tasks in their current clinical practice

Task	% (n) of participants who report never doing the task or only in the first consultation with their patients[a]						
	GP/FPs. (n = 79)	SPE. (n = 18)	CRE. (n = 21)	Nurses (n = 18)	Pharm. (n = 53)	Total (n = 189)	Significant differences[b]
Assess asthma control with spirometry	56% (n = 44)	17% (n = 3)	76% (n = 16)	50% (n = 9)	93% (n = 49)	64% (n = 121)	NV
Assess asthma symptoms and exacerbations with spirometry	54% (n = 43)	28% (n = 5)	62% (n = 13)	56% (n = 10)	94% (n = 50)	64% (n = 121)	NV

GP general practitioner, *FP* family physician, *SPE* specialist, *CRE* Certified Respiratory Educator, *Pharm* community pharmacist, *NV* Chi square not valid due to distribution

[a] Other nominal answer choices provided were "In most of my patients' consultations" and "Systematically in each of my patients' consultations"

[b] Significant differences between professions using Chi square (p < 0.05)

profession reporting a lesser use of spirometry for monitoring asthma symptoms and exacerbations (62% never doing it or only on first consultation), followed by nurses (56%), GP/FPs (54%), and specialists (28%).

Among GP/FPs, 43% selected "lack of access to spirometry in their practice setting" as an important barrier to providing optimal asthma care whereas 0% of SPE selected this item as an important barrier (p = 0.001, see Fig. 1). The need to have better access to spirometry for community family physicians was frequently mentioned by interviewed participants:

> *"The spirometry is not universally available in the community. What we do in our office is all of our tests are performed by respiratory therapists, which is quite expensive [...] I have sympathy for the primary care physicians that often they don't have the availability of the tools such as spirometry to help them."*
>
> -Specialist

Challenges with the individualisation of devices to patient needs

Over a third of nurses perceived that individualising the type of device based on their patient's preferences (39%) and assessing/demonstrating its proper use (also 39%) to not be necessary or to be necessary only in specific cases (see Table 4).

As shown in Table 6, sub-optimal skills selecting the device best adapted to a given patient were also reported in a higher proportion by nurses (61%) as compared to other participants (p = 0.029). Pharmacists had the lowest proportion of participants reporting a skill gap related to this task (20%).

Increasing variety of available type of devices was mentioned by interviewed participants as a contributor to the difficulty in selecting the most suitable device to the patient needs:

> *"There are about fifteen kinds [...] that's a lot... There's at least ten devices to use the inhaler, and it*

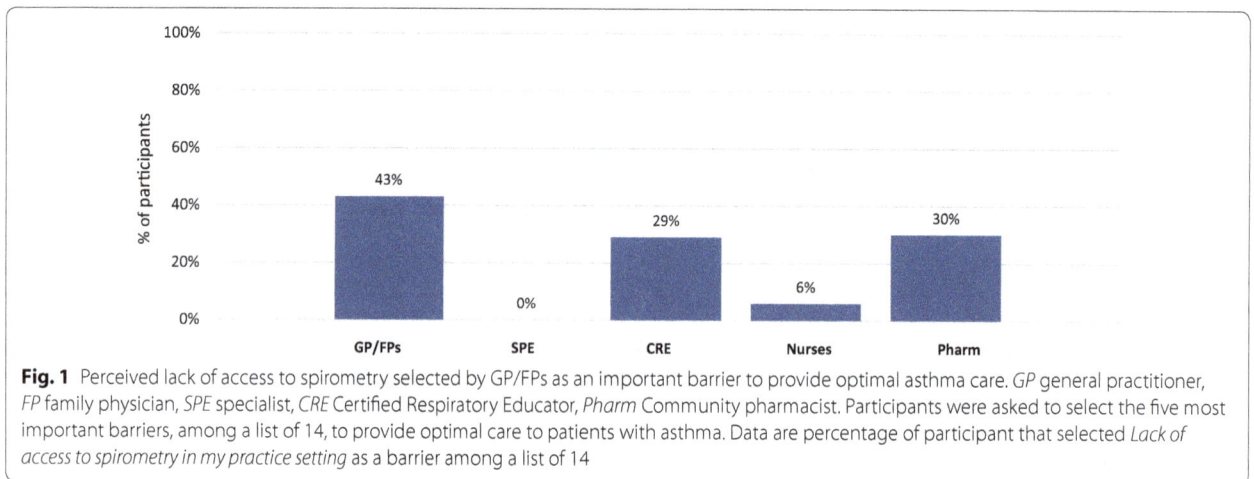

Fig. 1 Perceived lack of access to spirometry selected by GP/FPs as an important barrier to provide optimal asthma care. *GP* general practitioner, *FP* family physician, *SPE* specialist, *CRE* Certified Respiratory Educator, *Pharm* Community pharmacist. Participants were asked to select the five most important barriers, among a list of 14, to provide optimal care to patients with asthma. Data are percentage of participant that selected *Lack of access to spirometry in my practice setting* as a barrier among a list of 14

Table 6 Sub-optimal skills reported by healthcare providers

Skill	% (n) of participants who reported sub-optimal skills in relation to what it should be, given their professional role[a]						
	GP/FPs. (n = 79)	SPE. (n = 18)	CRE. (n = 21)	Nurses (n = 18)	Pharm. (n = 54)	Total (n = 190)	Significant differences[b]
Selecting/recommending the most adapted device to a given patient	33% (n = 26)	28% (n = 5)	29% (n = 6)	61%[c] (n = 11)	20% (n = 11)	31% (n = 59)	p = 0.029
Promoting self-management	17% (n = 13)	6% (n = 1)	14% (n = 3)	39% (n = 7)	28% (n = 15)	21% (n = 39)	NV

GP general practitioner, *FP* family physician, *SPE* specialist, *CRE* Certified Respiratory Educator, *Pharm* community pharmacist, *NV* Chi square not valid due to distribution

[a] Self-reported 1 to 3 on a 5-pt scale, with 1 = low, given my professional role 3 = acceptable, but could be improved, given my professional role and 5 = optimal, given my professional role

[b] Significant differences between professions using Chi square (p < 0.05)

[c] Post hoc test indicated for statistical difference

doesn't work with all the patients: people are more familiar with one or the other, and it needs to be tested".

-Specialist

Challenges with promotion of patient adherence and self-management

There was a perception from interviewed participants that lack of patient adherence is often explained by an overall disengagement of the patients from their condition, generating frustration within the health-care team. As detailed in Table 3, more than half of all participants (55%) agreed with the statement that "most patients with asthma do not proactively help themselves". Specialists agreed with this statement (67%), followed by pharmacists (61%) and GP/FPs (56%). In addition, a large majority of specialists (72%) agreed that managing adult patients with asthma is time-consuming and frustrating. Other professions also agreed with this statement although to a lesser extent (see Table 3).

Patient complacency toward their symptoms was the most often identified barrier to providing optimal care, selected by 70% of participants. As summarized in Fig. 2, pharmacists (74%) selected this most often, followed by nurses (72%) and GP/FPs (71%). In addition, patient overuse of rescue medication, a specific type of non-adherence, was the second being selected by 66% of participants, and especially by pharmacists (91%) (p = 0.001). The sense of frustration of healthcare providers when treating and managing asthma was reported to be especially high when providing care to young, busy adults:

"I would say probably a young healthy otherwise healthy asthmatic, especially male. I have quite a few patients between the ages of like twenty to thirty. They are hard to treat because of compliance and trying to get them to take their asthma seriously. The problem is compliance and getting them to book appointments if they work, as they have to take time off work. "

-CRE

As illustrated in Fig. 3, 47% of participants reported that providing a written action plan to patients is not at all necessary or only in certain cases. Specifically, near half of CRE (43%), GP/FPs (44%), and half of pharmacists (52%) perceived that providing a written plan as not necessary. Providing an oral action plan was perceived as more important than a written plan, although, 19% of participants reported that providing oral plan was not necessary at all, or only in specific cases.

A large majority of participants agreed they should be doing more when caring for patient with asthma (78%). As summarized in Table 3, the level of agreement reached 89% among nurses and 87% among pharmacists.

The overall lack of perceived importance by the healthcare team of providing the patient with a written plan, was also a main theme identified by multiple type of participants during the semi-structured interviews:

*"I do not [use a written action plan]. Because I show them. So, I will draw something on my examination paper on my room and I'll take a couple of puffs up to my fake inhaler and I'll do it that way. **But I do not give people a written plan.**"*

-FP/GP

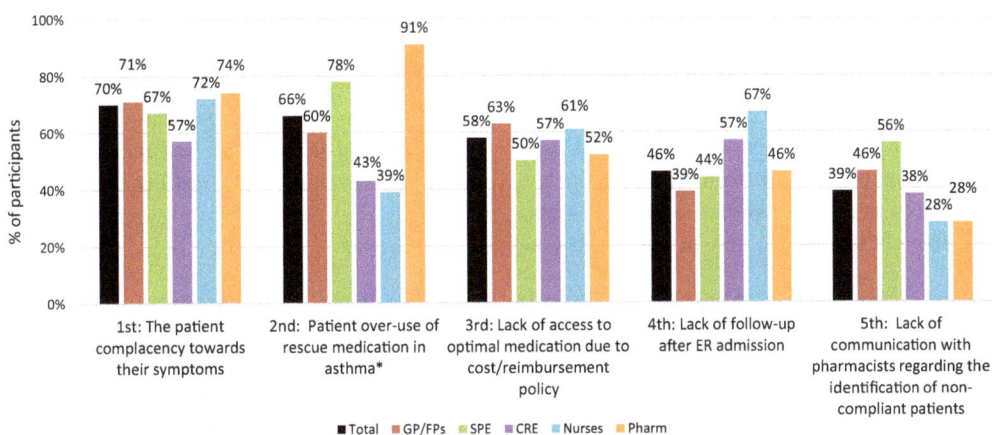

Fig. 2 Top 5 most often selected barriers to providing optimal care. *GP* general practitioner, *FP* family physician, *SPE* specialist, *CRE* Certified Respiratory Educator, *Pharm* Community pharmacist. Participants were asked to select the five most important barriers, among a list of 14, to providing optimal care to patients with asthma. Barriers presented are the top five most selected in total. Data are % of participants who selected that barrier

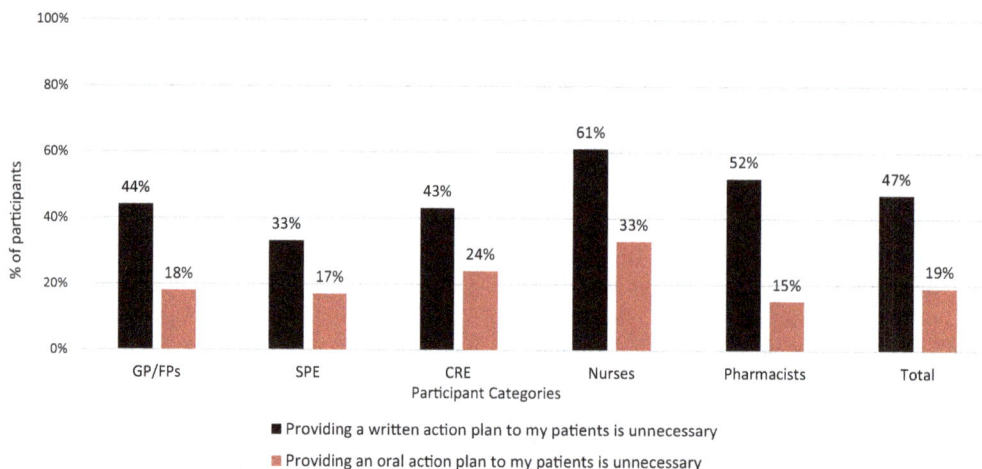

Fig. 3 Perceived importance of providing an oral versus a written action plan. *GP* general practitioner, *FP* family physician, *SPE* specialist, *CRE* Certified Respiratory Educator, *Pharm* community pharmacist. Question asked: Please indicate how necessary, in your professional role, are the following items in your practice with adult patients suffering from asthma. Scale: 1 = Not necessary at all, 3 = Only necessary in specific cases and 5 = Always necessary. Data are the percentage of participants that selected 1, 2 or 3

The following quote by an asthma clinic administrator illustrates how important providing a written plan should be to promote patient compliance:

*"That [written] asthma action plan is the bee's knees to me. **That's one thing that just lets the patient know when and why they would need to be concerned, and how they should be treating their asthma.** [...] If they've never gone through it [...] how would they know? They're just treating themselves as they think they should be."*

-Asthma clinic administrator

Sub-optimal sharing of roles and responsibilities among health-care team, especially regarding patient education

As shown in Table 2, almost half of nurses and pharmacists reported knowledge gaps of the roles of respective healthcare team members (44 and 41%). The lack of communication with pharmacists regarding the identification of non-compliant patients was among the top five barriers the most often selected among a list of 14 and was selected by 46% of GP/FPs and 56% of specialists (see Fig. 2).

This lack of clarity about team members' roles and responsibilities emerged as an important theme from the semi-structured interviews:

*"I think asthma care could be optimized if there was more education around what the specific role of each health professional (doctor, pharmacist) was in regards to asthma care. **I am not confident that all physicians are monitoring their asthma patients**

using spirometry/peak flow, and if pharmacists were aware of this gap in treatment they may make more of an effort to fill the gap."*

-Pharmacist

Participants in semi-structured interviews expressed the need to improve the clarity of roles and responsibilities of healthcare professionals, especially pharmacists, in the management of adult patients with asthma, with the objective of providing clear information to patient:

"Different information coming from a physician/ pharmacist and then information coming through me, if it's not the same. That would be probably one of the hardest, the biggest barriers to get over directly with a patient."

-CRE

"What works not so well, consistency between healthcare professionals. The patients are often getting mixed messages. I had mentioned the problem with a pharmacist earlier. That would be one example."

-Specialist

Discussion

This study provides evidence of clinical challenges experienced by healthcare providers in Canada in five areas related to treatment and management of patients with asthma in community settings. Challenges and their causes were identified in five specific areas: asthma practice guidelines, use of spirometry, individualisation of devices, patient adherence, and sharing of roles among the multidisciplinary team.

A main finding of this report is related to the poor integration of asthma guidelines into practice. This finding could be explained by a lack of exposure to guidelines among health care teams, as well as the lack of access to spirometry in primary care settings, combined with the widespread belief that spirometry is not necessary to diagnose or monitor asthma.

The resulting general underuse of spirometry in primary care settings, and its relationship to uncertainty surrounding asthma diagnoses, emerged as another important issue in this study, as it did in others conducted in the U.S., Asia, and Europe [20]. Health care teams simply may not perceive the value of incorporating these guidelines into practice, nor the consequences of failing to do so.

One of these consequences is a contribution to the over-diagnosis of asthma in Canada [21, 22]. For example, a recent Canadian study conducted among 613 asthma patients, reported that 33% of these patients were wrongly diagnosed [23]. It is critical to address the perceived low importance of spirometry, both for diagnosis and monitoring, since it may also lead to under-recognition of asthma as a diagnosis, overestimation of asthma control, as well as misdiagnoses when asthma-like symptoms are observed. Ultimately, this could lead to delayed referrals to specialists or unnecessary emergency admissions due to the non-identification of unresponsive or uncontrolled patients in a timely manner [11].

For improved long-term management of asthma patients, and to increase the knowledge of best practices and the perceived importance of spirometry, GPs, specialists, as well as allied healthcare providers (such as CRE and nurses) must become better familiarized with asthma guidelines. The development of clear and concise guidelines (especially those pertaining to asthma control), followed by a promotion of their use, value, and inclusion into medical education curricula, would help establish a working integration of those documents into practice.

Perceived contextual and systemic barriers to optimal asthma care were reported in this study. Lack of access to objective lung function test and to specific medications due to cost and lack of reimbursement from insurance, is likely hindering adherence to best practices and treatment recommendations. Providing better access to spirometry and medications in primary care settings, especially in communities where specialized centers and specialists are not readily available, appears essential to improve the current state of asthma care in Canada. It is possible that the difficulty accessing spirometry led family physicians to make alternative clinical decisions to rapidly relieve patients from asthma symptoms. Initiating a medication trial based on a suspected, yet unconfirmed diagnosis is an example of current practice, reported in this study by both GP/FPs and specialists that may be perceived as the only way to proceed in the absence of objective lung function tests, even if not aligned with current best practices [24]. Therefore, contextual and systemic barriers have direct influence on family physicians' practice habits and clinical decision-making. To verify the validity of this perception, or to identify the factors that could explain this perception, future research could examine family physicians' access to objective lung function tests in a community setting.

Findings from this study confirmed that the lack of patient adherence to treatment plans is perceived by healthcare providers as an important barrier to provide optimal asthma care and that there is a need to educate patients regarding recognition of symptoms, better adherence, complacency issues, and timely intervention. This is supported by a survey which has demonstrated that a high proportion of patients (97%) believed their asthma to be controlled, when according to guidelines, it would have been considered uncontrolled for 47% of them (4). This is also supported by the observation that patients often prefer living with slightly more severe symptoms, in order to reduce their medication intake [25].

Results of this study show that healthcare providers do not see the value of basic recommendations such as providing written action plan or individualizing type of device, which could suggest complacency or lack of education regarding their importance. Healthcare providers are likely overestimating the patient capacity to retain and follow a verbal plan. Despite the benefits of written action plans repeatedly reported in literature and guidelines, their underuse combined with inappropriate follow-ups to assess asthma control, contribute to a lack of patient adherence to their treatment plan [26–31]. Patients and healthcare providers often do not perceive asthma as a potentially life-threatening condition, despite the fact that 250 Canadians die from asthma complications each year [32]. This highlights a need to raise awareness among healthcare providers regarding consequences of poor asthma control, and to enhance the perceived value of using written as opposed to verbal action plans.

It has been demonstrated that prevention and control of chronic conditions is optimized by the presence of a multidisciplinary, collaborative care team, involving physicians and allied health-care providers [33]. Findings from this study indicated that there is confusion regarding the individual roles and responsibilities of the physician, the nurse, the CRE and the pharmacist. Each of these healthcare providers could play a specific role in the correction of these identified gaps.

A first step towards optimal multidisciplinary management of asthma would be to provide clear guidelines about "who does what and when". This would have to be applied to the individual community contexts since specialized personnel such as CREs may not be readily accessible leading to greater involvement by pharmacists and nurses. Previous studies suggested that pharmacists should routinely verify proper patient use of their device and provide education regarding medication and the patient treatment plan [34]. A recent survey among Canadian physicians reported that most practitioners were in favour of increasing pharmacists' involvement related to management of asthma patients [35]. A survey distributed among Canadian community pharmacists in 2006 revealed that less than 10% of those surveyed had assessed if their clients used their asthma devices properly [36]. It is known that patients who incorrectly use their devices are more likely to have poor asthma control, and visit emergency departments more frequently [37]. The pharmacist's role has already evolved to include this task in various healthcare locations and settings; however further research is needed to determine the educational needs of the pharmacists, as well as the best way to communicate and collaborate with physicians (e.g. reporting on compliance) and to increase their current scope of practice.

Government recognition and support for policies that would increase access to CREs, either through centralized asthma clinics or itinerant CRE, could certainly contribute to optimizing patient care as well as physician time and efficiency. Another potential solution to help achieve a clearer understanding of roles and responsibilities in multidisciplinary care would be to provide opportunities, within community practice settings, for interprofessional continuing education (IPCE) or interprofessional continuing development (IPCD) [38, 39]. However, evidence indicates that these programs have had little to no significant impact on professional practice [40]. It would therefore be important that future development of educational activities in asthma be designed around evidenced based needs, such as those identified by this needs assessment study.

Study limitations
Given the objectives of this needs assessment, the focus of this manuscript was on areas of improvement that could be targeted by educational interventions. Therefore, areas where care was reported to be optimal were not included. As all self-reported studies, there is the possibility of erroneous self-assessment bias. Participation of healthcare providers was voluntary, which could

introduce a selection bias. To mitigate potential bias, a purposive sampling, including multiple stakeholders having different years of practice was implemented to increase how representative the sample is in relation to the healthcare population working in community settings. Small sample sizes and skewed distribution in response to certain items did not allow for valid Chi square tests to assess differences between sub-groups; therefore, differences observed through valid Chi square tests only were reported. This study was conducted among community settings in the 4 largest Canadian provinces only. Respective roles and responsibilities of healthcare providers might differ in community settings of smaller provinces and therefore, findings should be generalized with caution.

Conclusion
This Canadian needs assessment identified gaps and challenges in the treatment and management of adults with asthma using the perspective of multiple stakeholders involved in asthma care. This study also reports many gaps that were identified more than a decade ago, but that are still currently present in community practice settings, despite several attempts and strategies to overcome them. Most importantly, this study leads to a better understanding of the specific causes that could explain the observed challenges and needs of healthcare providers and patients. Many of the deficiencies pertained to lack of knowledge, confidence, and skills to properly perform specific tasks for optimal treatment and management of asthma, which could be addressed through educational activities. Future continuing medical education needs to be adapted to the needs it aims to achieve (e.g. knowledge vs. skills gaps) to obtain concrete improvement in practice. Providers in community settings also require access to adequate materials, resources (e.g. spirometry), and training to support optimal care of adult patients with asthma.

Abbreviations
CTS: Canadian Thoracic Society; CRE: Certified Respiratory Educators; FP: family physicians; GINA: Global Initiative for Asthma; GP: general practitioners; IPCD: interprofessional continuing development; IPCE: interprofessional continuing education; SPE: specialists; SPSS: Statistical Package for the Social Sciences.

Authors' contributions
SM, the principal investigator, was involved in the study design, the development of the research tools, contributed to the analysis plan and interpretation of the findings. She took part in critical discussions around the manuscript content and reviewed the final manuscript. SL was involved in the study design, led the development of research tools, the data collection, the qualitative and quantitative analyses, the interpretation of findings, and developed a first draft of the manuscript. AK, KP and SW were part of an oversight committee which provided clinical expertise to help determine the areas of investigation, refine the study design and the research tools, and contextualize the interpretation of the findings. They critically reviewed content of the manuscript and approved the final version submitted. All co-authors have

contributed sufficiently to this article to be considered as authors, as per the authorship requirements detailed by the International Committee of medical Journal Editors (ICMJE). All authors read and approved the final manuscript.

Author details

[1] AXDEV Group Inc., 210-8, Place du Commerce, Brossard, QC J4W 3H2, Canada. [2] Department of Family and Community Medicine, University of Toronto, 500 University Ave, Toronto, ON M5G 1V7, Canada. [3] Winnipeg Regional Health Authority, Winnipeg, MB R2R 2S8, Canada. [4] Division of Clinical Immunology and Allergy, McMaster University, 1280 Main St West, HSC 3V49, Hamilton, ON L8S 4K1, Canada.

Acknowledgements

This study was conducted by AXDEV Group. The authors would also like to acknowledge the support provided by Patrice Lazure (Director of Research, AXDEV Group, Canada), and Sophie Péloquin (Director Performance Strategy, AXDEV Group, Canada), who supported the analysis and interpretation of the data, as well as Marc Distexhe (Project coordinator, AXDEV Group, Canada), who supported data collection, communications and other coordination aspects of the research. The authors would like to thank all the healthcare providers and other key stakeholders who took part in this study as participants.

Competing interests

SM and SL declare that they have no competing interests.

AK declares relationships with the following commercial interest: Advisory Board or Speakers bureau for Astra Zeneca, Boehrninger Ingelheim, GSK, Merck Frosst, Meda, Pfizer, Purdue, Novartis, Griffols, Teva, Trudel, Mylan, Paladdin and Johnson & Johnson. AK is co-chair of the Health Quality Ontario COPD Community Therapy program and the Chairperson of the Family Physician Airways Group of Canada.

KP declares relationships with the following commercial interests: Advisory Board and Speakers Bureau: Pfizer; Funding (Grants/Honoraria) by the Canadian Foundation For Pharmacy, University of Manitoba; Research/Clinical Trials honoraria: Canadian Asthma Study Jan–Sept 2017 (AXDEV); MANTRA IPC pilot project (August 2016–April 2017); Speaker/Consulting Fees: GSK, AZ, Pfizer, BI, Takeda, Teva, Novartis, Forest Labs, Trudell & Merck.

SW declares relationships with the following commercial interests: Honoraria for consultant: AstraZeneca, GSK, Merck, Nycomed, CSL Behring, Mylan, Shire, Meda, Novartis, Sanofi, Pfizer, Aralez, Pediapharm. SM is also an employee of McMaster University.

Funding

This study was financially supported with education research funds from TEVA Canada. The funding body had no role in the design of the study, in the collection, analysis, and interpretation of data. TEVA Canada reviewed the manuscript but final decision regarding the manuscript's content was the responsibility of the authors.

References

1. Statistics Canada. Asthma 2014. http://www.statcan.gc.ca/pub/82-625-x/2015001/article/14179-eng.htm. Accessed 3 Apr 2018.
2. Boulet LP, Devlin H, O'Donnell DE. The physicians' practice assessment questionnaire on asthma and COPD. Respir Med. 2011;105:8–14.
3. Cochrane MG, Bala MV, Downs KE, Mauskopf J, Ben-Joseph RH. Inhaled corticosteroids for asthma therapy: patient compliance, devices, and inhalation technique. Chest. 2000;117:542–50.
4. FitzGerald JM, Boulet LP, McIvor RA, Zimmerman S, Chapman KR. Asthma control in Canada remains suboptimal: the reality of asthma control (TRAC) study. Can Respir J. 2006;13:253–9.
5. Labrecque M, Lavallee M, Beauchesne MF, Cartier A, Boulet LP. Can access to spirometry in asthma education centres influence the referral rate by primary physicians for education? Can Respir J. 2006;13:427–31.
6. Licskai CJ, Sands TW, Paolatto L, Nicoletti I, Ferrone M. Spirometry in primary care: an analysis of spirometry test quality in a regional primary care asthma program. Can Respir J. 2012;19:249–54.
7. Juniper EF, Svensson K, Mork AC, Stahl E. Measuring health-related quality of life in adults during an acute asthma exacerbation. Chest. 2004;125:93–7.
8. Nunes C, Pereira AM, Morais-Almeida M. Asthma costs and social impact. Asthma Res Pract. 2017;3:1.
9. Ismaila AS, Sayani AP, Marin M, Su Z. Clinical, economic, and humanistic burden of asthma in Canada: a systematic review. BMC Pulm Med. 2013;13:70.
10. Statistic Canada. mortality, summary list of causes; 2009. https://www.statcan.gc.ca/pub/84f0209x/84f0209x2009000-eng.htm. Accessed 3 Apr 2018.
11. Hayes SM, Peloquin S, Menzies-Gow A, Rabe KF, Aubier M, Murray S, Waserman S. International perspectives on severe asthma: current and future challenges in patient care. Eur Respir J. 2016;48:PA3374.
12. Green JS, Eckstein JB. What is a needs assessment? Alliance for CME Almanac. 2003;25:4–5.
13. Olsen WK. Triangulation in social research: qualitative and quantitative methods can really be mixed. In: Holborn M, Haralambos M, editors. Developments in sociology. Ormskirk: Causeway Press; 2004.
14. Maudsley G. Mixing it but not mixed-up: mixed methods research in medical education (a critical narrative review). Med Teach. 2011;33:e92–104.
15. ESOMAR (European Society for Opinion and Marketing Research), ICC (International Chamber of Commerce). The ICC/ESOMAR international code on market, opinion and social research and data analytics. 2016. https://www.esomar.org/uploads/public/knowledge-and-standards/codes-and-guidelines/ICCESOMAR_Code_English_.pdf. Accessed 3 Apr 2018.
16. Palinkas LA, Horwitz SM, Green CA, Wisdom JP, Duan N, Hoagwood K. Purposeful sampling for qualitative data collection and analysis in mixed method implementation research. Adm Policy Ment Health. 2015;42:533–44.
17. Lazure P, Marshall JL, Hayes SM, Murray S. Challenges that hinder the translation of clinical advances into practice: results from an international assessment in colorectal cancer. Clin Colorectal Cancer. 2016;15:54–66.
18. Boyatzis RE. Thematic analysis and code development: transforming qualitative information. Thousand Oaks: Sage Publications; 1998.
19. Hsieh HF, Shannon SE. Three approaches to qualitative content analysis. Qual Health Res. 2005;15:1277–88.
20. Mannino DM, Buist AS, Petty TL, Enright PL, Redd SC. Lung function and mortality in the United States: data from the first national health and nutrition examination survey follow up study. Thorax. 2003;58:388–93.
21. Aaron SD, Vandemheen KL, Boulet LP, McIvor RA, Fitzgerald JM, Hernandez P, Lemiere C, Sharma S, Field SK, Alvarez GG, et al. Overdiagnosis of asthma in obese and nonobese adults. CMAJ. 2008;179:1121–31.
22. Stanbrook MB, Kaplan A. The error of not measuring asthma. CMAJ. 2008;179:1099–102.
23. Aaron SD, Vandemheen KL, FitzGerald JM, Ainslie M, Gupta S, Lemiere C, Field SK, McIvor RA, Hernandez P, Mayers I, et al. Reevaluation of diagnosis in adults with physician-diagnosed asthma. JAMA. 2017;317:269–79.
24. Kaplan AG, Balter MS, Bell AD, Kim H, McIvor RA. Diagnosis of asthma in adults. CMAJ. 2009;181:E210–20.
25. Haughney J, Barnes G, Partridge M, Cleland J. The living and breathing study: a study of patients' views of asthma and its treatment. Prim Care Respir J. 2004;13:28–35.
26. Wood-Baker R, McGlone S, Venn A, Walters EH. Written action plans in chronic obstructive pulmonary disease increase appropriate treatment for acute exacerbations. Respirology. 2006;11:619–26.
27. Bischoff EW, Hamd DH, Sedeno M, Benedetti A, Schermer TR, Bernard S, Maltais F, Bourbeau J. Effects of written action plan adherence on COPD exacerbation recovery. Thorax. 2011;66:26–31.

28. Trappenburg JC, Monninkhof EM, Bourbeau J, Troosters T, Schrijvers AJ, Verheij TJ, Lammers JW. Effect of an action plan with ongoing support by a case manager on exacerbation-related outcome in patients with COPD: a multicentre randomised controlled trial. Thorax. 2011;66:977–84.

29. Fan VS, Gaziano JM, Lew R, Bourbeau J, Adams SG, Leatherman S, Thwin SS, Huang GD, Robbins R, Sriram PS, et al. A comprehensive care management program to prevent chronic obstructive pulmonary disease hospitalizations: a randomized, controlled trial. Ann Intern Med. 2012;156:673–83.

30. McCurdy BR. Action plans for individuals with chronic obstructive pulmonary disease (COPD): a rapid review. health quality Ontario; 2013. http://www.hqontario.ca/Portals/0/Documents/evidence/rapid-reviews/action-plans-copd-130111-en.pdf. Accessed 3 Apr 2018.

31. Criner GJ, Bourbeau J, Diekemper RL, Ouellette DR, Goodridge D, Hernandez P, Curren K, Balter MS, Bhutani M, Camp PG, et al. Executive summary: prevention of acute exacerbation of COPD: american college of chest physicians and Canadian Thoracic Society Guideline. Chest. 2015;147:883–93.

32. Theriault L, Hermus G, Goldfarb D, Stonebridge C, Bounajm F: Cost risk analysis for chronic lung disease in Canada. Ottawa Conference Board of Canada; 2012. http://www.conferenceboard.ca/e-library/abstract.aspx?did=4585&AspxAutoDetectCookieSupport=1. Accessed 3 Apr 2018.

33. Chauhan BF, Jeyaraman M, Mann AS, Lys J, Skidmore B, Sibley KM, Abou-Setta A, Zarychanksi R. Behavior change interventions and policies influencing primary healthcare professionals' practice-an overview of reviews. Implement Sci. 2017;12:3.

34. Terrie YC. Managing Asthma: the pharmacist's role. In: Pharmacy times; 2014. http://www.pharmacytimes.com/publications/issue/2014/april 2014/managing-asthma-the-pharmacists-role. Accessed 3 Apr 2018.

35. Tilly-Gratton A, Lamontagne A, Blais L, Bacon SL, Ernst P, Grad R, Lavoie KL, McKinney ML, Desplats E, Ducharme FM. Physician agreement regarding the expansion of pharmacist professional activities in the management of patients with asthma. Int J Pharm Pract. 2017;25(5):335–42.

36. Rene-Henri N, Khamla Y, Nadaira N, Ouellet C, Blais L, Lalonde L, Collin J, Beauchesne MF. Community pharmacists' interventions in asthma care: a descriptive study. Ann Pharmacother. 2009;43:104–11.

37. Al-Jahdali H, Ahmed A, Al-Harbi A, Khan M, Baharoon S, Bin Salih S, Halwani R, Al-Muhsen S. Improper inhaler technique is associated with poor asthma control and frequent emergency department visits. Allergy Asthma Clin Immunol. 2013;9(1):8.

38. Reeves S. An overview of continuing interprofessional education. J Contin Educ Health Prof. 2009;29:142–6.

39. Lung Health Institute of Canada. RESPTREC—Respiratory Training & Educator Course. https://www.resptrec.org/. Accessed 3 Apr 2018.

40. Rouleau R, Beauchesne MF, Laurier C. Impact of a continuing education program on community pharmacists' interventions and asthma medication use: a pilot study. Ann Pharmacother. 2007;41:574–80.

18

Airway reversibility in asthma and phenotypes of Th2-biomarkers, lung function and disease control

Jianghong Wei[1], Libing Ma[1], Jiying Wang[1], Qing Xu[1], Meixi Chen[1], Ming Jiang[1], Miao Luo[1], Jingjie Wu[1], Weiwei She[1], Shuyuan Chu[1,2]* ⓘ and Biwen Mo[1,2]*

Abstract

Background: High bronchodilator reversibility in adult asthma is associated with distinct clinical characteristics. In this study, we aim to make a comparison with T-helper 2 (Th2)-related biomarkers, lung function and asthma control between asthmatic patients with high airway reversibility (HR) and low airway reversibility (LR).

Methods: Patients with asthma diagnosed by pulmonologist according to Global Initiative for Asthma guidelines were recruited from the outpatient department of our hospital from August 2014 to July 2017. Patients were divided into HR and LR subgroups based on their response to bronchodilators of lung function (HR = Δforced expiratory volume in one second (FEV1) postbronchodilator $\geq$ 20%). Blood eosinophil count and serum IgE level, which are biomarkers of T-helper (Th)-2 phenotypes, were detected for patients. Asthma Control Test (ACT) was used to assess asthma control after the first-month initial treatment.

Results: A total of 265 patients with asthma were followed 1 month after initial treatment. HR group shows a higher level of Th2-high biomarkers (blood eosinophil count (10^9/L): 0.49 ± 0.28 vs 0.36 ± 0.19, P < 0.01; IgE (ng/ml): 1306 ± 842 vs 413 ± 261, P < 0.01), lower baseline lung function (FEV1%pred: $51.91 \pm 19.34\%$ vs $60.42 \pm 19.22\%$, P < 0.01; forced expiratory flow (FEF)25–75: 0.76 ± 0.37 vs 1.00 ± 0.67, P < 0.01; FEF25–75%pred: $21.15 \pm 10.09\%$ vs $29.06 \pm 16.50\%$, P < 0.01), and better asthma control (ACT score: 22 ± 4 vs 20 ± 4, P = 0.01) than LR group. HR was associated with a decreased risk of uncontrolled asthma after the first-month initial treatment (adjusted OR: 0.12 [95% confidence intervals: 0.03–0.50]).

Conclusions: HR is a physiologic indicator of lower lung function and severe small airway obstruction, and is more related with an increased level of Th2-biomarkers than LR. Moreover, HR may indicate controlled asthma after the first-month initial treatment. This finding may contribute to identification of asthma endotype.

Keywords: Asthma, Airway reversibility, Th2-biomarkers, Lung function, Asthma control

Background

Airway bronchodilator reversibility is the characteristic that differentiates asthma population from patients with irreversible obstructive lung diseases [1]. It has been emerged as a characteristic to categorize asthma patients into different phenotype [2], and a physiologic biomarker associated with co-morbidities of asthma patients [3]. Interestingly, the high airway bronchodilator reversibility was found as a physiologic indicator for reduced lung function, and was associated with elevated Th2-biomarkers [4]. Thus, airway bronchodilator reversibility may be a crosslinking point in understanding the diversity of asthma endotype, and then identify profiles to guide treatment [5]. However, that previous study didn't investigate obstruction in small airway, or asthma control after the initial treatment according to the Global Initiative for Asthma guidelines (GINA)

*Correspondence: emilyyuanchu@163.com; 1042587352@qq.com
[1] Department of Respiratory and Critical Care Medicine, Affiliated Hospital of Guilin Medical University, Guilin 541001, Guangxi, China
Full list of author information is available at the end of the article

alone [1]. Therefore, we conducted this hospital-based cohort study to investigate immune pathway biomarkers, obstruction in small airway, and disease control after the initial treatment in asthma patients with high or low airway reversibility.

Methods

From August 2014 to July 2017, adult patients with asthma diagnosed by pulmonologists at the first time according to the definition of GINA [1] were recruited in the study from the Affiliated Hospital of Guilin Medical University, Guilin, China. Blood eosinophil count and serum IgE level were tested. Asthma control was assessed in terms of Asthma Control Test (ACT) after the first-month initial treatment with a face-to-face interview by pulmonologists [6, 7]. The study protocol was approved by the Institutional Review Board at the Affiliated Hospital of Guilin Medical University, and conformed to the declaration of Helsinki. Written informed consent was obtained from each subject.

Inclusion criteria in the present study were as following: (1) age between 18 and 65 years, (2) forced expiratory volume in one second (FEV1) % predicted less than 80%, (3) reversibility in FEV1 12% (and at least 200 ml) following administration of a short-acting β-agonist, (4) no evidence of active infection, (5) no medical conditions associated with immune suppression. Patients were excluded if they had chronic obstructive pulmonary disease (COPD) or asthma-COPD overlap [8], had a history of intubation within 3 years of enrollment, or had obstructive sleep apnea.

Subjects were classified into high airway reversibility (HR) group and low airway reversibility (LR) group. The HR group included patients with a $\geq 20\%$ increase in FEV1 following administration of a short-acting bronchodilator during screening and baseline pulmonary function testing. The LR group included those with reversibility below that level [2].

Group data were expressed as the mean $\pm$ standard deviation (SD). Significant differences were evaluated using independent-samples t test or Chi square test. The associations between asthma control and clinical characteristics were explored with unconditional logistic regression models with LOGISTIC procedure in SAS 9.4 (SAS Institute Inc., Cary, North Carolina, USA). The results were presented as odds ratios (OR) and 95% confidence intervals (CI). P values < 0.05 were considered to be statistically significant.

Results

Figure 1 shows the subject selection process. We excluded subjects if they had no record of lung function responding to bronchodilators, blood eosinophil count,

serum IgE level, or ACT score. A total of 265 subjects were selected for final analyses.

Demographics characteristics for all patients were summarized in Table 1. HR and LR groups were similar in percentages of male, smoker and subjects having history of allergy, age and body-mass index (BMI). All patients were received inhaled corticosteroid (ICS) combined long-acting inhaled β2-agonist (LABA) as initial treatment.

Moreover, Table 1 illustrates the difference of Th-2 phenotypes, lung function and asthma control between HR and LR groups. In HR group, eosinophil count in blood and IgE level in serum were higher than those in LR group (eosinophil count (10^9/L): 0.49 ± 0.28 vs 0.36 ± 0.19; IgE (ng/ml): 1306.0 ± 841.5 vs 413.4 ± 261.6. All P values < 0.01). Moreover, the base lung function in HR group was worse than that in LR group (FEV1%pred: $51.91 \pm 19.34\%$ vs $60.42 \pm 19.22\%$; forced expiratory flow (FEF)25–75: 0.76 ± 0.37 vs 1.00 ± 0.67; FEF25–75%pred: $21.15 \pm 10.09\%$ vs $29.06 \pm 16.50\%$. All P values < 0.01). In addition, HR group was showed better asthma control than LR group after the first-month initial treatment (ACT score: 22 ± 4 vs 20 ± 4, P = 0.01).

We further explored the association between HR and asthma control after the first-month initial treatment. Table 2 shows that HR was associated with a decreased

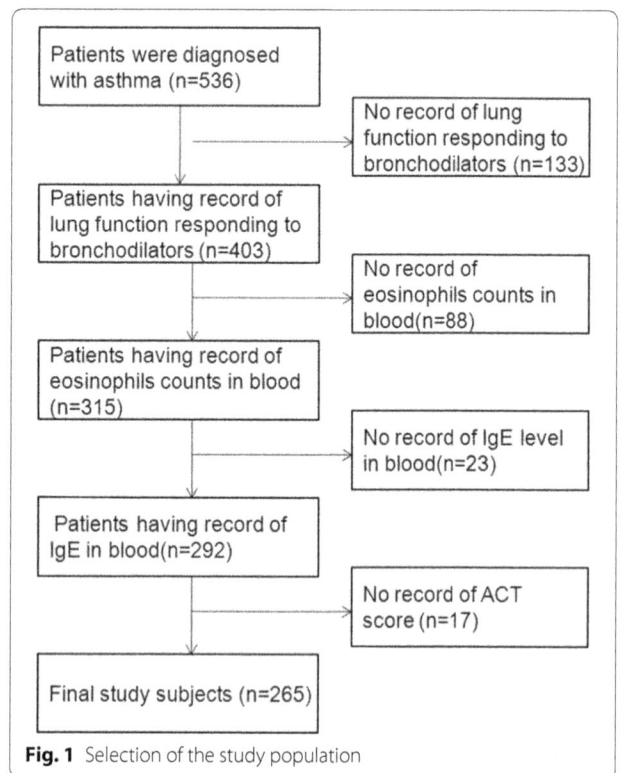

Fig. 1 Selection of the study population

Table 1 Comparison of patients between HR and LR groups

Variable	HR group (n = 60)	LR group (n = 205)	P value
Gender (male)	30 (50.0%)	82 (40.0%)	0.17
Age (years)	45 ± 10	47 ± 13	0.23
BMI (kg/m2)	22.80 ± 3.34	23.50 ± 4.07	0.23
Smoker (yes)	21 (35.0%)	90 (43.9%)	0.22
Self-reported history of allergy (yes)	7 (11.7%)	42 (20.5%)	0.12
Eosinophil count in blood (10^9/L)	0.49 ± 0.28	0.36 ± 0.19	< 0.01
IgE in blood (ng/ml)	1306.0 ± 841.5	413.4 ± 261.6	< 0.01
High-dose ICS+LABA	2 (3.3%)	3 (1.5%)	0.69
Lung function test			
Pre inhaling short-acting bronchodilator			
FVC (L)	3.01 ± 2.62	2.69 ± 0.84	0.14
FEV1 (L)	1.52 ± 0.62	1.69 ± 0.65	0.08
FEV1%pred (%)	51.91 ± 19.34	60.42 ± 19.22	< 0.01
FEV1/FVC (%)	55.43 ± 11.97	61.94 ± 12.59	< 0.01
PEF (L/s)	3.60 ± 1.49	3.88 ± 1.61	0.23
PEF%pred	43.70 ± 16.80	50.59 ± 18.86	0.01
FEF50 (L/s)	0.97 ± 0.50	1.23 ± 0.75	< 0.01
FEF50%pred (%)	23.05 ± 12.18	30.75 ± 17.26	< 0.01
FEF75 (L/s)	0.39 ± 0.40	0.69 ± 1.07	< 0.01
FEF75%pred (%)	19.05 ± 9.16	25.96 ± 16.08	< 0.01
FEF25–75	0.76 ± 0.37	1.00 ± 0.67	< 0.01
FEF25–75%pred (%)	21.15 ± 10.09	29.06 ± 16.50	< 0.01
Post inhaling short-acting bronchodilator			
FVC (L)	2.73 ± 0.99	2.79 ± 0.85	0.67
FEV1 (L)	2.11 ± 0.98	1.84 ± 0.68	0.02
FEV1%pred (%)	72.45 ± 32.46	67.56 ± 26.88	0.23
FEV1/FVC (%)	81.69 ± 38.48	65.73 ± 16.38	< 0.01
PEF (L/s)	4.12 ± 1.54	4.12 ± 1.69	0.98
PEF%pred	50.09 ± 17.85	53.12 ± 18.96	0.27
FEF50 (L/s)	1.38 ± 0.75	1.46 ± 0.81	0.51
FEF50%pred (%)	33.12 ± 16.20	36.69 ± 18.64	0.15
FEF75 (L/s)	0.58 ± 0.59	0.76 ± 0.97	0.08
FEF75%pred (%)	27.84 ± 14.14	31.28 ± 18.86	0.13
FEF25-75	1.15 ± 0.65	1.50 ± 4.40	0.28
FEF25–75%pred (%)	30.99 ± 16.96	44.60 ± 136.36	0.17
FEV1 change[a]	30.13 ± 9.69	8.83 ± 9.11	< 0.01
ACT score	22 ± 4	20 ± 4	0.01

HR high airway reversibility, *LR* low airway reversibility, *BMI* body mass index, *ICS* inhaled corticosteroid, *LABA* long-acting b-agonist, *FEV1* forced expiratory volume in 1 s, *FVC* forced vital capacity, *PEF* peak expiratory flow, *FEF* forced expiratory flow, *%pred* % predicted, *ACT* asthma control test

[a] FEV1 change between pre- and post-inhaling short-acting bronchodilator

risk of uncontrolled asthma after the first-month initial treatment (adjusted OR for ACT score < 20: 0.12 [95% CI 0.03–0.50]). We furthermore assessed the association between asthma control and obstruction in small airway after inhaling short-acting bronchodilator. We found that FEF25–75 was associated with a decreased risk of uncontrolled or partly controlled asthma (adjusted OR

for ACT score < 20: 0.07 [95% CI 0.01–0.73]; adjusted OR for ACT score 20–24: 0.03 [95% CI 0.01–0.71]).

Discussions

In our study, HR was more frequently associated with a higher level of Th2-biomarkers, lower lung function in baseline, and better asthma control after the first-month initial treatment than LR. Furthermore, HR and high

Table 2 Adjusted and unadjusted relative risks of asthma control after the first-month initial treatment

Exposure categories	Unadjusted OR	95% CI	P values	Adjusted OR	95% CI	P values
Asthma uncontrolled (n = 105)						
HR[a]	0.36	0.16–0.82	0.02	0.12	0.03–0.50	< 0.01
Eosinophil count in blood (10^9/L)[a]	1.10	0.18–6.58	0.92	2.36	0.23–23.96	0.47
IgE in blood (ng/ml)[a]	1.00	0.99–1.00	0.29	1.00	0.99–1.00	0.89
FEF75 (L/s)[b, c]	1.31	0.77–2.24	0.32	0.82	0.41–1.63	0.57
FEF75%pred (%)[b, c]	1.01	0.99–1.04	0.24	1.01	0.96–1.06	0.81
FEF25–75[b, c]	1.57	0.91–2.73	0.11	0.07	0.01–0.73	0.03
FEF25–75%pred (%)[b, c]	1.02	1.02–1.05	0.04	1.09	1.01–1.18	0.02
Asthma partly controlled (n = 120)						
HR[a]	0.59	0.27–1.28	0.18	0.35	0.10–1.22	0.10
Eosinophil count (10^9/L)[a]	1.79	0.32–9.97	0.51	2.85	0.31–26.12	0.36
IgE (ng/ml)[a]	1.00	0.99–1.00	0.93	1.00	0.99–1.001	0.93
FEF75 (L/s)[b, c]	1.30	0.76–2.20	0.34	0.84	0.42–1.65	0.60
FEF75%pred (%)[b, c]	1.02	0.99–1.04	0.18	1.01	0.95–1.06	0.82
FEF25–75[b, c]	1.52	0.87–2.62	0.14	0.03	0.01–0.71	0.03
FEF25–75%pred (%)[b, c]	1.02	1.00–1.04	0.06	1.07	1.00–1.15	0.06

HR high airway reversibility, ACT asthma control test, FEF forced expiratory flow, %pred % predicted, FEV1 forced expiratory volume in 1 s, FVC forced vital capacity

Asthma uncontrolled: ACT < 20, Asthma partly controlled: 20 ≤ ACT ≤ 24, Asthma controlled: ACT = 25

[a] Adjusted for age, BMI, eosinophil count, IgE, HR, FEV1, FEV1%pred, FVC, FEV1/FVC, FEV1-post inhaling short-acting bronchodilator, FVC-post inhaling short-acting bronchodilator, FEV1/FVC-post inhaling short-acting bronchodilator

[b] Adjusted for age, BMI, eosinophil count, IgE, HR, FEF50, FEF50%pred, FEF75, FEF75%pred, FEF25–75, FEF25–75%pred

[c] Lung function after inhaling short-acting bronchodilator

FEF25–75 after inhaling short-acting bronchodilator were respectively associated with better asthma control. It may contribute to identifying the endotype of asthma by further clarifying the relationship between airway bronchodilator reversibility, obstruction in small airway, Th2-biomarkers and disease control after initial treatment.

In the present study, asthmatic patients with HR were showed a higher level of Th2-biomarkers than LR group. That finding was similar with previous report [4]. Moreover, in comparison with that previous study, we found that not only serum IgE level but also blood eosinophil count of patients with HR was higher than those with LR. That may be mainly due to different characteristics of our subjects from that previous study. In our study, all patients received ICS combined LABA treatment. ICS could affect circulating eosinophil counts and cytokine expression [9]. In addition, Chinese demographics and clinical characteristics of populations in our study may partly contribute to our different findings. In our study, Chinese patients were showed a lower baseline lung function, a higher level of Th2-biomarkers than Europeans in previous study [4]. Thus, Th2-biomarkers may be more related with HR endotype than LR in Chinese patients with asthma.

Interestingly, it didn't find an association between Th2 biomarker and asthma control after the first-month initial treatment in our study. Previous study found that asthmatic patients with higher blood eosinophil counts fared poorer asthma control [10]. However, that study followed subjects for a long term, and didn't combine with the phenotype of HR. Thus, our study suggested that for patients with HR, higher Th2-biomarkers may not indicate poorer disease control after a short-term initial treatment. Blood eosinophil counts as a biomarker of asthma control in patients with HR phenotype may be combined with other biomarkers. Future study with larger sample size is needed to confirm our findings.

FEF50, FEF75 and FEF25–75 in baseline of patients with HR were less than those with LR in our study. FEF75 and FEF25–75 could accurately reflect flow at low lung volumes, which is helpful to showing small airway obstruction in early stage of obstructive lung disease [11, 12]. Particularly, FEF25–75 is a sensitive indicator for obstructive small airway disease [13]. Thus, asthmatic patients with HR may have a higher risk for small airway obstruction than those with LR. Furthermore, we assessed the association between asthma control after initial treatment and FEF75 or FEF25–75 post-inhaling bronchodilator. We found that FEF25–75 post-inhaling bronchodilator was associated with a decreased risk of poor asthma control, suggesting that high FEF25–75 post-inhaling bronchodilator may indicate better asthma control. Since FEF25–75 is an effective indicator for asthma control [14], FEF25–75 post-inhaling bronchodilator may be a desirable indicator for asthma control after short-term initial treatment in the endotype of HR.

Furthermore, the present study showed that HR was associated with a decreased risk of poor asthma control after the first-month initial treatment. In contrast, previous study found that patients with higher airway reversibility were showed worse controll of asthma at 12 month-follow-up [15]. These findings suggested that asthmatic patients with HR may have a better response than those with LR at the beginning of initial treatment with ICS combined with LABA. However, the long-term response to that treatment may be not good in patients with HR as previous reported [15]. The factors are not well clarified. It may be partly related with complex pathogenesis and progress of asthma, variously adjustment in therapeutic strategies during long-term treatment, or patients' incompliance with treatment. Thus, for patients with HR, it may be particularly important to regularly monitor disease control and then adjust therapeutic strategy in a long term.

We acknowledge that our study has limitations. The patients were followed only 1 month after initial treatment. Although we can't explore asthma control of HR group in a long-term, previous study reported different findings on asthma control in patients with HR for a long-term from a short-term [15]. Those indicated that there may be dynamic changes of asthma control during a long period of treatment. Moreover, atopy test was absent in our study. Thus, we couldn't explore the relationship between atopy and HR endotype. Even though, the self-reported history of allergy was not significant different between HR and LR groups when demographic characteristics were well matched.

Conclusions

In conclusion, HR is a physiologic indicator of lower lung function, particularly small airway obstruction, and is more related with an increased level of Th2-biomarkers than LR. Moreover, HR indicates well asthma control after the first-month initial treatment. Those findings may be help to identify the endotype of asthma.

Abbreviations
GINA: Global Initiative for Asthma guidelines; ACT: Asthma Control Test; FEV1: forced expiratory volume in one second; Th2: T-helper 2; COPD: chronic obstructive pulmonary disease; HR: high airway reversibility; LR: low airway reversibility; OR: odds ratios; CI: confidence intervals; SD: standard deviation; BMI: body-mass index; ICS: inhaled corticosteroid; LABA: long-acting inhaled β2-agonist; FEF: forced expiratory flow.

Authors' contributions
JW, BM and SC designed the study. JW, LM, JW, QX, MC, MJ, ML, WJ and WS coordinated the overall undertaking of the study. JW and SC performed statistical analyses. JW and SC wrote the manuscript. All authors contributed to the revision. All authors read and approved the final manuscript.

Author details
[1] Department of Respiratory and Critical Care Medicine, Affiliated Hospital of Guilin Medical University, Guilin 541001, Guangxi, China. [2] Laboratory of Respiratory Diseases, Affiliated Hospital of Guilin Medical University, Guilin 541001, Guangxi, China.

Competing interests
The authors declare that they have no competing interests.

Funding and acknowledgements
This work was supported by grants from the National Natural Science Foundation of China (Nos. 81460005 and 81760008), the Guangxi Natural Science Foundation (Nos. 2012GXNSFDA053020 and 2015GXNSFAA139107).

References
1. Global strategy for asthma management and prevention 2014. Global Initiative for Asthma website. http://www.ginasthma.org/. Accessed 1 Aug 2014.
2. Busse WW, Holgate S, Kerwin E, Chon Y, Feng J, Lin J, et al. Randomized, double-blind, placebo-controlled study of brodalumab, a human anti-IL-17 receptor monoclonal antibody, in moderate to severe asthma. Am J Respir Crit Care Med. 2013;188(11):1294–302.
3. Nadeau M, Boulay MÈ, Milot J, Lepage J, Bilodeau L, Maltais F, et al. Comparative prevalence of co-morbidities in smoking and non-smoking asthma patients with incomplete reversibility of airway obstruction, non-smoking asthma patients with complete reversibility of airway obstruction and COPD patients. Respir Med. 2017;125:82–8.
4. Busse WW, Holgate ST, Wenzel SW, Klekotka P, Chon Y, Feng J, et al. Biomarker profiles in asthma with high vs low airway reversibility and poor disease control. Chest. 2015;148(6):1489–96.
5. Agache IO. From phenotypes to endotypes to asthma treatment. Curr Opin Allergy Clin Immunol. 2013;13(3):249–56.
6. Vega JM, Badia X, Badiola C, López-Viña A, Olaguíbel JM, Picado C, et al. Validation of the Spanish version of the Asthma Control Test (ACT). J Asthma. 2007;44(10):867–72.
7. Jia CE, Zhang HP, Lv Y, Liang R, Jiang YQ, Powell H, et al. The Asthma Control Test and Asthma Control Questionnaire for assessing asthma control: systematic review and meta-analysis. J Allergy Clin Immunol. 2013;131(3):695–703.
8. Diagnosis of diseases of chronic airflow limitation: asthma, COPD and asthma COPD overlap syndrome. Global initiative for chronic obstructive lung disease website. http://www.goldcopd.org/uploads/users/fles/AsthmaCOPDOverlap.pdf. Accessed 25 Aug 2014.
9. Anderson WJ, Short PM, Jabbal S, Lipworth BJ. Inhaled corticosteroid dose response in asthma: should we measure inflammation? Ann Allergy Asthma Immunol. 2017;118(2):179–85.
10. Price DB, Rigazio A, Campbell JD, Bleecker ER, Corrigan CJ, Thomas M, et al. Blood eosinophil count and prospective annual asthma disease burden: a UK cohort study. Lancet Respir Med. 2015;3(11):849–58.
11. Pereira CA, Barreto SP, Simões JG, Pereira FW, Gerstler JG, Nakatani J. Valores de referência para espirometria em uma amostra da população brasileira adulta. J Pneumol. 1992;18(1):10–22.
12. Rodrigues MT, Fiterman-Molinari D, Barreto SS, Fiterman J. The role of the FEF50%/0.5FVC ratio in the diagnosis of obstructive lung diseases. J Bras Pneumol. 2010;36(1):44–50.
13. Simon MR, Chinchilli VM, Phillips BR, Sorkness CA, Lemanske RF Jr, Szefler SJ, et al. Forced expiratory flow between 25 and 75% of vital capacity and FEV1/forced vital capacity ratio in relation to clinical and physiological parameters in asthmatic children with normal FEV1 values. J Allergy Clin Immunol. 2010;126(3):527-34.e1-8.
14. Lutfi MF. Patterns of changes and diagnostic values of FEF50%, FEF25%–75% and FEF50%/FEF25%–75% ratio in patients with varying control of bronchial asthma. Int J Health Sci (Qassim). 2016;10(1):3–11.
15. Khusial RJ, Sont JK, Loijmans RJB, Snoeck-Stroband JB, Assendelft PJJ, Schermer TRJ, et al. Longitudinal outcomes of different asthma phenotypes in primary care, an observational study. NPJ Prim Care Respir Med. 2017;27(1):55.

19

Oral immunotherapy with the ingestion of house dust mite extract in a murine model of allergic asthma

Yao-Tung Wang[1,2†], Hsu-Chung Liu[2,3,4†], Hui-Chen Chen[5], Yen-Ching Lee[4], Tung-Chou Tsai[4], Hsiao-Ling Chen[6], Hueng-Chuen Fan[7,8,9*] and Chuan-Mu Chen[4,10,11*]

Abstract

Background: Allergen-specific immunotherapy (ASIT) has the potential to modify allergic diseases, and it is also considered a potential therapy for allergic asthma. House dust mite (HDM) allergens, a common source of airborne allergen in human diseases, have been developed as an immunotherapy for patients with allergic asthma via the subcutaneous and sublingual routes. Oral immunotherapy with repeated allergen ingestion is emerging as another potential modality of ASIT. The aim of this study was to evaluate the therapeutic efficacy of the oral ingestion of HDM extracts in a murine model of allergic asthma.

Methods: BABL/c mice were sensitized twice by intraperitoneal injection of HDM extracts and $Al(OH)_3$ on day 1 and day 8. Then, the mice received challenge to induce airway inflammation by intratracheal instillation of HDM extracts on days 29–31. The treatment group received immunotherapy with oral HDM extracts ingestion before the challenge. All the mice were sacrificed on day 32 for bronchoalveolar inflammatory cytokines, mediastinal lymph node T cells, lung histology, and serum HDM-specific immunoglobulins analyses.

Results: Upon HDM sensitization and following challenge, a robust Th2 cell response and eosinophilic airway inflammation were observed in mice of the positive control group. The mice treated with HDM extracts ingestion had decreased eosinophilic airway inflammation, suppressed HDM-specific Th2 cell responses in the mediastinal lymph nodes, and attenuated serum HDM-specific IgE levels.

Conclusions: Oral immunotherapy with HDM extracts ingestion was demonstrated to have a partial therapeutic effect in the murine model of allergic asthma. This study may serve as the basis for the further development of oral immunotherapy with HDM extracts in allergic asthma.

Keywords: Allergen-specific immunotherapy, House dust mite, Allergic asthma, Oral immunotherapy, Airway inflammation

*Correspondence: fanhuengchuen@yahoo.com.tw; chchen1@dragon.nchu.edu.tw

†Yao-Tung Wang and Hsu-Chung Liu contributed equally to this work

[4] Department of Life Sciences, College of Life Sciences, National Chung Hsing University, No. 250, Kuo-Kuang Road, Taichung 402, Taiwan

[7] Department of Pediatrics, Tungs'Taichung Metroharbor Hospital, No. 699, Sec. 8, Taiwan Blvd., Wuchi, Taichung 435, Taiwan

Full list of author information is available at the end of the article

Background

Allergic asthma, an allergic disease, is characterized by Th2 cell-mediated airway inflammation and a hypersensitive reaction to allergen exposure. Allergen-specific immunotherapy (ASIT) is the repeated administration of specific, relevant allergens to treat IgE-mediated allergic disease. It is predicted that ASIT has the potential to modify the disease course of allergic asthma [1]. In the past 100 years, many studies regarding ASIT have promoted the development of many modalities of immunotherapy in allergic diseases [2]. Because the house dust mite (HDM) is an important airborne allergen source associated with asthma attacks in the domestic environment, many ASIT studies have been conducted using HDM extracts to treat asthma. There are two major immunotherapy modalities for the clinical application of allergic asthma, subcutaneous immunotherapy (SCIT) [3] and sublingual immunotherapy (SLIT) [4].

In addition, the induction of immune tolerance through repeated ingestion of allergens, called oral immunotherapy, is a novel modality of immunotherapy [5]. Although murine models of allergic asthma have been used to analyze disease mechanisms and to develop new therapies in past decades [6, 7], there have been few animal studies evaluating ASIT with an oral administration route of the HDM allergens in allergic asthma. In a study by Hsu et al. [8], the oral administration of recombinant *Dermatophagoides pteronyssinus* allergen 5 (Dp 5), produced by plants, was demonstrated to down-regulate allergen-induced airway inflammation in mice [8]. In our previous studies, oral ingestion of transgenic milk containing recombinant *D. pteronyssinus* allergen 2 (Dp 2) was demonstrated to partially protect mice from subsequent development of allergic airway inflammation [9]. These two studies used single isolated HDM allergens as airway inflammation irritants and as the oral ingestion formula. However, the whole mite extract is a complex compound and more representative of real-life aeroallergen exposure in humans [10]. There were only few experimental asthma studies focusing on the oral ingestion of HDM extracts. The aim of this study was to evaluate the therapeutic efficacy of oral HDM extracts ingestion as an immunotherapy modality for allergic asthma in the murine model.

Methods

An murine model of allergic airway inflammation

Commercial HDM extracts with low endotoxin content (*D. pteronyssinus* protein 39.6 mg/vial; endotoxin 25,500 EU/vial) were used in an animal model of HDM-specific allergic airway inflammation. They were purchased from Greer Laboratories (Lenoir, North Carolina, USA). The HDM extracts were dissolved in sterile phosphate-buffered saline (PBS; 2.5 mg protein weight/mL) before being used for intraperitoneal sensitization, intratracheal challenge, and oral ingestion.

Six-week-old female BALB/c mice were obtained from the animal-breeding center of the College of Medicine, at National Taiwan University. All mice were housed under specific pathogen-free and dust mite-free conditions. The body weight of mice was controlled within a 5% variation of 25 g. The animal trials in this study were approved by the Institutional Animal Care and Use Committee of National Chung Hsing University, Taiwan (IACUC No.104-123). Initially, these mice received sensitization (intraperitoneal injection) twice on days 1 and 8 with 25 µg of HDM extracts and 2 mg of $Al(OH)_3$ in 200 µL of PBS. Alum, $Al(OH)_3$ (Alu-gel-S, Serva, Heidelberg, Germany), was used as an adjuvant for the promotion of T helper cell 2 (Th2) immunologic response in mice [11]. Mice were divided into three experimental groups: (A) the normal control (NC) group, composed of unsensitized mice fed formula who did not receive intraperitoneal injections of the HDM extracts; (B) the positive control (PC) group, composed of HDM-sensitized mice that received sensitization and following challenge with HDM extracts to induce allergic airway inflammation and that served as the inflammation control; and (C) the treatment (HDM) group, composed of HDM-treated mice that received HDM extracts orally daily from day 15 to day 31 and that served as the intervention group. To induce allergic airway inflammation [11–13], the mice in groups B and C received allergen challenges by intratracheal (i.t.) instillation with 100 µg HDM extracts in 50 µL of PBS under light anesthesia three times on three consecutive days (day 29–day 31). The mice of group A only received i.t. challenge with PBS. The timeline of the animal trial is shown in Fig. 1.

Analysis of inflammatory cell counts and cytokine expression levels in BAL fluids

After i.t. challenge, the experimental mice were sacrificed for the collection of bronchoalveolar lavage (BAL) fluid at day 32. BAL fluid collection and the analysis of inflammatory cells were performed as previous reported [14]. One milliliter of Hanks' balanced salts (HBSS) free of ionized calcium and magnesium but supplemented with 0.05 mmol/L sodium EDTA was instilled four times via the tracheal cannula and recovered by gentle manual aspiration. The recovered fluids were centrifuged (700*g* for 10 min at 4 °C). The cell pellets were washed twice and finally resuspended in 1 mL of HBSS. The percentage of leukocytes among the BAL cells was determined with a hemocytometer (VWR, Lutterworth, UK). The cytospin preparation of 100 µL of BAL fluids was followed by staining with Liu stain. The differential counts

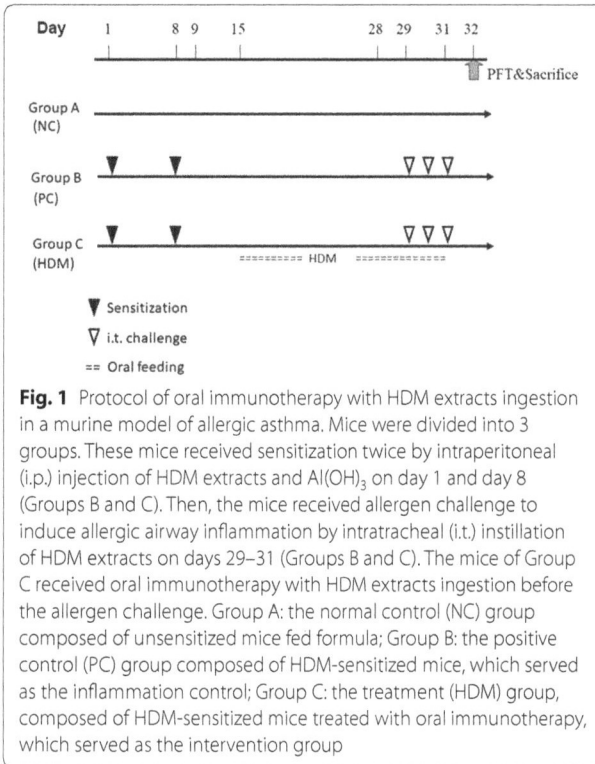

Fig. 1 Protocol of oral immunotherapy with HDM extracts ingestion in a murine model of allergic asthma. Mice were divided into 3 groups. These mice received sensitization twice by intraperitoneal (i.p.) injection of HDM extracts and Al(OH)$_3$ on day 1 and day 8 (Groups B and C). Then, the mice received allergen challenge to induce allergic airway inflammation by intratracheal (i.t.) instillation of HDM extracts on days 29–31 (Groups B and C). The mice of Group C received oral immunotherapy with HDM extracts ingestion before the allergen challenge. Group A: the normal control (NC) group composed of unsensitized mice fed formula; Group B: the positive control (PC) group composed of HDM-sensitized mice, which served as the inflammation control; Group C: the treatment (HDM) group, composed of HDM-sensitized mice treated with oral immunotherapy, which served as the intervention group

of BAL cells (eosinophil, neutrophil, lymphocyte) were performed under a microscope, and 200 total cells were counted. In addition, the supernatants of the BAL fluid were aspirated and stored at −80 °C until the detection of the cytokine levels. The analysis of the cytokine levels in the BAL fluids was done via paired antibodies for murine IFN-γ, IL-4, and IL-5 in standardized sandwich ELISAs according to the manufacturer's protocol [15].

Cytokine assays of mediastinal lymph node T cells after HDM re-stimulation

After BAL, the mediastinal lymph nodes were dissected and placed separately into 4 °C HBSS. The mediastinal lymph nodes were digested with collagenase I (Gibco Invitrogen, Grand Island, NY, USA) and DNase (Roche Applied Science, Mannheim, Germany) for 30 min at 37 °C. We filtered the cell suspensions through a 70-μm cell strainer and depleted them of red blood cells using red blood cell lysis buffer. The recovered cells were filtered through a 70-μm nylon sieve (BD Falcon, San Jose, CA, USA), washed twice, resuspended in complete media, and counted with a hemocytometer. We pooled cells from each group and cultured 1.5×10^6 lymph node cells in triplicate for 72 h in medium with or without HDM extracts (100 μg/mL) in 96-well plates, respectively. The culture medium was RPMI 1640 (Perbio, Waltham, MA, USA) containing 5% heat-inactivated

fetal calf serum (FCS), 50 mM 2-mercaptoethanol and penicillin–streptomycin (Gibco Invitrogen, Grand Island, NY, USA) [16]. The supernatants were analyzed for the expression levels of IFN-γ (Th1 cytokine) and IL-5 (Th2 cytokine) by ELISAs [17].

Lung tissue histology and scoring of pulmonary inflammation

The left lungs were fixed in formalin. Paraffin-embedded sections were stained with hematoxylin and eosin (H&E) for histological analysis and comparison. Pieces from all lung lobes are used for histological examination. Sections of 2.5-μm thickness are cut and stained with H&E [18, 19]. A scoring and grading method of lung inflammation was used as in previous studies [14]. A value from 0 to 3 criterion was scored for each tissue section. Two separate scoring criteria were documented for pulmonary inflammation: peribronchial inflammation and perivascular inflammation. A value of 0 was assigned when no inflammation was detectable, a value of 1 was assigned when occasional cuffing with inflammatory cells was observed, a value of 2 was assigned when most bronchi or vessels were surrounded by a thin layer (one to five cells) of inflammatory cells, and a value of 3 was assigned when most bronchi or vessels were surrounded by a thick layer (more than 5 cells) of inflammatory cells. In total, 10 tissue sections per mouse were scored in high power fields (×400), and the inflammation scores were expressed mean values and compared between groups.

Measurements of serum HDM-specific immunoglobulins

Blood was collected from the hearts of the mice after they were sacrificed. The blood was centrifuged at 2500 rpm for 20 min. The serum was collected and stored at −80 °C before analysis. The serum HDM-specific IgE, IgG1, and IgG2a levels were determined by using ELISA kits, and the measurements were done according to the manufacture's protocol [20].

Analysis of regulatory T (Treg) cell populations

We pooled the cells from the mediastinal lymph nodes in each group and cultured 4×10^6 T cells in 96-well plates [16]. For intracellular staining, we incubated cells with 100 μg/mL HDM extracts and 1 μg/mL anti-CD28 antibody (Becton–Dickinson, East Rutherford, NJ, USA) for 6 h. Brefeldin A (5 mg/mL; Sigma-Aldrich, St. Louis, MO, USA) was added during the last 4 h. Then, we stained the cells with a monoclonal antibody (mAb) against CD4, fixed the cells, permeabilized them with the Cytofix/ Cytoperm reagent (Becton–Dickinson, East Rutherford, NJ, USA), and stained them with an antibody against CD40L (Becton–Dickinson, East Rutherford, NJ, USA) and mAb against Foxp3 (eBioscience, San Diego, CA, USA). Finally, we analyzed them by fluorescence activated cell sorting (FACS; Beckman Coulter Inc., Brea, CA, USA).

Statistical analysis

To assess the different levels of airway inflammation, a repeated measure ANOVA was performed to compare between groups. A value of $P < 0.05$ was used to indicate statistical significance.

Results

Therapeutic effect of HDM extracts ingestion on allergic airway inflammation

To determine the therapeutic effect of HDM extracts on the inflammatory response, the differential cell counts in the BAL fluids of mice were measured to evaluate the extent of airway inflammation. The HDM group had fewer eosinophil cells in BAL fluids than PC group (Fig. 2). The PC group had obvious inflammatory cell infiltration in both bronchi (Fig. 3b) and the lung parenchyma (Fig. 3e). However, the HDM group had less infiltration of inflammatory cells (Figs. 3c, f) than the PC group. Furthermore, the peribronchial and perivascular pulmonary inflammation were scored according to the inflammatory scoring criteria. Both the peribronchial and perivascular inflammatory scores of the HDM group were lower than those of the PC group (Fig. 4).

These findings suggest that oral immunotherapy the ingestion of HDM extracts could suppress eosinophilic airway inflammation in mice with established HDM-specific sensitization and following a challenge.

The Th2 cytokine levels, such as IL-4 and IL-5, were also measured in these BAL fluids. The results showed

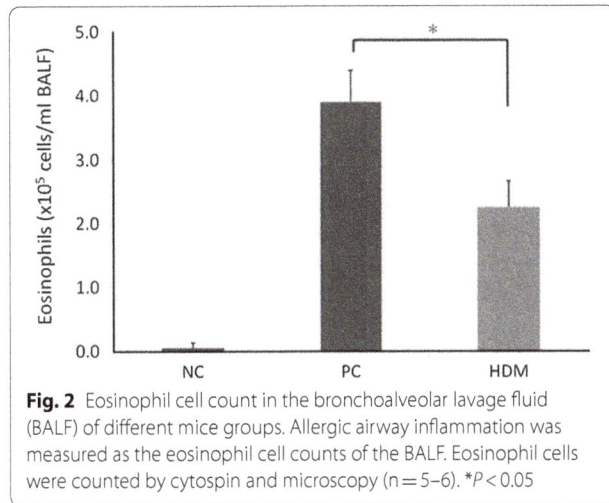

Fig. 2 Eosinophil cell count in the bronchoalveolar lavage fluid (BALF) of different mice groups. Allergic airway inflammation was measured as the eosinophil cell counts of the BALF. Eosinophil cells were counted by cytospin and microscopy (n = 5–6). *$P < 0.05$

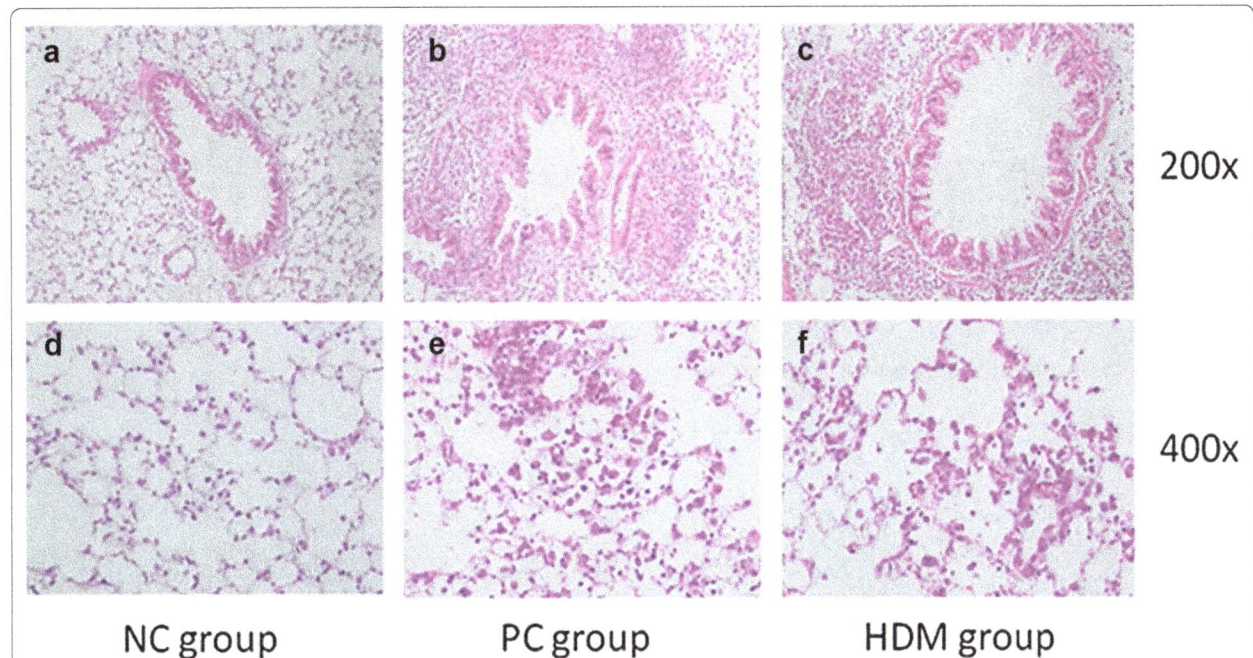

Fig. 3 Histological analysis of allergic airway inflammation by immunohistochemical (IHC) staining. **a**, **d** Image representative of the negative control from normal mice. **b**, **e** Image representative of the positive control from the HDM-sensitized mice that received following challenge with HDM extractrs. **c**, **f** Image representative of the HDM group that HDM-sensitized mice received oral immunotherapy with HDM extracts ingestion before the challenge. There were numerous inflammatory cells that had infiltrated beneath the tracheal epithelium in the PC and HDM groups. Representative photomicrographs of different groups are shown; n = 5 mice per group

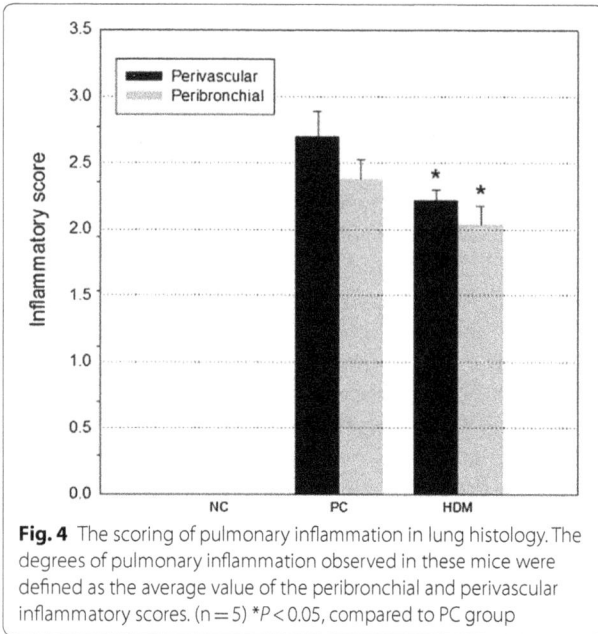

Fig. 4 The scoring of pulmonary inflammation in lung histology. The degrees of pulmonary inflammation observed in these mice were defined as the average value of the peribronchial and perivascular inflammatory scores. (n = 5) *P < 0.05, compared to PC group

that there were no significant differences between the HDM group and the PC group (Figs. 5a, b). The Th1 cytokine level of INF-γ was also tested in the BAL fluids, but the levels were undetectable in all three groups (data not shown).

Effect of HDM extracts ingestion on T cell function of the lymph nodes

The mediastinal lymph node T cells were collected from the individual mice. These cells were co-cultured in triplicate with 100 μg/mL HDM extracts for a reaction of re-stimulation. The supernatants were analyzed for the levels of IL-4 (Th2 cytokine) and INF-γ (Th1 cytokine) 72 h later. The results showed that the HDM group had a significantly lower IL-4 level than the PC group (Fig. 5c). However, the INF-γ level in the HDM group was not significantly different than that of the PC group (Fig. 5d). These findings suggested that the ingestion of HDM extracts could suppress the HDM-specific response of Th2 cells in the mediastinal lymph nodes.

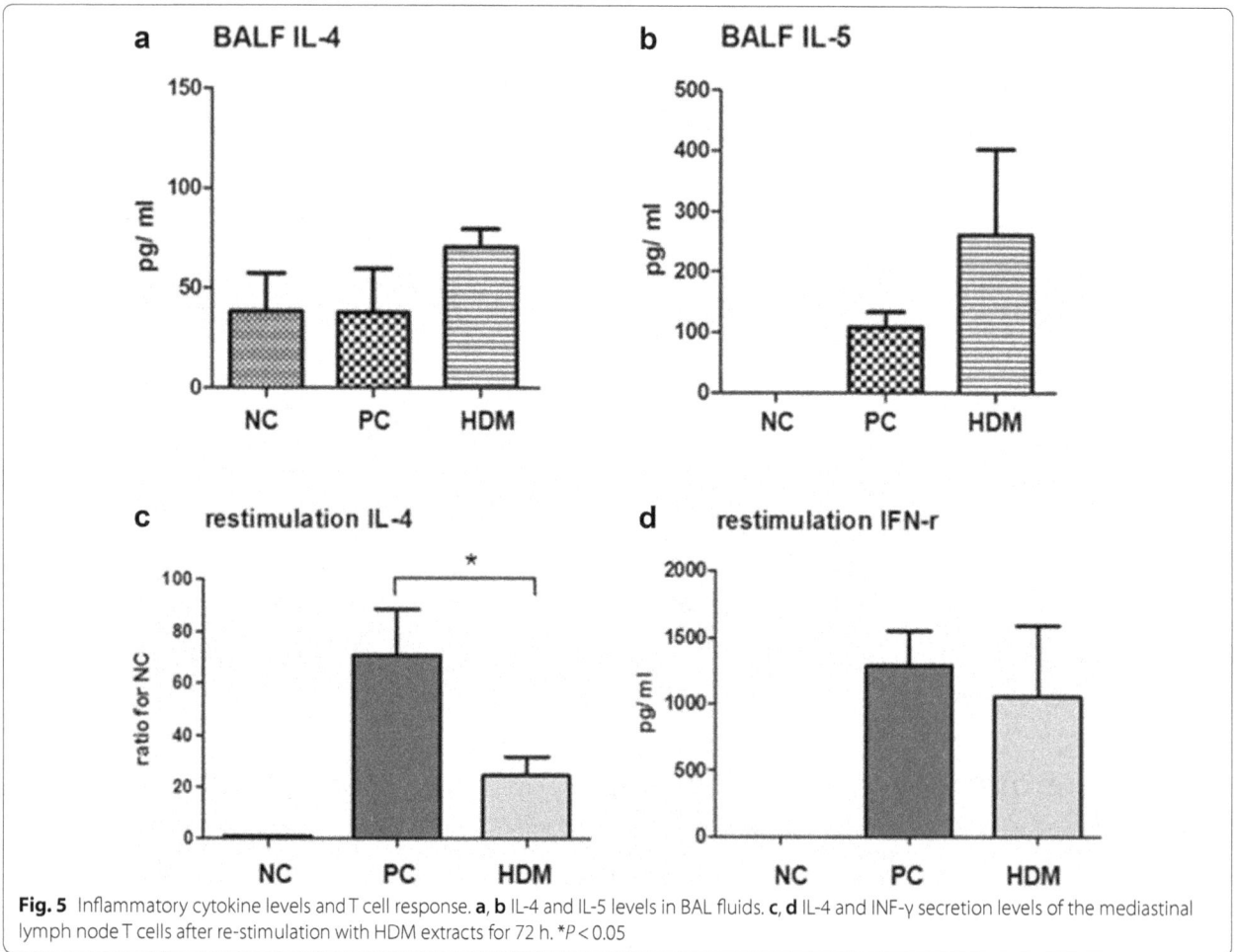

Fig. 5 Inflammatory cytokine levels and T cell response. **a, b** IL-4 and IL-5 levels in BAL fluids. **c, d** IL-4 and INF-γ secretion levels of the mediastinal lymph node T cells after re-stimulation with HDM extracts for 72 h. *P < 0.05

Therapeutic effect of HDM extracts ingestion on serum HDM-specific IgE

The serum levels of HDM-specific immunoglobulin were analyzed by ELISA. The HDM group had lower serum HDM-specific IgE and IgG2a levels than the PC group (Fig. 6). There was no statistical difference in the level of HDM-specific IgG1 between the HDM group and the PC group. These data suggested that the ingestion of HDM extracts could suppress the Th2 response and, subsequently, the HDM-specific IgE level in these HDM-sensitized mice.

The regulatory T cells (Treg) population from the mediastinal lymph nodes

The mediastinal lymph node cells were collected and pooled in vitro with HDM extracts (100 μg/mL). After 24 h of HDM extracts stimulation, the cells were stained for CD4 and Foxp3. The percentage of CD4+Foxp3+ Treg cells in the CD4+ T cell population from the three experimental groups are shown in the upper right quadrant of Fig. 7. The results showed that there was no significant increase in the Treg cell percentage in the HDM group compared with the PC group. This finding suggested that the therapeutic effect of HDM extracts ingestion in this model may not be directly mediated by the up-regulation of Treg cells.

Discussion

In this murine study of allergic asthma, the intra-peritoneally HDM-sensitized mice developed eosinophilic airway inflammation after the intra-tracheal challenge with HDM extracts. The oral ingestion of HDM extracts was demonstrated to have a therapeutic effect; it decreased eosinophilic airway inflammation, suppressed the HDM-specific Th2 cell response in the mediastinal lymph node, and attenuated the serum HDM-specific IgE level. However, the histological and bronchoalveolar lavage analysis showed that the HDM group still had an obvious inflammatory reaction when compared with the NC group. This result reveals that the allergic airway inflammation seems to be not completely resolved by this oral immunotherapy. The commercial HDM extracts used in this study are composed of various allergens and non-allergenic peptides from *D. pteronyssinus*. Some of the components have been proven to have intrinsic enzymatic activity or to have ability to induce the inflammatory response [6, 21], which implies that the exposure to HDM extracts in the airway could induce a complex Th1/Th2 inflammatory response. The confounding factor of intrinsic enzymatic activity may be one explanation for the remaining obvious inflammatory infiltrates in the histologic analysis and elevated cytokine level in the bronchoalveolar lavage in the HDM group.

Several possible underlying mechanisms of ASIT have been proposed, including tachyphylaxis, the induction of T cell anergy, switching from a Th2 to a Th1 response, and Treg cells [2]. It has been proposed that the shift from an allergen-specific effector T cell response to a Treg cell response appears to be a key event in the induction of tolerance in patients undergoing ASIT [22]. However, our analysis of the Treg cell population in the mediastinal lymph nodes showed no significant up-regulation of Treg cells in mice received treatment with HDM extracts ingestion. The absence of up-regulated Treg cells in this study may be related to the treatment dose of the HDM extracts. It is thought that low doses of antigen ingestion favor tolerance driven by Treg cells, whereas high doses of antigen ingestion favor tolerance mediated

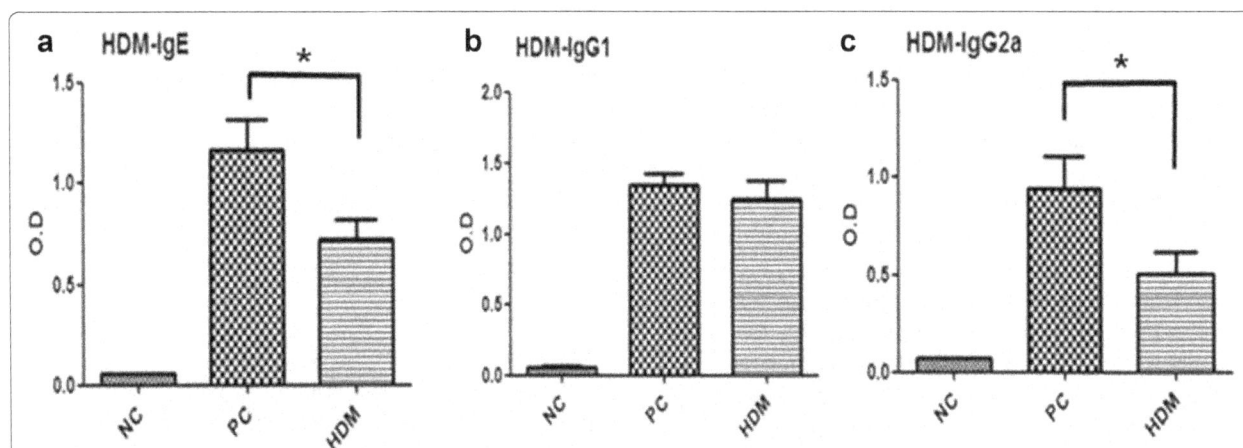

Fig. 6 Serum HDM-specific immunoglobulin levels. Serum samples from mice in the three experimental groups were analyzed to determine the HDM-specific IgE levels (**a**), HDM-specific IgG1 levels (**b**), and HDM-specific IgG2a levels (**c**) by ELISA. The data are expressed as the mean ± SD of the values obtained for the individual mice. n = 5–6 mice per group. *$P < 0.05$

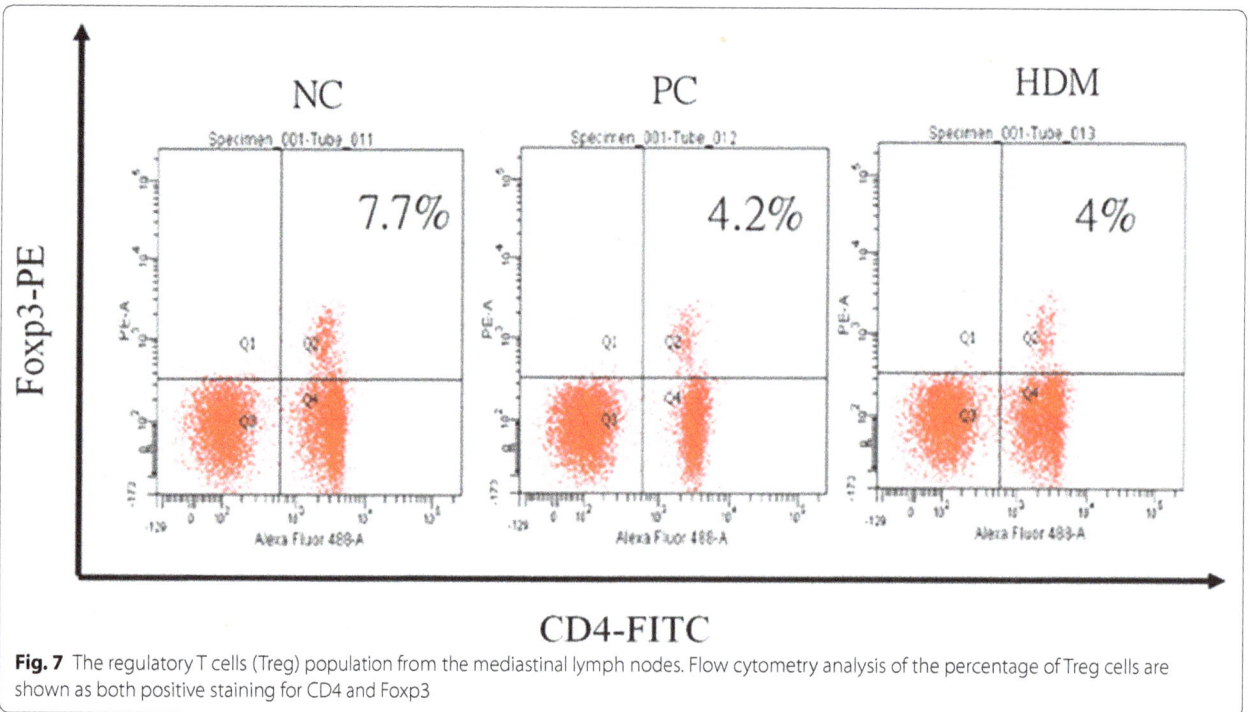

Fig. 7 The regulatory T cells (Treg) population from the mediastinal lymph nodes. Flow cytometry analysis of the percentage of Treg cells are shown as both positive staining for CD4 and Foxp3

by lymphocyte anergy [5]. Therefore, anergy-driven tolerance could be a more possible mechanism to explain the therapeutic effect of oral immunotherapy with HDM extracts ingestion in this study.

From clinical studies in patients with asthma and HDM allergy, both subcutaneous immunotherapy or sublingual immunotherapy with HDM extracts have been demonstrated to have therapeutic effects on reducing symptoms and the use of medication [3, 23]. Although there is a mild to moderate potential benefit, the concern of the risk of adverse effects and the inconvenience in receiving prolonged course of immunotherapy impede patient preferences for this treatment modality. Therefore, ASIT is considered to have weak evidence and limited application in clinical asthma management guideline [24]. In comparison to the subcutaneous and sublingual routes of allergen administration, oral allergen ingestion has the advantage of being more convenient in practice. It has been well established from previous studies in both animals and humans that repeated allergen exposure in the gut mucosa can induce immune tolerance [5, 25]. This study demonstrated that oral immunotherapy with HDM extracts ingestion could be a potential alternative immunotherapy modality in treating allergic asthma. However, further clinical studies are needed to compare the efficacy and safety among oral immunotherapy and the relative well-established models of SCIT and SLIT.

It is well known that mice could not spontaneously develop allergic asthma. Several allergen challenge models in mice have been developed for studying asthma and they could reproduce airway inflammatory features mimicking allergic asthma. Our sensitization and challenge protocol using intraperitoneal allergen injection and intratracheal instillation was according to the basic rules of acute allergen challenge models described in previous studies [6, 7]. A successful sensitization usually requires multiple systemic administration of target allergen with the coincidences of adjuvant. Aluminum hydroxide $Al(OH)_3$ are common adjuvant used to promote a Th2 phenotype inflammation in mice when they are mixed with antigen via intraperitoneal administration. Because asthma is defined as a chronic inflammatory disease of airways, murine experiments of allergen challenge models have some disparity indeed both in immunology and anatomy when comparing with clinical asthma. The findings in this acute allergen challenge model still have limitations when extrapolating the results to the human disease.

Conclusions

In summary, oral immunotherapy with HDM extracts ingestion in the murine model of allergic asthma demonstrated a partial therapeutic effect. This study provides helpful information on the further development of oral immunotherapy in allergic asthma.

Abbreviations
ASIT: allergen-specific immunotherapy; BAL: bronchoalveolar lavage; Dp2: group 2 allergen from *Dermatophagoides pteronyssinus*; Dp5: group 5 allergen from *Dermatophagoides pteronyssinus*; ELISA: enzyme-linked immunosorbent assay; HBSS: Hanks' balanced salts; HDMs: house dust mites; H&E: hematoxylin and eosin; SCIT: subcutaneous injection immunotherapy; SLIT: sublingual immunotherapy; Th2: T helper cell 2; Treg: regulatory T cells.

Authors' contributions
CMC, YTW, HCF and HCL designed the experiments. HCC, YCL, TCT and HCL performed the experiments. YTW, HLC, HCF and CMC performed data analysis. YTW, HCL and CMC prepared the manuscript and figures. CMC, HCL and HCF contributed the revising and correcting manuscript. CMC provided project leadership. All authors contributed to the final manuscript. All authors read and approved the final manuscript.

Author details
[1] Division of Pulmonary Medicine, Department of Internal Medicine, Chung Shan Medical University Hospital, Taichung, Taiwan. [2] School of Medicine, Chung Shan Medical University, Taichung, Taiwan. [3] Division of Chest Medicine, Department of Internal Medicine, Cheng Ching Hospital, Taichung, Taiwan. [4] Department of Life Sciences, College of Life Sciences, National Chung Hsing University, No. 250, Kuo-Kuang Road, Taichung 402, Taiwan. [5] Department of Microbiology and Immunology, School of Medicine, China Medical University, Taichung, Taiwan. [6] Department of Bioresources, Da-Yeh University, Changhwa, Taiwan. [7] Department of Pediatrics, Tungs'Taichung Metroharbor Hospital, No. 699, Sec. 8, Taiwan Blvd., Wuchi, Taichung 435, Taiwan. [8] Department of Medical Research, Tungs'Taichung Metroharbor Hospital, No. 699, Sec. 8, Taiwan Blvd., Wuchi, Taichung 435, Taiwan. [9] Department of Rehabilitation, Jen-Teh Junior College of Medicine, Nursing and Management, Miaoli, Taiwan. [10] The iEGG and Animal Biotechnology Center, National Chung Hsing University, Taichung, Taiwan. [11] Rong Hsing Research Center for Translational Medicine, National Chung Hsing University, Taichung, Taiwan.

Acknowledgements
The authors would like to thank Dr. Cheng-Wei Lai in the Molecular Embryology & DNA Methylation Laboratory for his discussions and help with technical issues.

Competing interests
The authors declare that they have no competing interests.

Funding
This research was supported by a research project of Chung Shan Medical University Hospital (Project Number: CSH-2014-C-037), Chung-Kang Branch, Cheng-Ching General Hospital Research Fund (Grant Number CH10600208B) and Grant MOST-104-2313-B-005-043-MY3 from the Ministry of Science and Technology, Taiwan, and financially supported by the iEGG and Animal Biotechnology Center from the Feature Areas Research Center Program within the framework of the Higher Education Sprout Project by the Ministry of Education (MOE) in Taiwan. The funders had no role in study design, data collection and analysis, decision to publish, or preparation of the manuscript.

References
1. Nagata M, Nakagome K. Allergen immunotherapy in asthma: current status and future perspectives. Allergol Int. 2010;59:15–9.
2. Ring J, Gutermuth J. 100 years of hyposensitization: history of allergen-specific immunotherapy (ASIT). Allergy. 2011;66:713–24.
3. Abramson MJ, Puy RM, Weiner JM. Injection allergen immunotherapy for asthma. Cochrane Database Syst Rev. 2010;2010:CD001186.
4. Normansell R, Kew KM, Bridgman AL. Sublingual immunotherapy for asthma. Cochrane Database Syst Rev. 2015;2015:CD011293.
5. Burks AW, Laubach S, Jones SM. Oral tolerance, food allergy, and immunotherapy: implications for future treatment. J Allergy Clin Immunol. 2008;121:1344–50.
6. Nials AT, Uddin S. Mouse models of allergic asthma: acute and chronic allergen challenge. Dis Model Mech. 2008;1:213–20.
7. Bates JH, Rincon M, Irvin CG. Animal models of asthma. Am J Physiol Lung Cell Mol Physiol. 2009;297:L401–10.
8. Hsu CH, Lin SS, Liu FL, Su WC, Yeh SD. Oral administration of a mite allergen expressed by zucchini yellow mosaic virus in cucurbit species downregulates allergen-induced airway inflammation and IgE synthesis. J Allergy Clin Immunol. 2004;113:1079–85.
9. Liu HC, Pai SY, Cheng WT, et al. Ingestion of milk containing the Dp2 peptide, a dust mite allergen, protects mice from allergic airway inflammation and hyper-responsiveness. Allergy Asthma Clin Immunol. 2013;9(1):21.
10. Cates EC, Fattouh R, Wattie J, et al. Intranasal exposure of mice to house dust mite elicits allergic airway inflammation via a GM-CSF-mediated mechanism. J Immunol. 2004;173(10):6384–92.
11. Agua-Doce A, Graca L. Prevention of house dust mite induced allergic airways disease in mice through immune tolerance. PLoS ONE. 2011;6(7):e22320.
12. Canonica GW, Virchow JC, Zieglmayer P, et al. Efficacy and safety of SQ house dust mite (HDM) SLIT-tablet treatment of HDM allergic asthma. Expert Rev Clin Immunol. 2016;12(8):805–15.
13. Liu HC, Pai SY, Chen HL, et al. Recombinant Derp5 secreted in the milk leading by aS1-casein signal peptide protects against dust mite allergen-induced airway inflammation. J Dairy Sci. 2014;97(11):6792–803.
14. Tournoy KG, Kips JC, Schou C, Pauwels RA. Airway eosinophilia is not a requirement for allergen-induced airway hyperresponsiveness. Clin Exp Allergy. 2000;30(1):79–85.
15. Tung YT, Tsai TC, Kuo YH, et al. Comparison of solid-state-cultured and wood-cultured *Antrodia camphorata* in anti-inflammatory effects using NF-κB/luciferase inducible transgenic mice. Phytomedicine. 2014;21(12):1708–16.
16. Verhasselt V, Milcent V, Cazareth J, et al. Breast milk-mediated transfer of an antigen induces tolerance and protection from allergic asthma. Nat Med. 2008;14(2):170–5.
17. Chen HL, Yen CC, Wang SM, et al. Aerosolized bovine lactoferrin reduces lung injury and fibrosis in mice exposed to hyperoxia. Biometals. 2014;27(5):1057–68.
18. Lai CW, Chen HL, Tsai TC, et al. Sexually dimorphic expression of eGFP transgene in the *Akr1A1* locus of mouse liver regulated by sex hormone-related epigenetic remodeling. Sci Rep. 2016;6:e24023.
19. Lai CW, Chen HL, Tu MY, et al. A novel osteoporosis model with ascorbic acid deficiency in *Akr1A1* gene knockout mice. Oncotarget. 2017;8(5):7357–69.
20. Noble A, Zhao J. Follicular helper T cells are responsible for IgE responses to Der p 1 following house dust mite sensitization in mice. Clin Exp Allergy. 2016;46(8):1075–82.
21. Epton MJ, Smith W, Hales BJ, et al. Non-allergenic antigen in allergic sensitization: responses to the mite ferritin heavy chain antigen by allergic and non-allergic subjects. Clin Exp Allergy. 2002;32(9):1341–7.
22. Akdis CA, Akdis M. Mechanisms of allergen-specific immunotherapy. J Allergy Clin Immunol. 2011;127(1):18–27.
23. Tao L, Shi B, Shi G, Wan H. Efficacy of sublingual immunotherapy for allergic asthma: retrospective meta-analysis of randomized, double-blind and placebo-controlled trials. Clin Respir J. 2014;8(2):192–205.
24. Bateman ED, Hurd SS, Barnes PJ, et al. Global strategy for asthma management and prevention: GINA executive summary. Eur Respir J. 2008;31(1):143–78.
25. Vickery BP, Burks AW. Immunotherapy in the treatment of food allergy: focus on oral tolerance. Curr Opin Allergy Clin Immunol. 2009;9(4):364–70.

20

Asthma

Jaclyn Quirt[1*], Kyla J. Hildebrand[2], Jorge Mazza[3], Francisco Noya[4] and Harold Kim[1,3]

Abstract

Asthma is the most common respiratory disorder in Canada. Despite significant improvement in the diagnosis and management of this disorder, the majority of Canadians with asthma remain poorly controlled. In most patients, however, control can be achieved through the use of avoidance measures and appropriate pharmacological interventions. Inhaled corticosteroids (ICS) represent the standard of care for the majority of patients. Combination ICS/long-acting beta$_2$-agonist inhalers are preferred for most adults who fail to achieve control with ICS therapy. Biologic therapies targeting immunoglobulin E or interleukin-5 are recent additions to the asthma treatment armamentarium and may be useful in select cases of difficult to control asthma. Allergen-specific immunotherapy represents a potentially disease-modifying therapy for many patients with asthma, but should only be prescribed by physicians with appropriate training in allergy. In addition to avoidance measures and pharmacotherapy, essential components of asthma management include: regular monitoring of asthma control using objective testing measures such as spirometry, whenever feasible; creation of written asthma action plans; assessing barriers to treatment and adherence to therapy; and reviewing inhaler device technique. This article provides a review of current literature and guidelines for the appropriate diagnosis and management of asthma in adults and children.

Background

Asthma remains the most common chronic respiratory disease in Canada, affecting approximately 10% of the population [1]. It is also the most common chronic disease of childhood [2]. Although asthma is often believed to be a disorder localized to the lungs, current evidence indicates that it may represent a component of systemic airway disease involving the entire respiratory tract, and this is supported by the fact that asthma frequently coexists with other atopic disorders, particularly allergic rhinitis [3].

Despite significant improvements in the diagnosis and management of asthma over the past decade, as well as the availability of comprehensive and widely-accepted national and international clinical practice guidelines for the disease, asthma control in Canada remains suboptimal. Results from the Reality of Asthma Control in Canada study suggest that over 50% of Canadians with asthma have uncontrolled disease [4]. Poor asthma control contributes to unnecessary morbidity, limitations to daily activities and impairments in overall quality of life [1].

This article provides an overview of diagnostic and therapeutic guideline recommendations from the Global Initiative for Asthma (GINA) and the Canadian Thoracic Society and as well as a review of current literature related to the pathophysiology, diagnosis, and appropriate treatment of asthma.

Definition

Asthma is defined as a chronic inflammatory disease of the airways. The chronic inflammation is associated with airway hyperresponsiveness (an exaggerated airway-narrowing response to specific triggers such as viruses, allergens and exercise) that leads to recurrent episodes of wheezing, breathlessness, chest tightness and/or coughing that can vary over time and in intensity. Symptom episodes are generally associated with widespread, but variable, airflow obstruction within the lungs that is usually reversible either spontaneously or with appropriate asthma treatment such as a fast-acting bronchodilator [5].

*Correspondence: jaclyn.quirt@medportal.ca
[1] McMaster University, Hamilton, ON, Canada
Full list of author information is available at the end of the article

Epidemiology

The 2003 Canadian Community Health Survey found that 8.4% of the Canadian population ≥ 12 years of age had been diagnosed with asthma, with the prevalence being highest among teens ($> 12\%$) [6]. Between 1998 and 2001, close to 80,000 Canadians were admitted to hospital for asthma, and hospitalization rates were highest among young children and seniors. However, the survey also found that mortality due to asthma has fallen sharply since 1985. In 2001, a total of 299 deaths were attributed to asthma. Seven of these deaths occurred in persons under 19 years of age, while the majority (62%) occurred in those over 70 years of age [6].

More recent epidemiological evidence suggests that that the prevalence of asthma in Canada is rising, particularly in the young population. A population-based cohort study conducted in Ontario found that the age- and sex-standardized asthma prevalence increased from 8.5% in 1996 to 13.3% in 2005, a relative increase of 55% [7]. The age-standardized increase in prevalence was greatest in adolescents and young adults compared with other age groups, and the gender-standardized increase in prevalence was greater in males compared with females. Compared with females, males experienced higher increases in prevalence in adolescence and young adulthood and lower increases at age 70 years or older.

Another recent study of over 2800 school-aged children in Toronto that assessed parental reports of asthma by questionnaire found the prevalence of asthma to be approximately 16% in this young population [8]. The results of these studies suggest that effective clinical and public health strategies are needed to prevent and manage asthma in the Canadian population.

Pathophysiology and etiology

Asthma is associated with T helper cell type-2 (Th2) immune responses, which are typical of other atopic conditions. Asthma triggers may include allergic (e.g., house dust mites, cockroach residue, animal dander, mould, and pollens) and non-allergic (e.g., viral infections, exposure to tobacco smoke, cold air, exercise) stimuli, which produce a cascade of events leading to chronic airway inflammation. Elevated levels of Th2 cells in the airways release specific cytokines, including interleukin (IL)-4, IL-5, IL-9 and IL-13, and promote eosinophilic inflammation and immunoglobulin E (IgE) production. IgE production, in turn, triggers the release of inflammatory mediators, such as histamine and cysteinyl leukotrienes, that cause bronchospasm (contraction of the smooth muscle in the airways), edema, and increased mucous secretion, which lead to the characteristic symptoms of asthma [5, 9].

The mediators and cytokines released during the early phase of an immune response to an inciting trigger further propagate the inflammatory response (late-phase asthmatic response) that leads to progressive airway inflammation and bronchial hyperreactivity [9]. Over time, the airway remodeling that occurs with frequent asthma exacerbations leads to greater lung function decline and more severe airway obstruction [10]. This highlights the importance of frequent assessment of asthma control and the prevention of exacerbations.

Evidence suggests that there may be a genetic predisposition for the development of asthma. Several chromosomal regions associated with asthma susceptibility have been identified, such as those related to the production of IgE antibodies, expression of airway hyperresponsiveness, and the production of inflammatory mediators. However, further study is required to determine specific genes involved in asthma as well as the gene-environment interactions that may lead to expression of the disease [5, 9].

An extensive literature review undertaken as part of the development of the Canadian Healthy Infant Longitudinal Development (CHILD) study (an ongoing multicentre national observational study) examined risk factors for the development of allergy and asthma in early childhood [11]. Prenatal risk factors linked to early asthma development include: maternal smoking, use of antibiotics and delivery by caesarean section. With respect to prenatal diet and nutrition, a higher intake of fish or fish oil during pregnancy, and higher prenatal vitamin E and zinc levels have been associated with a lower risk of development of wheeze in young children. Later in childhood, risk factors for asthma development include: allergic sensitization (particularly house dust mite, cat and cockroach allergens), exposure to environmental tobacco smoke, breastfeeding (which may initially protect and then increase the risk of sensitization), decreased lung function in infancy, antibiotic use and infections, and gender. Future results from CHILD may help further elucidate risk factors for asthma development.

Asthma phenotypes

Although asthma has long been considered a single disease, recent studies have increasingly focused on its heterogeneity [12]. The characterization of this heterogeneity has led to the concept that asthma consists of various "phenotypes" or consistent groupings of characteristics. Using a hierarchical cluster analysis of subjects from the Severe Asthma Research Program (SARP), Moore and colleagues [13] have identified five distinct clinical phenotypes of asthma which differ in lung function, age of asthma onset and duration, atopy and sex.

In children with asthma, three wheeze phenotypes have been identified: (1) transient early wheezing; (2) non-atopic wheezing; and (3) IgE-mediated (atopic) wheezing [14]. The transient wheezing phenotype is associated with symptoms that are limited to the first 3–5 years of life; it is not associated with a family history of asthma or allergic sensitization. Risk factors for this phenotype include decreased lung function that is diagnosed before any respiratory illness has occurred, maternal smoking during pregnancy, and exposure to other siblings or children at daycare centres. The non-atopic wheezing phenotype represents a group of children who experience episodes of wheezing up to adolescence that are not associated with atopy or allergic sensitization. Rather, the wheezing is associated with a viral respiratory infection [particularly with the respiratory syncytial virus (RSV)] experienced in the first 3 years of life. Children with this phenotype tend to have milder asthma than the atopic phenotype. IgE-mediated (atopic) wheezing (also referred to as the "classic asthma phenotype") is characterized by persistent wheezing that is associated with atopy, early allergic sensitization, significant loss of lung function in the first years of life, and airway hyperresponsiveness.

Classifying asthma according to phenotypes provides a foundation for improved understanding of disease causality and the development of more targeted and personalized approaches to management that can lead to improved asthma control [13]. Research on the classification of asthma phenotypes and the appropriate treatment of these phenotypes is ongoing.

Diagnosis

The diagnosis of asthma involves a thorough medical history, physical examination, and objective assessments of lung function in those ≥ 6 years of age (spirometry preferred, both before and after bronchodilator) to document variable expiratory airflow limitation and confirm the diagnosis (see Table 1). Bronchoprovocation challenge testing and assessing for markers of airway inflammation may also be helpful for diagnosing the disease, particularly when objective measurements of lung function are normal despite the presence of asthma symptoms [5, 15, 16].

The importance of labeling asthma properly in children and preschoolers cannot be overemphasized since recurrent preschool wheezing has been associated with significant morbidity that can impact long-term health [17]. According to a recent position statement by the Canadian Paediatric Society and the Canadian Thoracic Society, asthma can be appropriately diagnosed as such in children 1–5 years of age, and terms that denote

either a suggestive pathophysiology (e.g., 'bronchospasm' or 'reactive airway disease') or vague diagnoses (e.g., 'wheezy bronchitis' or 'happy wheezer') should be abandoned in medical records [17].

Medical history

Important questions to ask when taking the medical history of patients with suspected asthma are summarized in Table 2. The diagnosis of asthma should be suspected in patients with recurrent cough, wheeze, chest tightness and/or shortness of breath. Symptoms that are variable, occur upon exposure to triggers such as allergens or irritants, that often worsen at night and that respond to appropriate asthma therapy are strongly suggestive of asthma [5, 16]. Alternative causes of suspected asthma symptoms should be excluded (see "Differential diagnosis" section in this article).

A positive family history of asthma or other atopic diseases and/or a personal history of atopic disorders, particularly allergic rhinitis, can also be helpful in identifying patients with asthma. During the history, it is also important to enquire for possible triggers of asthma symptoms, such as cockroaches, animal dander, moulds, pollens, exercise, and exposure to tobacco smoke or cold air. When possible, objective testing for these triggers should be performed. Exposure to agents encountered in the work environment can also cause asthma. If work-related asthma is suspected, details of work exposures and improvements in asthma symptoms during holidays should be explored. It is also important to assess for comorbidities that can aggravate asthma symptoms, such as allergic rhinitis, sinusitis, obstructive sleep apnea and gastroesophageal reflux disease [16].

The diagnosis of asthma in children is often more difficult since episodic wheezing and cough are commonly associated with viral infections, and children can be asymptomatic with normal physical examinations between exacerbations. In addition, spirometry is often unreliable in patients under 6 years of age, although it can be performed in some children as young as 5 years. A useful method of confirming the diagnosis in young children is a trial of treatment (8–12 weeks of a daily ICS and a short-acting bronchodilator as needed for rescue medication). Marked clinical improvement during the treatment period, as reflected by a reduction in daytime or nocturnal symptoms of asthma, a reduction in the use of rescue bronchodilator medication, absence of acute care visits (e.g., same-day physician appointments or emergency room visits) and hospitalizations for asthma exacerbations, and the absence of rescue oral corticosteroids are all indicators that the daily ICS therapy is working and that a diagnosis of asthma is likely [5, 18, 19]. In a young child who is

Table 1 Diagnosis of asthma based on medical history, physical examination and objective measurements [5, 15, 16]

Medical history
- Assess for classic symptoms of asthma:
  - Wheezing
  - Breathlessness
  - Chest tightness
  - Cough (with our without sputum)
- Assess for symptom patterns suggestive of asthma:
  - Recurrent/episodic
  - Occur/worsen at night or early in the morning
  - Occur/worsen upon exposure to allergens (e.g., animal dander, pollen, dust mites) or irritants (e.g., exercise, cold air, tobacco smoke, infections)
  - Respond to appropriate asthma therapy
- Assess for family or personal history of atopic disease (particularly allergic rhinitis)

Physical examination
- Examine for wheezing on auscultation
- Examine upper respiratory tract and skin for signs of other atopic conditions

Objective measures for confirming variable expiratory airflow limitation (spirometry preferred)
- Documented airflow limitation:
  - *Diagnostic criteria:* at least once during diagnostic process when FEV_1 is low, confirm that FEV_1/FVC is reduced (normally > 0.75–0.80 in adults, > 0.90 in children)

AND

- Documented excessive variability in lung function using one or more of the tests below (the greater the variations, or the more occasions excess variation is seen, the more confident the diagnosis):

	Diagnostic criteria
■ Positive bronchodilator (BD) reversibility test[a] (more likely to be positive if BD is withheld before test: SABA ≥ 4 h, LABA ≥ 15 h)	→ *Adults* increase in FEV_1 of > 12% and > 200 mL from baseline, 10–15 min after 200–400 μg albuterol or equivalent (greater confidence if increase is > 15% and > 400 mL) → *Children* increase in FEV_1 of > 12% predicted
■ Excessive variability in twice-daily PEF over 2 weeks[a]	→ *Adults* average daily diurnal PEF variability > 10%[b] → *Children* average daily diurnal PEF variability > 13%[b]
■ Significant increase in lung function after 4 weeks of anti-inflammatory treatment	→ *Adults* increase in FEV_1 by > 12% and > 200 mL (or PEF[c] by > 20%) from baseline after 4 weeks of treatment, outside respiratory infections
■ Positive exercise challenge test[a]	→ *Adults* fall in FEV_1 of > 10% and > 200 mL from baseline → *Children* fall in FEV_1 of > 12% predicted, or PEF > 15%
■ Positive bronchial challenge test (usually only performed in adults)	→ Fall in FEV_1 from baseline of ≥ 20% with standard doses of methacholine or histamine, or ≥ 15% with standardized hyperventilation, hypertonic saline or mannitol challenge
■ Excessive variation in lung function between visits (less reliable)[a]	→ *Adults* variation in FEV_1 of > 12% and > 200 mL between visits, outside of respiratory infections → *Children* variation in FEV_1 of > 12% or > 15% in PEF[c] between visits (may include respiratory infections)

Allergy testing
- Perform skin tests to assess allergic status and identify possible triggers

FVC forced vital capacity, *FEV₁* forced expiratory volume in 1 s, *PEF* peak expiratory flow (highest of three readings), *BD* bronchodilator (short-acting SABA or rapid-acting LABA), *LABA* long-acting beta₂-agonist, *SABA* short-acting beta₂-agonist

[a] These tests can be repeated during symptoms or in the early morning

[b] Daily diurnal PEF variability is calculated from twice daily PEF as ([day's highest minus day's lowest]/mean of day's highest and lowest), and averaged over 1 week

[c] For PEF, use the same meter each time, as PEF may vary by up to 20% between different meters. BD reversibility may be lost during severe exacerbations or viral infections. If bronchodilator reversibility is not present at initial presentation, the next step depends on the availability of other tests and the urgency of the need for treatment. In a situation of clinical urgency, asthma treatment may be commenced and diagnostic testing arranged within the next few weeks, but other conditions that can mimic asthma should be considered, and the diagnosis of asthma confirmed as soon as possible

symptomatic with cough, wheeze, or increased difficulty breathing, a physical examination both before and after administration of a bronchodilator is of extreme value and can be used as a diagnostic tool. If the respiratory symptoms resolve within 10–15 min of bronchodilator administration, a diagnosis of asthma may be established by a physician or other healthcare provider.

The modified Asthma Predictive Index (mAPI) is a useful tool for identifying young children with recurrent wheeze who may be at high risk of developing asthma (see Table 3; also available online at: https://www.mdcalc.com/modified-asthma-predictive-index-mapi). A positive mAPI in the preschool years has been found to be highly predictive of future school-age asthma [20].

Table 2 Key questions to ask when taking the medical history of patients with suspected asthma

- Asthma symptoms (cough, wheeze, increased work of breathing)?
- Age of onset of symptoms?
- Timing of symptoms (day vs. night)?
- Is there a seasonal component to the worsening of symptoms?
- Possible triggers (viral infections, animal exposures, pollens, tobacco smoke, emotion)?
- Severity of symptoms (often reflected by unscheduled physician appointments at a walk-in clinic or emergency room, hospital admissions, and need for rescue oral corticosteroids)?
- Past investigations including chest X-rays, spirometry, allergy testing, sweat chloride testing?
- Other co-morbidities (e.g., food allergy, venom allergy)?
- Current and past treatments? Duration of use? Reasons for discontinuation?
- Barriers to treatment (cost of medication, proximity to health care providers)?
- Exposure to second- and third-hand (i.e., the lingering smell of tobacco smoke on clothing or in vehicles) tobacco smoke?
- Presence of household pets?
- Impact of the symptoms on the patient/family quality of life (missed time from activities, school or work due to asthma symptoms)?

Table 3 Modified Asthma Predictive Index [20]

≥4 wheezing episodes in a year	
AND	
At least 1 major criteria:	OR **at least 2 minor criteria:**
• Parental physician-diagnosed asthma	• Wheezing unrelated to colds
• Physician-diagnosed atopic dermatitis	• Eosinophils ≥ 4% in circulation
• Allergic sensitization to at least 1 aeroallergen	• Allergic sensitization to milk, egg, or peanuts

Physical examination

Given the variability of asthma symptoms, the physical examination of patients with suspected asthma can often be unremarkable. Physical findings may only be evident if the patient is symptomatic. Therefore, the absence of physical findings does not exclude a diagnosis of asthma. The most common abnormal physical findings are a prolonged expiratory phase and wheezing on auscultation, which confirm the presence of airflow limitation [5]. Auscultating the chest before and after bronchodilator treatment can be informative as well, with improved breath sounds noted once the small airways undergo bronchodilation.

Among children with asthma, persistent cough is also a positive finding on physical examination since not all children with asthma wheeze. Physicians should also examine the upper respiratory tract (nose, pharynx) and

skin for signs of concurrent atopic conditions such as allergic rhinitis, dermatitis, and nasal polyps (also seen in cystic fibrosis) [16].

In pediatric patients, a scoring rubric called the Pediatric Respiratory Assessment Measure (PRAM) has been developed to assess a patient's acute asthma severity using a combination of scalene muscle contraction, suprasternal retractions, wheezing, air entry and oxygen saturation (see Table 4) [21, 22]. This tool has been validated in children 0–17 years of age, and is most commonly used in acute care settings such as emergency departments, pediatric intensive care units and inpatient units.

Objective measurements to confirm variable expiratory airflow limitation

In a patient with typical respiratory symptoms, obtaining objective evidence of excessive variability in expiratory airflow limitation is essential to confirming the diagnosis of asthma (see Table 1) [5]. The greater the variations in lung function, or the more times excess variation is seen, the more likely the diagnosis is to be asthma. Spirometry is the preferred objective measure to assess for airflow limitation and excessive variability in lung function. It is recommended for all patients over 6 years of age who are able to undergo lung function testing [5, 15].

Spirometry measures airflow parameters such as the forced vital capacity (FVC, the maximum volume of air that can be exhaled) and the forced expiratory volume in 1 s (FEV_1). Lung volumes are not measured with spirometry, and instead require full pulmonary function testing. The ratio of FEV_1 to FVC provides a measure of airflow obstruction. In the general population, the FEV_1/FVC ratio is usually greater than 0.75–0.80 in adults, and 0.90 in children. Any values less than these suggest airflow limitation and support a diagnosis of asthma [5, 23]. Because of the variability of asthma symptoms, patients will not exhibit reversible airway obstruction at every visit and a negative spirometry result does not rule out a diagnosis of asthma. This is particularly true for children who experience symptoms predominantly with viral infections, or who are well controlled on asthma medications. Therefore, to increase sensitivity, spirometry should be repeated, particularly when patients are symptomatic [15, 16].

Once airflow obstruction has been confirmed, obtaining evidence of excessive variability in expiratory lung function is an essential component of the diagnosis of asthma. In general, an increase in FEV_1 of > 12% and, in adults, a change of > 200 mL from baseline after administration of a rapid-acting bronchodilator is accepted as being consistent with asthma [5, 23].

Table 4 PRAM scoring table [21, 22]

Criterion	Description	Score
O$_2$ saturation (%)	≥ 95	0
	92–94	1
	< 92	2
Suprasternal retraction	Absent	0
	Present	2
Scalene muscle	Absent	0
contraction	Present	2
Air entry[a]	Normal	0
	↓ at the base	1
	↓ at the apex and the base	2
	Minimal or absent	3
Wheezing[b]	Absent	0
	Expiratory only	1
	Inspiratory (± expiratory)	2
	Audible without stethoscope or silent chest (minimal or no air entry)	3
PRAM score: (max. 12)		

Score	0–3	4–7	8–12
Severity	Mild	Moderate	Severe

On-line tool is available at https://www.mdcalc.com/pediatric-respiratory-asses
sment-measure-pram-asthma-exacerbation-severity

PRAM Pediatric Respiratory Assessment Measure, *RUL* right upper lobe, *RML* right middle lobe, *RLL* right lower lobe, *LUL* left upper lobe, *LLL* left lower lobe, O$_2$ oxygen

[a] In case of asymmetry, the most severely affected (apex-base) lung field (right or left, anterior or posterior) will determine the rating of the criterion

[b] In case of asymmetry, the two most severely affected auscultation zones, irrespectively of their location (RUL, RML, RLL, LUL, LLL), will determine the rating of the criterion

Other criteria for demonstrating excessive variability in expiratory lung function are listed in Table 1.

Spirometry must be performed according to standardized protocols (such as those proposed by the American Thoracic Society) by trained personnel. It is commonly performed in pulmonary function laboratories, but can also be performed in the outpatient clinical setting. During spirometry, the patient is instructed to take the deepest breath possible and then to exhale hard and fast and as fully as possible into the mouthpiece of the spirometer for a total of 6 s. Calibration of the spirometer should be performed daily.

Peak expiratory flow (PEF) monitoring is an acceptable alternative *when spirometry is not available*, and can also be useful for diagnosing occupational asthma and/or monitoring response to asthma treatments. However, PEF is not recommended for diagnosing asthma in children. PEF is usually measured in the morning and in the evening. A diurnal variation in PEF of more than 20% or an improvement of at least 60 L/min or at least 20% after inhalation of a rapid-acting bronchodilator suggests asthma [15]. Although simpler to perform than spirometry, PEF is more effort-dependent and much less reliable. Therefore, as mentioned earlier, spirometry is the preferred method of documenting variable expiratory airflow limitation and confirming the diagnosis of asthma.

The importance of objective measures for confirming the diagnosis of asthma cannot be overemphasized. The results of a recent multicentre study that included 613 adults with physician-diagnosed asthma from across Canada found that the diagnosis of current asthma was ruled out in 33% of patients; these subjects were not using daily asthma medications or had been weaned off medication [24]. Compared to subjects whose current asthma diagnosis was confirmed, those in whom the diagnosis was ruled out were less likely to have undergone testing for airflow limitation in the community at the time of the initial diagnosis. These findings suggest that re-evaluation of an asthma diagnosis may be warranted.

Tests of bronchial hyperreactivity

When spirometry is normal, but symptoms and the clinical history are suggestive of asthma, measurement of airway responsiveness using direct airway challenges to inhaled bronchoconstrictor stimuli (e.g., methacholine or histamine) or indirect challenges (e.g., with mannitol or exercise) may help confirm a diagnosis of asthma.

Tests of bronchial hyperreactivity should be conducted in accordance with standardized protocols in a pulmonary function laboratory or other facility equipped to manage acute bronchospasm. Bronchopovocation testing involves the patient inhaling increasing doses or concentrations of an inert stimulus until a given level of bronchoconstriction is achieved, typically a 20% fall in FEV$_1$. An inhaled rapid-acting bronchodilator is then provided to reverse the obstruction. Test results are usually expressed as the provocative dose (PD) or provocative concentration (PC) of the provoking agent that causes the FEV$_1$ to drop by 20% (the PD$_{20}$ or PC$_{20}$, respectively). For methacholine, most pulmonary function laboratories use a PC$_{20}$ value less than 4-8 mg/mL as the threshold for a positive result indicative of airway hyperreactivity, supporting a diagnosis of asthma. However, positive challenge tests are not specific to asthma and may occur with other conditions such as allergic rhinitis and chronic obstructive pulmonary disease (COPD). Therefore, tests of bronchial hyperreactivity may be most useful for ruling out asthma among individuals who are symptomatic. A negative test result in a symptomatic patient not receiving anti-inflammatory therapy is highly sensitive [16].

In order to properly assess lung function, patients who have been prescribed a combination of an ICS and a LABA must discontinue these long-acting medications 24 h prior to tests of airway hyperreactivity or testing with spirometry. Tests of bronchial hyperreactivity are contraindicated in patients with FEV_1 values less than 60–70% of the normal predicted value (since bronchoprovocation could cause significant bronchospasm), in patients with uncontrolled hypertension or in those who recently experienced a stroke or myocardial infarction [25].

Non-invasive markers of airway inflammation

The measurement of inflammatory markers such as sputum eosinophilia (proportion of eosinophils in the cell analysis of sputum) or levels of exhaled nitric oxide (a gaseous molecule produced by some cells during an inflammatory response) can also be useful for diagnosing asthma. Evidence suggests that exhaled nitric oxide levels can be supportive of the diagnosis of asthma, and may also be useful for monitoring patient response to asthma therapy [16]. It is still not accepted as a standard test for the diagnosis of asthma. Although these tests have been studied in the diagnosis and monitoring of asthma, they are not yet widely available in Canada.

Allergy skin testing

Allergy skin prick (epicutaneous) testing is recommended to identify possible environmental allergic triggers of asthma, and is helpful in identifying the asthma phenotype of the patient. Testing is typically performed using the allergens relevant to the patient's geographic region. Although allergen-specific IgE tests that provide an in vitro measure of a patient's specific IgE levels for specific allergens have been suggested as an alternative to skin tests, these tests are less sensitive, more invasive (requires venipuncture), and more expensive than skin prick tests [5, 15]. There is no minimum age at which skin prick testing can be performed.

Differential diagnosis

Conditions that should be considered in the differential diagnosis of adults with suspected asthma may include: COPD, bronchitis, gastrointestinal reflux disease, recurrent respiratory infections, heart disease, and vocal cord dysfunction. Distinguishing asthma from COPD can be particularly difficult as some patients have features of both disorders. The term asthma-COPD overlap syndrome (ACOS), though not a single disease entity, has been adopted to describe these patients. A recent population-based cohort study

Table 5 Differential diagnosis of recurrent respiratory symptoms in children [31, 36]

Infections	Congenital problems
• Recurrent respiratory tract infections	• Tracheomalacia
• Chronic rhino-sinusitis	• Tracheo-esophageal fistula
• Tuberculosis	• Cystic fibrosis
Mechanical problems	• Bronchopulmonary dysplasia
• Foreign body aspiration	• Congenital malformation causing narrowing of the intrathoracic airways
• Gastroesophageal reflux	
• Vocal cord dysfunction	• Primary ciliary dyskinesia syndrome
	• Immune deficiency
	• Congenital heart disease

conducted in Ontario suggests that the prevalence of concurrent asthma and COPD is increasing, particularly in women and young adults [26].

The differential diagnosis of asthma is unique for infants and young children and includes anatomic defects (laryngo- or tracheomalacia, congenital heart defects), physiological defects (primary ciliary dyskinesia) and genetic conditions such cystic fibrosis and primary immunodeficiency, to name just a few conditions. A chest X-ray may be considered in the work-up of a child with suspected asthma, particularly if the diagnosis is unclear or if the child is not responding as expected to treatment. Table 5 lists conditions to consider in the differential diagnosis of recurrent respiratory symptoms in children.

Management

The primary goal of asthma management is to achieve and maintain control of the disease in order to prevent exacerbations (abrupt and/or progressive worsening of asthma symptoms that often require immediate medical attention and/or the use of oral steroid therapy) and reduce the risk of morbidity and mortality. Other goals of therapy are to minimize the frequency and severity of asthma symptoms, decrease the need for reliever medications, normalize physical activity, and improve lung function as well as overall quality of life. The level of asthma control should be assessed at each visit using

Table 6 Criteria for assessing asthma control [5, 15]

No exacerbations

Fewer than 3 doses/week of a rapid-acting beta$_2$-agonist bronchodilator

Daytime symptoms < 3 days/week

No nighttime symptoms

Normal physical activity

No absenteeism from work or school

FEV_1 or PEF at least 90% of personal best

FEV$_1$ forced expiratory volume in 1 s, PEF peak expiratory flow

the criteria in Table 6, and treatment should be tailored to achieve control. In most asthma patients, control can be achieved using both trigger avoidance measures and pharmacological interventions. The pharmacologic agents commonly used for the treatment of asthma can be classified as controllers (medications taken daily on a long-term basis that achieve control primarily through anti-inflammatory effects) and relievers (medications used on an as-needed basis for quick relief of bronchoconstriction and symptoms). Controller medications include ICSs, leukotriene receptor antagonists (LTRAs), LABAs in combination with an ICS, long-acting muscarinic receptor antagonists (LAMAs), and biologic agents including anti-IgE therapy and anti-IL-5 therapy. Reliever medications include rapid-acting inhaled beta₂-agonists and inhaled anticholinergics

[5, 15, 16]. Allergen-specific immunotherapy may also be considered in most patients with allergic asthma, but must be prescribed by physicians who are adequately trained in the treatment of allergies (see *Allergen-specific immunotherapy* article in this supplement) [27–30]. Systemic corticosteroid therapy may also be required for the management of acute asthma exacerbations. A simplified, stepwise algorithm for the treatment of asthma is provided in Fig. 1.

The goal of asthma therapy is to treat individuals using the least amount of medications required to control asthma symptoms and maintain normal daily activities. When asthma control has been achieved, ongoing monitoring and follow-up are essential to monitor for side effects, preserve lung function over time, observe for new triggers, and establish the minimum maintenance

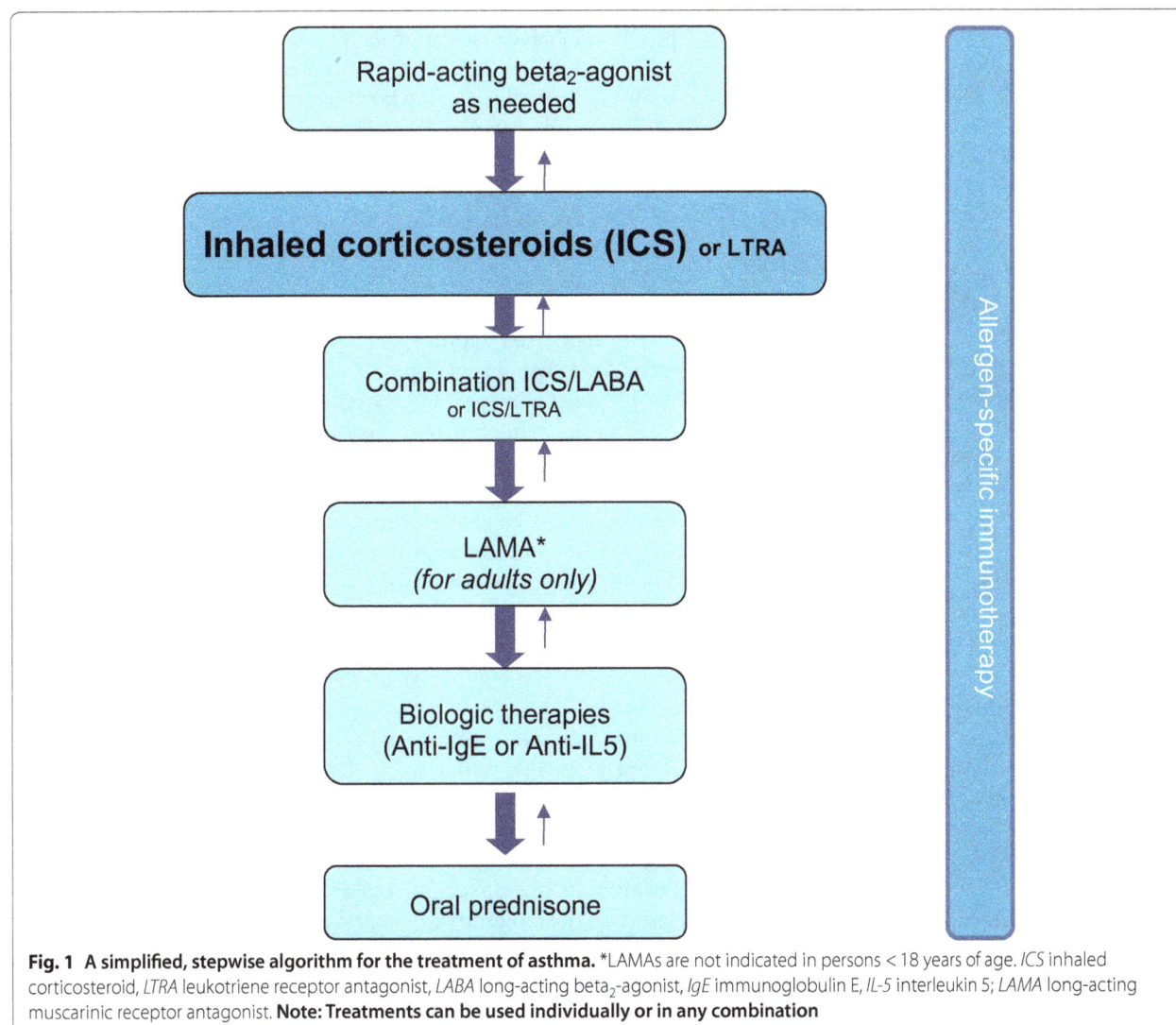

Fig. 1 A simplified, stepwise algorithm for the treatment of asthma. *LAMAs are not indicated in persons < 18 years of age. *ICS* inhaled corticosteroid, *LTRA* leukotriene receptor antagonist, *LABA* long-acting beta₂-agonist, *IgE* immunoglobulin E, *IL-5* interleukin 5; *LAMA* long-acting muscarinic receptor antagonist. **Note: Treatments can be used individually or in any combination**

doses required to maintain control. However, because asthma is a variable disease, treatment may need to be adjusted periodically in response to loss of control (as indicated by failure to meet the control criteria in Table 6) [5]. It is also imperative that all asthma patients be empowered to take an active role in the management of their disease. This can be accomplished by providing patients with a personalized written action plan for disease management and by educating the patient about the nature of the disease, the role of medications, the importance of adhering to controller therapy, and the appropriate use of inhaler devices [16]. Once a written action plan for management is provided, ongoing follow up should include:

- Reviewing the asthma action plan at each visit to determine if modifications are required based on level of asthma control;
- Observation of inhaler device technique at each visit;
- Counselling patients or caregivers who smoke on smoking cessation;
- Measuring height and weight of children and adolescents to monitor growth velocity and potential corticosteroid side effects;
- Screening for signs and symptoms of adrenal suppression for individuals requiring moderate- to high-dose ICS;
- Asking about food or venom allergies and ensuring that patients with these allergies are prescribed an epinephrine autoinjector and provided with a written anaphylaxis plan. Patients with poorly controlled asthma and food/venom allergy are at greater risk for anaphylaxis upon accidental exposure to their known allergen (see *Anaphylaxis* article in this supplement).
- Referring individuals who have difficulty achieving asthma control to an asthma specialist (respirologist, allergist or certified asthma educator) for further assessment (see "Indications for referral" section in this article).

Avoidance measures

Avoidance of exposure to tobacco smoke is important for all patients with asthma. Avoidance of other relevant allergens/irritants is also an important component of asthma management. Patients allergic to house dust mites should be instructed to use allergen-impermeable covers for bedding and to keep the relative humidity in the home below 50% (to inhibit mite growth). Pollen exposure can be reduced by keeping windows closed, using an air conditioner, and limiting the amount of time spent outdoors during peak pollen seasons. For patients allergic to animal dander, removal of the animal from the home is recommended and usually results in a

significant reduction in symptoms within 4–6 months. However, compliance with this recommendation is poor and, therefore, the use of high-efficiency particulate air (HEPA) filters and restricting the animal from the bedroom or to the outdoors may be needed to help decrease allergen levels. Measures for reducing exposure to mould allergens include cleaning with fungicides, de-humidification to less than 50%, and HEPA filtration [16].

Since these avoidance strategies can be labour-intensive, patient adherence is usually suboptimal. Frequent reassessments, encouragement and empowerment by the treating physician are often required to help promote adherence to these strategies. Furthermore, patients should be advised to use a combination of avoidance measures for optimal results, since single-strategy interventions have demonstrated no measurable benefits in asthma control [16].

Inhaled medication delivery devices

Inhaled asthma medications come in a variety forms including pressurized metered-dose inhalers (pMDIs) and dry powder inhalers (DPIs) (Turbuhaler, Diskus, Twisthaler, Ellipta). Not all medications are available in the same delivery devices. Also, some devices have dose counters included and others, such as pMDIs, do not. The most important factor in selecting a medication delivery device is to ensure that the patient uses it properly.

In children, it is recommended that pMDIs always be used with a spacer device since they are as effective as nebulizers; a pMDI with spacer is also preferred over nebulizers [31]. A spacer with face mask is recommended for children 2–4 years of age, while a spacer with mouthpiece is recommended for children 4–6 years of age. To transition to a spacer with mouthpiece, children must be able to form a seal around the mouthpiece and breathe through their mouths. For children 6 years of age or over, a pMDI plus spacer with mouthpiece or DPI is recommended. Since children must have sufficient inspiratory force to use a DPI, these devices are generally not recommended for children under 6 years of age.

Reliever medications

Inhaled rapid-acting beta$_2$-agonists are the preferred reliever medications for the treatment of acute symptoms, and should be prescribed to all patients with asthma. In Canada, several short-acting beta$_2$-agonists (SABAs; e.g., salbutamol, terbutaline) and one LABA (formoterol) are approved for this indication. SABAs should only be taken on an as needed basis for symptom relief. Use of an as-needed SABA in the absence of a controller therapy should be reserved for patients with symptoms less than twice per month, without nocturnal wakening in the past month, or an exacerbation within the past year. In children with well controlled asthma, a SABA should be used less than three times per week.

Unlike other LABAs, formoterol has a rapid onset of action and, therefore, can be used for acute symptom relief. Given that LABA monotherapy has been associated with an increased risk of asthma-related morbidity and mortality, formoterol should only be used as a reliever in patients 12 years of age or older who are on regular controller therapy with an ICS [5, 15, 16, 23].

Short-acting anticholinergic bronchodilators, such as ipratropium bromide, may also be used as reliever therapy. These agents appear to be less effective than inhaled rapid-acting beta$_2$-agonists and, therefore, should be reserved as second-line therapy for patients who are unable to use SABAs. They may also be used in addition to SABAs in patients experiencing moderate to severe asthma exacerbations. Short-acting anticholinergic bronchodilator therapy is not recommended for use in children [15].

Controller medications
Inhaled corticosteroids (ICSs)
ICSs are the most effective anti-inflammatory medications available for the treatment of asthma and represent the mainstay of therapy for most patients with the disease. Low-dose ICS monotherapy is recommended as first-line maintenance therapy for most children and adults with asthma. Regular ICS use has been shown to reduce symptoms and exacerbations, and improve lung function and quality of life. ICSs do not, however, "cure" asthma, and symptoms tend to recur within weeks to months of ICS discontinuation. Most patients will require long-term, if not life-long, ICS treatment [5, 15, 16].

Since ICSs are highly effective when used optimally, factors other than treatment efficacy need to be considered if ICS therapy is unsuccessful in achieving asthma control. These factors include: misdiagnosis of the disease, poor adherence to ICS therapy, improper inhaler technique, continued trigger exposure or the presence of other comorbidities. If, after addressing such factors, patients fail to achieve control with low-to-moderate ICS doses, then treatment should be modified. For most children, ICS dose escalation (to a moderate dose) is the preferred approach to achieve control, while the addition of another class of medications (usually a LABA) is recommended for patients over 12 years of age [15, 16, 23]. Low, medium and high doses of ICS therapy varies by age and are summarized in Table 7. Children who fail to achieve control on a moderate ICS dose should be referred to an asthma specialist, such a respirologist, an allergist, an immunologist or a pediatrician. It is also

recommended that children receiving daily ICS therapy do not increase their daily ICS dose with the onset of a viral illness [23].

Side effects The most common local adverse events associated with ICS therapy are oropharyngeal candidiasis (also known as oral thrush) and dysphonia (hoarseness, difficulty speaking). Rinsing and expectorating (spitting) after each treatment and the use of a spacer with pMDI devices can help reduce the risk of these side effects. Systemic adverse effects with ICS therapy are rare, but may occur at high doses, such as >500 µg of fluticasone propionate equivalent, and include changes in bone density, cataracts, glaucoma and growth retardation [5]. Patients using high ICS doses should also be monitored for adrenal suppression [32]. It is important to note that the potential for side effects with ICS therapy needs to be considered in the context of other steroids (i.e., systemic, intranasal and topical) that may be prescribed for other atopic conditions such as allergic rhinitis or atopic dermatitis.

Combination ICS/LABA inhalers
LABA monotherapy is not recommended in patients with asthma as it does not impact airway inflammation and is associated with an increased risk of morbidity and mortality. LABAs are only recommended when used in combination with ICS therapy. The combination of a LABA and ICS has been shown to be highly effective in reducing asthma symptoms and exacerbations, and is the preferred treatment option in adolescents or adults whose asthma is inadequately controlled on low-dose ICS therapy, or in children over 6 years of age who are uncontrolled on moderate ICS doses [15, 23]. Although there is no apparent difference in efficacy between ICSs and LABAs given in the same or in separate inhalers, combination ICS/LABA inhalers are preferred because they preclude use of the LABA without an ICS, are more convenient and may enhance patient adherence. Four combination ICS/LABA inhalers are available in Canada: fluticasone propionate/salmeterol, budesonide/formoterol, mometasone/formoterol and fluticasone furoate/vilanterol (see Table 7). Combination budesonide/formoterol has been approved for use as a single inhaler for both daily maintenance (controller) and reliever therapy in individuals 12 years of age and older. It should only be used in patients whose asthma is not adequately controlled with low-dose ICS who warrant treatment with combination therapy [5, 15, 23].

Leukotriene receptor antagonists
The LTRAs, montelukast and zafirlukast, are also effective for the treatment of asthma and are generally considered to be safe and well tolerated. Because these

Table 7 Overview of the main controller therapies used for the treatment of asthma [23, 31]

	Usual adult dose	Pediatric dose information	
		< 6 years of age	6–18 years of age
ICSs			
Beclomethasone (Qvar, generics)	pMDI: 100–800 µg/day, divided bid	pMDI • *Low* 50 µg bid • *Med* 100 µg bid • *High* refer to specialist *Approved age by Health Canada ≥ 5 years*	pMDI • *Low* 50–100 µg bid • *Med* > 100 µg bid • *High* > 200 µg bid
Budesonide (Pulmicort)	DPI: 400–2400 µg/day, divided bid Nebules: 1–2 mg bid	DPI not recommended for children < 6 years	DPI • *Low* 100 µg bid • *Med* 200–400 µg bid • *High* > 400 µg bid *Approved age by Health Canada ≥ 6 years*
		Nebules: 0.25–0.5 mg bid (for children 3 months to 12 years)	
Ciclesonide (Alvesco)	pMDI: 100–800 µg/day	pMDI: • *Low* 100 µg once daily • *Med* 200 µg daily • *High* refer to specialist	pMDI: • *Low* 100 µg once daily • *Med* 200–400 µg daily • *High* > 400 µg daily *Approved age by Health Canada ≥ 6 years*
Fluticasone propionate (Flovent HFA, Flovent Diskus)	pMDI/DPI: 100–500 µg bid	pMDI/DPI • *Low* 50 µg bid • *Med* 100–125 µg bid • *High* refer to specialist *Approved age by Health Canada ≥ 1 year for pMDI, ≥ 4 years for Diskus (DPI)*	pMDI/DPI • *Low* ≤ 100 µg bid • *Med* > 100–200 µg bid • *High* ≥ 200 µg bid
Mometasone (Asmanex)	DPI: 200–400 µg/day	DPI not recommended for children < 6 years	DPI • *Low* ≤ 200 µg daily • *Med* > 100–200 µg bid • *High* > 200 µg bid *Approved age by Health Canada ≥ 12 years*
Fluticasone furoate (Arnuity Ellipta)	DPI: 100–200 µg/day	Not indicated for children < 12 years	
Combination ICS/LABA inhalers			
Budesonide/formoterol (Symbicort)	DPI (maintenance): 100/6 µg or 200/6 µg, 1–2 puffs od or bid; max 4 puffs/day DPI (maintenance and reliever): 100/6 µg or 200/6 µg, 1–2 puffs bid or 2 puffs od; plus 1 puff prn for relief of symptoms (no more than 6 puffs on any single occasion); max 8 puffs/day	Refer to specialist	DPI • *Low* 100/6 µg 1 dose bid • *Med* 100/6 µg 2 doses bid, 200/6 µg 1–2 doses bid • *High* > 200/6 µg 2 doses bid *Approved age by Health Canada ≥ 12 years*
Fluticasone furoate/salmeterol (Advair pMDI, Advair Diskus)	pMDI: 125/25 µg or 250/25 µg, 2 puffs bid Diskus: 100/50 µg, 250/50 µg or 500/50 µg: 1 puff bid	Refer to specialist *Approved age by Health Canada ≥ 4 years for Diskus (DPI)*	DPI/pMDI • *Low* 100/50 µg bid • *Med* > 100–200 µg bid • *High* ≥ 250/50 µg bid *Approved age by Health Canada ≥ 12 years for pMDI*
Mometasone/formoterol (Zenhale)	For patients previously treated with Low-dose ICS: 50/5 µg, 2 puffs bid Medium-dose ICS: 100/5 µg, 2 puffs bid High-dose ICS: 200/5 µg, 2 puffs bid	Refer to specialist	pMDI • *Low* 50/5–100/5 µg 1 dose bid • *Med* 100/5 µg 2 doses bid, 200/5 µg 1–2 doses bid • *High* > 200/5 µg *Approved age by Health Canada ≥ 12 years*
Fluticasone furoate/vilanterol (Breo Ellipta)	DPI: 100/25 µg/day or 200/25 µg/day	Not indicated for children < 18 years of age	

Table 7 (continued)

	Usual adult dose	Pediatric dose information	
		< 6 years of age	6–18 years of age
LTRAs			
Montelukast (Singulair)	10 mg tablet od (taken in the evenings)	4 mg po daily *Approved age by Health Canada ≥2 years*	5 mg po daily (6–14 years) 10 mg po daily (≥ 15 years)
Zafirlukast (Accolate)	20 mg tablet bid, at least 1 h before or 2 h after meals	Refer to specialist	20 mg tablet bid, at least 1 h before or 2 h after meals *Approved age by Health Canada ≥ 12 years*
LAMAs			
Tiotropium (Spiriva Respimat)	1.25 µg, 2 puffs od	Not indicated for children < 18 years	
Anti-IgE therapy			
Omalizumab (Xolair)	150–375 mg sc every 2–4 weeks (based on patient's weight and pre-treatment serum IgE level)	Not indicated for children < 6 years	75–375 mg sc every 2–4 weeks (based on patient's weight and pre-treatment serum IgE level)
Anti-IL5 therapy			
Mepolizumab (Nucala)	100 mg sc every 4 weeks	Not indicated for children < 18 years	
Reslizumab (Cinqair)	3 mg/kg IV every 4 weeks	Not indicated for children < 18 years	
Benralizumab (Fasenra)	30 mg sc every 4 weeks for the first 3 doses, then every 8 weeks thereafter	Not indicated for children < 18 years	

Pediatric dose information adapted from BCGuidelines.ca Guidelines & Protocols Advisory Committee, 2015 [31]

ICS inhaled corticosteroid, *pMDI* pressurized metered-dose inhaler, *DPI* dry powder inhaler, *LTRA* leukotriene receptor antagonists, *IgE* immunoglobulin E, *IL-5* interleukin 5, *bid* twice daily, *sc* subcutaneously, *IV* intravenously, *LABA* long acting beta agonist, *LAMA* long-acting muscarinic receptor antagonist, *po* oral, *prn* as needed

agents are less effective than ICS treatment when used as monotherapy, they are usually reserved for patients who are unwilling or unable to use ICSs. LTRAs can also be used as add-on therapy if asthma is uncontrolled despite the use of low-to-moderate dose ICS therapy or combination ICS/LABA therapy. It is important to note, however, that LTRAs are considered to be less effective than LABAs as add-on therapy in adults [5, 15, 23]. In children, if medium-dose ICS therapy is ineffective, LTRAs are considered the next-line treatment option [23]. If, however, the child has persistent airway obstruction, the addition of a LABA may be preferred.

Long-acting muscarinic receptor antagonists
The LAMA, tiotropium, administered by mist inhaler can be used as add-on therapy for patients with a history of exacerbations despite treatment with ICS/LABA combination therapy. It is only indicated for patients 12 years of age and older.

Theophylline
Theophylline is an oral bronchodilator with modest anti-inflammatory effects. Given its narrow therapeutic window and frequent adverse events (e.g., gastrointestinal symptoms, loose stools, seizures, cardiac arrhythmias, nausea and vomiting), its use is generally reserved

for patients over 12 years of age who are intolerant to or continue to be symptomatic despite other add-on therapies [5, 15].

Biologic therapies
The anti-IgE monoclonal antibody, omalizumab, has been shown to reduce the frequency of asthma exacerbations by approximately 50%. The drug is administered subcutaneously once every 2–4 weeks and is approved in Canada for the treatment of moderate to severe, persistent allergic asthma in patients 6 years of age or older. At present, omalizumab is reserved for patients with difficult to control asthma who have documented allergies, an elevated serum IgE level, and whose asthma symptoms remain uncontrolled despite ICS therapy in combination with a second controller medication [15].

Two monoclonal antibodies to IL-5 have been approved in Canada for patients aged 18 years or older with severe eosinophilia: mepolizumab and reslizumab. These are given every 4 weeks by subcutaneous injection and intravenous infusion, respectively, and are indicated in patients who are uncontrolled despite treatment with high-dose ICS therapy and an additional controller therapy, such as a LABA, and who have elevated blood eosinophils [5]. Recently, benralizumab, a monoclonal antibody against the IL-5 receptor has also been approved in Canada for the treatment of adult patients with severe eosinophilic asthma.

Table 7 provides a list of the commonly used controller therapies and their recommended dosing regimens. It is important to note that long-term compliance with controller therapy is poor because patients tend to stop therapy when their symptoms subside. Therefore, regular follow-up visits are important to help promote treatment adherence.

Systemic corticosteroids

Systemic corticosteroids, such as oral prednisone, are generally used for the acute treatment of moderate to severe asthma exacerbations. While chronic systemic corticosteroid therapy may also be effective for the management of difficult to control asthma, prolonged use of oral steroids are associated with well-known and potentially serious adverse effects and, therefore, their routine or long-term use should be avoided if at all possible, particularly in children [23]. Adverse events with short-term, high-dose oral prednisone are uncommon, but may include: reversible abnormalities in glucose metabolism, increased appetite, edema, weight gain, rounding of the face, mood alterations, hypertension, peptic ulcers and avascular necrosis of the hip [5].

Bronchial thermoplasty

Bronchial thermoplasty involves the treatment of airways with a series of radiofrequency pulses. This treatment may be considered for adult patients with severe asthma despite pharmacotherapy [5].

Allergen-specific immunotherapy

Allergen-specific immunotherapy involves the subcutaneous or sublingual administration of gradually increasing quantities of the patient's relevant allergens until a dose is reached that is effective in inducing immunologic tolerance to the allergen. Although it has been widely used to treat allergic asthma, it is not universally accepted by all clinical practice guideline committees due to the potential for serious anaphylactic reactions with this form of therapy [28].

A Cochrane review of 88 randomized controlled trials examining the use of allergen-specific immunotherapy in asthma management confirmed its efficacy in reducing asthma symptoms and the use of asthma medications, and improving airway hyperresponsiveness [27]. Similar benefits have been noted with sublingual immunotherapy [33], which is now available for use in Canada for grass and ragweed allergies, as well as house dust mite-induced allergic rhinitis (see *Allergen-specific immunotherapy*

article in this supplement). Evidence also suggests that allergen-specific immunotherapy may prevent the onset of asthma in atopic individuals [34, 35].

At present, allergen-specific immunotherapy should be considered on a case-by-case basis. Allergen-specific subcutaneous immunotherapy may be considered as add-on therapy in patients using ICS monotherapy, combination ICS/LABA inhalers, ICS/LTRAs and/ or omalizumab if asthma symptoms are controlled. It should not be initiated in patients with uncontrolled asthma or an $FEV_1 < 70\%$ of predicted. For subcutaneous immunotherapy, asthma must be controlled at the time of each injection, and it must be administered in clinics that are equipped to manage possible life-threatening anaphylaxis where a physician is present. Since allergen-specific immunotherapy carries the risk of anaphylactic reactions, it should only be prescribed by physicians who are specialists in allergy [5].

Indications for referral

In older children, adolescents and adults, referral to a specialist in asthma care (e.g., respirologist, allergist) is recommended when:

* Atypical asthma symptoms are present or the diagnosis of asthma is in question;
* The patient has poor asthma control (poor lung function, persistent asthma symptoms) or severe asthma exacerbations (≥ 1 course of systemic steroids per year or hospitalization) despite moderate doses of ICS (with proper technique and good compliance);
* The patient requires a detailed assessment for and management of potential environmental triggers;
* The patient has been admitted to the intensive care unit (ICU) for asthma.

In young children 1–5 years of age, referral to an asthma specialist is recommended when there is diagnostic uncertainty or suspicion of comorbidity; poor symptom and exacerbation control despite ICS at daily doses of 200–250 µg; a life-threatening event (requiring ICU admission and/or intubation); and/or for allergy testing to assess the possible role of environmental allergens [17].

Conclusion

Asthma is the most common respiratory disorder in Canada, and contributes to significant morbidity and mortality. A diagnosis of asthma should be suspected in patients with recurrent cough, wheeze, chest tightness and dyspnea, and should be confirmed using objective measures of lung function (spirometry preferred). Allergy testing is also recommended to identify possible triggers of asthma symptoms.

In most patients, asthma control can be achieved using avoidance measures and appropriate pharmacological interventions. ICSs represent the standard of care for the majority of asthma patients. For those who fail to achieve control with low-to-moderate ICS doses, combination therapy with a LABA and ICS is the preferred treatment choice in most adults. LTRAs can also be used as add-on therapy if asthma is uncontrolled despite the use of low-to-moderate dose ICS therapy, particularly in patients with concurrent allergic rhinitis. LAMAs or biologic therapies targeting IgE or IL-5 may be useful in select cases of difficult to control asthma. Allergen-specific immunotherapy is a potentially disease-modifying therapy, but should only be prescribed by physicians with appropriate training in allergy. All patients with asthma should have regular follow-up visits during which criteria for asthma control, adherence to therapy and proper inhaler technique should be reviewed.

Key take-home messages

- A clinical diagnosis of asthma should be suspected in patients with intermittent symptoms of wheezing, coughing, chest tightness and breathlessness.
- Objective measurements of lung function, preferably using spirometry, are needed to confirm the diagnosis. The best time to perform this testing is when the patient is symptomatic. Spirometry can generally be performed in children 6 years of age and older.
- In children <6 years of age who are unable to perform spirometry, a trial of therapy (8–12 weeks in duration) and monitoring of symptoms can act as a surrogate method to diagnose asthma.
- All asthma patients should be prescribed a rapid-acting bronchodilator to be used as needed for relief of acute symptoms.
- ICS therapy is the standard of care for most patients with asthma.
- Combination ICS/LABA inhalers are recommended for most adult patients who fail to achieve control with low-to-moderate ICS doses.
- LTRAs can also be used as add-on therapy if asthma is uncontrolled despite the use of low-to-moderate ICS doses.
- Tiotropium by mist inhaler can be added in patients 12 years of age or older with an exacerbation history despite ICS/LABA treatment.

- Biologic therapy targeting IgE or IL-5 may be useful in select cases of difficult to control asthma.
- Allergen-specific immunotherapy is a potentially disease-modifying therapy that can be considered in most cases of allergic asthma.
- Regular monitoring of asthma control every 3–4 months, adherence to therapy and inhaler technique are important components of asthma management.

Abbreviations

ICS: inhaled corticosteroid; LABA: long-acting beta$_2$-agonist; IgE: immunoglobulin E; IL: interleukin; GINA: Global Initiative for Asthma; Th2: T helper cell type-2; BMI: body mass index; FEV$_1$: forced expiratory volume in one second; FVC: forced vital capacity; LTRA: leukotriene receptor antagonist; LAMA: long-acting muscarinic receptor antagonist; pMDI: pressurized metered dose inhalers; DPI: dry powder inhaler; PD: provocative dose; PC: provocative concentration; PEF: peak expiratory flow; COPD: chronic obstructive pulmonary disease; ACOS: asthma-COPD overlap syndrome; CHILD: Canadian Healthy Infant Longitudinal Development; SARP: Severe Asthma Research Program; PRAM: Pediatric Respiratory Assessment Measure; HEPA: high-efficiency particulate air; SABA: short-acting beta$_2$-agonist; ICU: intensive care unit; RSV: respiratory syncytial virus; mAPI: modified Asthma Predictive Index.

Declarations

Authors' contributions All authors wrote and/or edited sections of the manuscript. All authors read and approved the final manuscript.

Author details

[1] McMaster University, Hamilton, ON, Canada. [2] University of British Columbia, Vancouver, BC, Canada. [3] Western University, London, ON, Canada. [4] McGill University, Montreal, QC, Canada.

Acknowledgements

This article is an update to the Asthma article that originally appeared in the supplement entitled, *Practical Guide to Allergy and Immunology in Canada*, which was published in *Allergy, Asthma & Clinical Immunology* in 2011 (available at: https://aacijournal.biomedcentral.com/articles/supplements/volume-7-supplement-1). The authors would like to thank Julie Tasso for her editorial services and assistance in the preparation of this manuscript.

Competing interests

Dr. Jaclyn Quirt has received honoraria from AstraZeneca, Merck, Meda Pharmaceuticals and Sanofi. Dr. Kyla J. Hildebrand is the Section Chair of Pediatrics for the Canadian Society of Allergy and Clinical Immunology, and was an expert panel member for the development of the BCGuidelines.ca publication, Asthma in Children—Diagnosis and Management (2015). Dr. Jorge Mazza has received consulting fees and honoraria from AstraZeneca, GlaxoSmithKline, Graceway Pharmaceuticals and Novartis. Dr. Francisco Noya has received honoraria from Sanofi Pasteur and Pediapharm, and clinical trial grants from Sanofi Pasteur. Dr. Harold Kim is Vice President of the Canadian Society of Allergy and Clinical Immunology, Past President of the Canadian Network for Respiratory Care, and Co-chief Editor of *Allergy, Asthma and Clinical Immunology*. He has received consulting fees and honoraria for continuing medical education from AstraZeneca, Aralez, Boehringer Ingelheim, CSL Behring, Kaleo, Merck, Novartis, Pediapharm, Sanofi, Shire and Teva.

Funding
Publication of this supplement has been supported by AstraZeneca, Boehringer Ingelheim, CSL Behring Canada Inc., MEDA Pharmaceuticals Ltd., Merck Canada Inc., Pfizer Canada Inc., Shire Pharma Canada ULC, Stallergenes Greer Canada, Takeda Canada, Teva Canada Innovation, Aralez Tribute and Pediapharm.

About this supplement
This article has been published as part of *Allergy, Asthma & Clinical Immunology* Volume 14 Supplement 2, 2018: Practical guide for allergy and immunology in Canada 2018. The full contents of the supplement are available online at https://aacijournal.biomedcentral.com/articles/supplements/volume-14-supplement-2.

References
1. Public Health Agency of Canada. Life and breath: respiratory disease in Canada. Ottawa, Ontario; 2007. http://www.phac-aspc.gc.ca/publicat/2007/lbrdc-vsmrc/index-eng.php. Accessed 15 July 2010.
2. Akinbami LJ, Moorman JE, Garbe PL, Sondik EJ. Status of childhood asthma in the United States, 1980–2007. Pediatrics. 2009;123(Suppl 3):S131–45.
3. Bourdin A, Gras D, Vachier I, Chanez P. Upper airway 1: allergic rhinitis and asthma: united disease through epithelial cells. Thorax. 2009;64(11):999–1004.
4. FitzGerald JM, Boulet LP, McIvor RA, Zimmerman S, Chapman KR. Asthma control in Canada remains suboptimal: the Reality of Asthma Control (TRAC) study. Can Respir J. 2006;13(5):253–9.
5. Global Initiative for Asthma (GINA). Global strategy for asthma management and prevention. Updated 2017. http://www.ginasthma.org. Accessed 19 Feb 2017.
6. Statistics Canada. Asthma. Health Reports. 2005;16(2). http://publications.gc.ca/Collection-R/Statcan/82-003-XIE/0020482-003-XIE.pdf. Accessed 6 June 2017.
7. Gershon AS, Guan J, Wang C, To T. Trends in asthma prevalence and incidence in Ontario, Canada, 1996–2005: a population study. Am J Epidemiol. 2010;172(6):728–36.
8. Yang CL, To T, Foty RG, Stieb DM, Dell SD. Verifying a questionnaire diagnosis of asthma children using health claims data. BMC Pulm Med. 2011;11:52.
9. Lemanske RF, Busse WW. Asthma: clinical expression and molecular mechanisms. J Allergy Clin Immunol. 2010;125:S95–102.
10. Bai TR, Vonk JM, Postma DS, Boezen HM. Severe exacerbations predict excess lung function decline in asthma. Eur Respir J. 2007;30(3):452–6.
11. Subbarao P, Mandhane PJ, Sears MR. Asthma: epidemiology, etiology and risk factors. CMAJ. 2009;181(9):E181–90.
12. Wenzel SE. Asthma phenotypes: the evolution from clinical to molecular approaches. Nat Med. 2012;18(5):716–25.
13. Moore WC, Meyers DA, Wenzel SE, Teague WG, Li H, Li X, D'Agostino R Jr, Castro M, Curran-Everett D, Fitzpatrick AM, Gaston B, Jarjour NN, Sorkness R, Calhoun WJ, Chung KF, Comhair SA, Dweik RA, Israel E, Peters SP, Busse WW, Erzurum SC, Bleecker ER. National Heart, Lung, and Blood Institute's Severe Asthma Research Program. Identification of asthma phenotypes using cluster analysis in the Severe Asthma Research Program. Am J Respir Crit Care Med. 2010;181(4):315–23.
14. Stein RT, Martinez FD. Asthma phenotypes in childhood: lessons from an epidemiological approach. Paediatr Respir Rev. 2004;5(2):155–61.
15. Lougheed MD, Lemière C, Dell SD, Ducharme FM, Fitzgerald JM, Leigh R, Licskai C, Rowe BH, Bowie D, Becker A, Boulet LP. Canadian Thoracic Society asthma management continuum: 2010 consensus summary for children six years of age and over, and adults. Can Respir J. 2010;17(1):15–24.
16. Kaplan AG, Balter MS, Bell AD, Kim H, McIvor RA. Diagnosis of asthma in adults. Can Med Assoc J. 2009;181:E210–20.
17. Ducharme FM, Dell SD, Radhakrishnan D, Grad RM, Watson WT, Yang CL, Zelman M. Diagnosis and management of asthma in preschoolers: a Canadian Thoracic Society and Canadian Paediatric Society position paper. Can Respir J. 2015;22(3):135–43.
18. Kovesi T, Schuh S, Spier S, Bérubé D, Carr S, Watson W, McIvor RA. Achieving control of asthma in preschoolers. Can Med Assoc J. 2010;182(4):E172–83.
19. Becker A, Lemière C, Bérubé D, Boulet LP, Ducharme FM, FitzGerald M, Kovesi T. Asthma Guidelines Working Group of the Canadian Network For Asthma Care Summary of recommendations from the Canadian asthma consensus guidelines, 2003 and Canadian pediatric asthma consensus guidelines, 2003. Can Med Assoc J. 2005;173(6 Suppl):S1–56.
20. Chang TS, Lemanske RF Jr, Guilbert TW, Gern JE, Coen MH, Evans MD, Gangnon RE, Page CD, Jackson DJ. Evaluation of the modified Asthma Predictive Index in high-risk preschool children. J Allergy Clin Immunol Pract. 2013;1(2):152–6.
21. Chalut DS, Ducharme FM, Davis GM. The Preschool Respiratory Assessment Measure (PRAM): a responsive index of acute asthma severity. J Pediatr. 2000;137(6):762–8.
22. Ducharme FM, Chalut D, Plotnick L, Savdie C, Kudirka D, Zhang X, Meng L, McGillivray D. The Pediatric Respiratory Assessment Measure: a valid clinical score for assessing acute asthma severity from toddlers to teenagers. J Pediatr. 2008;152(4):476–80.
23. Lougheed MD, Lemiere C, Ducharme FM, Licskai C, Dell SD, Rowe BH, Fitzgerald M, Leigh R, Watson W, Boulet LP, Canadian Thoracic Society Asthma Clinical Assembly. Canadian Thoracic Society 2012 guideline update: diagnosis and management of asthma in preschoolers, children and adults. Can Respir J. 2012;19(2):127–64.
24. Aaron SD, Vandemheen KL, FitzGerald JM, Ainslie M, Gupta S, Lemière C, Field SK, McIvor RA, Hernandez P, Mayers I, Mulpuru S, Alvarez GG, Pakhale S, Mallick R, Boulet LP, Canadian Respiratory Research Network. Reevaluation of diagnosis in adults with physician-diagnosed asthma. JAMA. 2017;317(3):269–79.
25. Crapo RO, Casaburi R, Coates AL, Enright PL, Hankinson JL, Irvin CG, MacIntyre NR, McKay RT, Wanger JS, Anderson SD, Cockcroft DW, Fish JE, Sterk PJ. Guidelines for methacholine and exercise challenge testing—1999. This official statement of the American Thoracic Society was adopted by the ATS Board of Directors July 1999. Am J Respir Crit Care Med. 2000;161(1):309–29.
26. Kendzerska T, Sadatsafavi M, Aaron SD, To TM, Lougheed MD, FitzGerald JM, Gershon AS, Canadian Respiratory Research Network. Concurrent physician-diagnosed asthma and chronic obstructive pulmonary disease: a population study of prevalence, incidence and mortality. PLoS ONE. 2017;12(3):e0173830.
27. Abramson MJ, Puy RM, Weiner JM. Injection allergen immunotherapy for asthma. Cochrane Database Syst Rev. 2010;8:001186.
28. Frew AJ. Allergen immunotherapy. J Allergy Clin Immunol. 2010;125(Suppl 2):S306–13.
29. Canadian Society of Allergy and Clinical Immunology. Immunother Manual. 2016. http://csaci.ca/wp-content/uploads/2017/12/IT-Manual-2016-5-July-2017-rev.pdf. Accessed 12 July 2018.
30. Cox L, Nelson H, Lockey R, Calabria C, Chacko T, Finegold I, Nelson M, Weber R, Bernstein DI, Blessing-Moore J, Khan DA, Lang DM, Nicklas RA, Oppenheimer J, Portnoy JM, Randolph C, Schuller DE, Spector SL, Tilles S, Wallace D. Allergen immunotherapy: a practice parameter third update. J Allergy Clin Immunol. 2011;127(1 Suppl):S1–55.
31. BCGuidelines.ca Guidelines & Protocols Advisory Committee. Asthma in children: diagnosis and management. October 28, 2015. http://www2.gov.bc.ca/assets/gov/health/practitioner-pro/bc-guidelines/asthma-children-full-guideline.pdf. Accessed 19 June 2017.
32. Issa-El-Khoury K, Kim H, Chan ED, Vander Leek T, Noya F. CSACI position statement: systemic effect of inhaled corticosteroids on adrenal suppression in the management of pediatric asthma. Allergy Asthma Clin Immunol. 2015;11(1):9.
33. Calamita Z, Saconato H, Pela AB, Atallah AN. Efficacy of sublingual immunotherapy in asthma: systematic review of randomized clinical trials using the Cochrane Collaboration method. Allergy. 2006;61(10):1162–72.
34. Grembiale RD, Camporota L, Naty S, Tranfa CM, Djukanovic R, Marsico SA. Effects of specific immunotherapy in allergic rhinitic individuals with bronchial hyperresponsiveness. Am J Respir Crit Care Med. 2000;162(6):2048–52.
35. Niggemann B, Jacobsen L, Dreborg S, Ferdousi HA, Halken S, Høst A, Koivikko A, Koller D, Norberg LA, Urbanek R, Valovirta E, Wahn U, Möller C, PAT Investigator Group. Five-year follow-up on the PAT study: specific immunotherapy and long-term prevention of asthma in children. Allergy. 2006;61(7):855–9.

21

Characterization of tenascin-C as a novel biomarker for asthma: utility of tenascin-C in combination with periostin or immunoglobulin E

Mina Yasuda[1,2], Norihiro Harada[1,3,4]* (iD), Sonoko Harada[1,4], Ayako Ishimori[1], Yoko Katsura[1], Yukinari Itoigawa[1], Kei Matsuno[1,3], Fumihiko Makino[1], Jun Ito[1,3], Junya Ono[5], Kazunori Tobino[1,2], Hisaya Akiba[6], Ryo Atsuta[1], Kenji Izuhara[7] and Kazuhisa Takahashi[1,3]

Abstract

Background: Extracellular matrix proteins tenascin-C (TNC) and periostin, which were identified as T-helper cell type 2 cytokine-induced genes in human bronchial epithelial cells, accumulate in the airway basement membrane of asthmatic patients. Although serum periostin has been accepted as a type 2 biomarker, serum TNC has not been evaluated as a systemic biomarker in asthma. Therefore, the objective of this study was to evaluate whether serum TNC can serve as a novel biomarker for asthma.

Methods: We evaluated 126 adult patients with mild to severe asthma. Serum TNC, periostin, and total IgE concentrations were quantified using enzyme-linked immunosorbent assays.

Results: Serum TNC levels were significantly higher in patients with severe asthma and high serum total IgE levels. Patients with both high serum TNC (> 37.16 ng/mL) and high serum periostin (> 95 ng/mL) levels (n $=20$) or patients with both high serum TNC and high serum total IgE (> 100 IU/mL) levels (n $=36$) presented higher disease severity and more severe airflow limitation than patients in other subpopulations.

Conclusions: To our knowledge, this is the first study to show that serum TNC levels in asthmatic patients are associated with clinical features of asthma and that the combination of serum TNC and periostin levels or combination of serum TNC and total IgE levels were more useful for asthma than each single marker, suggesting that serum TNC can serve as a novel biomarker for asthma.

Keywords: Tenascin-C, Periostin, Asthma, Type 2 biomarker, Immunoglobulin E

Background

Although the mechanisms of heterogeneous chronic inflammatory disorders of the airway, including bronchial asthma, are not fully clarified, airway inflammation and remodeling typically occur in these pathologies [1–3]. Asthma is characterized by inflammation of the airways associated with excessive deposition of the extracellular matrix, including basement membrane thickening, mucous cell metaplasia, epithelial shedding, angiogenesis, inflammatory cell infiltration, and smooth muscle cell and lung fibroblast proliferation [4]. An increase in the number of lung fibroblasts characterized by collagen synthesis and in both tenascin and periostin deposition within the basement membrane matrix may occur in response to allergen challenge in asthmatic patients [5, 6].

Although a variety of cell types are involved in allergic airway inflammation, antigen-specific CD4+

*Correspondence: nor@juntendo.ac.jp
[1] Department of Respiratory Medicine, Juntendo University Faculty of Medicine and Graduate School of Medicine, 3-1-3 Hongo, Bunkyo-ku, Tokyo 113-8431, Japan
Full list of author information is available at the end of the article

T-helper cell type 2 (Th2) and type 2 innate lymphoid cells, which secrete Th2 cytokines such as interleukin (IL)-4 and IL-13, are believed to drive asthma pathobiology [7, 8]. Previous microarray analyses identified tenascin-C (TNC) and periostin as IL-4- or IL-13-induced genes in human bronchial epithelial cells [9–13]. Both TNC and periostin are glycoproteins that are secreted into the extracellular matrix. Previous studies suggested that periostin may promote eosinophil infiltration into the asthmatic airway during inflammation and serum periostin may be a systemic biomarker for eosinophilic airway inflammation and disease severity in asthmatic patients [6, 14–18]. It has also been reported that serum periostin has the potential as a prognostic biomarker to predict the risk of a decline in forced expiratory volume in 1 s (FEV$_1$) in late-onset and eosinophil-dominant asthmatic patients [19–21].

TNC is prototypic of the TN family and supports the migration of inflammatory cells from the interstitium to the airspace. TNC is highly expressed in human lung during embryonic development, and its expression is especially strong in the extracellular matrix underlying the airway epithelium during the gestational stages [22, 23]. Although TNC expression is less abundant and more restricted in normal adult tissues, TNC expression in the airway subepithelial reticular basement membrane in asthmatic patients is prominently increased after allergen challenge and is a histopathological subepithelial marker to detect disease activity in asthma [24–26]. The thickness of TNC deposition was correlated with the number of eosinophils, T-lymphocytes, and IL-4-positive cells in bronchial mucosa of atopic asthmatics [27]. Previous studies using TNC-deficient mice suggested that TNC provides protection against ovalbumin-induced Th2-driven airway inflammation [28]. Moreover, treating asthmatics with mepolizumab, an anti-IL-5 monoclonal antibody for severe asthma, significantly decreased airway eosinophil numbers and significantly reduced TNC deposition in the airway subepithelial reticular basement membrane when compared with placebo [25]. Furthermore, one report has been demonstrated that serum TNC levels were significantly higher in patients with refractory asthma than in non-refractory asthma and normal volunteers [29]. Although these reports indicated that TNC in asthmatic patients may play a key role in Th2/type 2 airway inflammation, serum TNC has not been evaluated as a potential biomarker of Th2/type 2 airway inflammation and asthma. Therefore, in the present study, we evaluate whether serum TNC levels can serve as a novel biomarker for asthma.

Methods

Patients

Consecutive patients with mild to severe asthma, who were aged 20 years or older, were recruited with informed consent from our outpatient clinic at Juntendo University Hospital (Tokyo, Japan). Asthma was diagnosed by a clinical history of episodic symptoms with airflow limitation and by either variation in pulmonary function monitored by forced expiratory volume in 1 s (FEV$_1$) or peak expiratory flow (PEF) in accordance with the Global Initiative for Asthma (GINA) guidelines [30]. The disease severity was also assessed in accordance with the GINA guidelines [30]. The present study was reviewed and approved by the Juntendo University Research Ethics Committee (Tokyo, Japan). Written informed consent was obtained from each patient before their participation in the study. This study was registered in the UMIN Clinical Trial Registry (UMIN000009968) on February 5, 2013 (http://www.umin.ac.jp/). Patients having any of the following criteria were excluded: a diagnosis of chronic obstructive pulmonary disease defined by the Global Initiative for Chronic Obstructive Lung Disease guidelines [31] and any current respiratory disorder other than asthma.

The asthma control test (ACT) score, pulmonary function parameters, and fractional exhaled nitric oxide (FeNO) levels were measured. FeNO levels were measured in accordance with the American Thoracic Society recommendations at a constant flow of 0.05 L/s against an expiratory resistance of 20 cm water with a chemiluminescence analyzer (NOA 280i; Sievers, Boulder, CO, USA). On the same day these clinical examination and venous blood sampling were performed.

Quantification of serum periostin and TNC levels

The sera of patients were collected after density-gradient centrifugation of blood samples and frozen at −80 °C. Periostin levels were measured with an enzyme-linked immunosorbent assay (ELISA) (Shino test, Sagamihara, Japan), as described previously [32]. TNC was simultaneously quantified in thawed serum using the human TNC ELISA kit (IBL Co. Ltd, Gunma, Japan) [33, 34].

Statistical analysis

Sample normality was examined using the D'Agostino–Pearson test. Differences in parameters between populations were analyzed for significance using Student's t test, the Mann–Whitney U test, the Chi square test, and Fisher's exact test as appropriate. For correlation between variables, the Pearson's correlation coefficient and Spearman's rank correlation coefficient, which is denoted as r_s for a sample statistic, were used where appropriate. One-way ANOVA followed by the Tukey test and Kruskal–Wallis test followed by the Dunn test were used for multigroup analysis. Differences were statistically significant when P values were 0.05 or less. Statistical analyses were performed using Graph Pad Prism version 6 software (GraphPad Software, Inc., La Jolla, CA, USA). A Th2-high subgroup was defined as both a serum total immunoglobulin

E (IgE) level of > 100 IU/mL and a peripheral blood eosinophil count of $\geq 0.14 \times 10^9$ cells/L [13, 35, 36].

Results

Baseline characteristics

We first determined the baseline characteristics of asthmatic patients (Table 1). This study enrolled 126 patients with mild to severe asthma, including 13 (10.3%) in GINA treatment steps 1 and 2, 32 (25.4%) in step 3, 57

Table 1 Baseline characteristics of the study population

	Total n = 126	GINA step 1–3 n = 45	GINA step 4 + 5 n = 81	P value
Sex (M/F), n (%)	43 (34.1)/83 (65.9)	21 (46.7)/24 (53.3)	22 (27.2)/59 (72.8)	0.032*
Age (years)	53.91 ± 15.86	55.47 ± 15.66	53.05 ± 16.01	0.415
Age at asthma onset (years)	35.08 ± 22.05	36.87 ± 22.46	34.09 ± 21.90	0.437
Duration of asthma (years)	18.83 ± 15.95	18.60 ± 17.20	18.96 ± 15.32	0.613
BMI (kg/m²)	24.00 ± 4.88	23.30 ± 4.08	24.38 ± 5.26	0.317
Smoking history (never/ex/current), n (%)	79 (62.7)/42 (33.3)/5 (4.0)	20 (44.4)/23 (51.1)/2 (4.4)	59 (72.8)/19 (23.4)/3 (3.7)	0.006*
Pack year smoking history (pack year)	5.63 ± 10.79	9.00 ± 13.74	3.75 ± 8.25	0.003*
Atopic predisposition, n (%)	99 (78.6)	33 (73.3)	66 (81.5)	0.365
AERD, n (%)	12 (9.5)	1 (2.2)	11 (13.6)	0.055
Atopic dermatitis, n (%)	27 (21.4)	10 (22.2)	17 (21.0)	1.000
Allergic rhinitis, n (%)	66 (52.4)	24 (53.3)	42 (51.9)	1.000
Chronic sinusitis, n (%)	38 (30.2)	13 (28.9)	25 (30.9)	0.843
Daily dose of ICS (FP equivalent dose, μg)	584.13 ± 383.49	177.78 ± 92.05	809.88 ± 283.99	< 0.001*
Daily dose of OCS (PSL equivalent dose, mg)	0.35 ± 1.41	0.00 ± 0.00	0.55 ± 1.73	0.014*
ACT score, n = 125	23.20 ± 2.82	24.29 ± 1.47	22.59 ± 3.20	< 0.001*
FeNO (ppb)	55.04 ± 43.69	65.31 ± 53.19	49.34 ± 36.53	0.037*
Peripheral neutrophils (cells/μL)	4022.36 ± 1492.54	3696.30 ± 1115.92	4203.51 ± 1644.02	0.113
Peripheral eosinophils (cells/μL)	263.54 ± 236.05	231.11 ± 180.79	281.55 ± 261.08	0.775
Serum IgE (IU/mL)	616.37 ± 1686.39	467.19 ± 718.39	699.24 ± 2034.77	0.731
Th2-high[†], n (%)	53 (42.1)	21 (46.7)	32 (39.5)	0.457
Serum periostin (ng/mL)	87.65 ± 34.49	94.62 ± 30.83	83.78 ± 35.96	0.012*
Serum TNC (ng/mL)	39.49 ± 25.18	30.95 ± 16.69	44.23 ± 27.82	0.002*
FVC (L)	3.22 ± 0.95	3.51 ± 0.87	3.06 ± 0.96	0.004*
%FVC (predicted, %)	103.06 ± 16.22	107.16 ± 14.69	100.80 ± 16.59	0.013*
FEV₁ (L)	2.38 ± 0.79	2.55 ± 0.70	2.29 ± 0.82	0.079
%FEV₁ (predicted, %)	90.98 ± 18.37	93.80 ± 15.93	89.41 ± 19.51	0.201
FEV₁/FVC ratio (%)	73.46 ± 10.30	72.56 ± 8.29	73.97 ± 11.28	0.189
PEF (L/s)	7.23 ± 2.06	7.74 ± 1.94	6.95 ± 2.08	0.037*
%PEF (predicted, %)	103.28 ± 21.12	105.46 ± 19.00	102.07 ± 22.23	0.389
MMF (L)	1.95 ± 1.07	1.93 ± 0.95	1.95 ± 1.13	0.951
%MMF (predicted, %)	58.93 ± 27.49	57.98 ± 22.69	59.46 ± 29.95	0.773

Data are presented as the mean ± standard deviation unless otherwise indicated

Comparisons performed by Student's t test, the Mann–Whitney U test, the Chi square test, and Fisher's exact test as appropriate

ACT asthma control test, *AERD* aspirin-exacerbated respiratory disease, *BMI* body mass index, *FeNO* fractional exhaled nitric oxide, *FEV1* forced expiratory volume in 1 s, *FP* fluticasone propionate, *FVC* forced vital capacity, *GINA* Global Initiative for Asthma, *ICS* inhaled corticosteroid, *IgE* immunoglobulin E, *MMF* mid-maximal flow rate, *OCS* oral corticosteroids, *PEF* peak expiratory flow, *PSL* prednisolone, *Th2* T-helper cell type 2, *TNC* tenascin-C

*$P < 0.05$, GINA treatment steps 1–3 group versus GINA treatment steps 4 + 5

[†] Th2-high: total IgE level of more than 100 IU/mL and a peripheral blood eosinophil count of 0.14×10^9 cells/L or more

(45.2%) in step 4, and 24 (19.0%) in step 5. The male to female ratio was 43:83, and the median age was 53 years (range 20–86 years). The mean (±standard deviation) duration of asthma was 18.83 ± 15.95 years, and the mean FEV_1/forced vital capacity (FVC) ratio was $73.46 \pm 10.3\%$ (Table 1). We also compared the characteristics of 45 patients (35.7%) included in GINA treatment steps 1–3 (GINA step 1–3 group) and 81 patients (64.3%) included in GINA treatment steps 4 and 5 (GINA step 4+5 group) (Table 1). In the GINA step 4+5 group, the male to female ratio ($P=0.032$), smoking history (in pack-years) ($P=0.003$), ACT score ($P<0.001$), FVC ($P=0.004$), percent predicted FVC (%FVC) ($P=0.013$), PEF ($P=0.037$), FeNO levels ($P=0.037$), and serum periostin concentrations ($P=0.012$) were significantly lower than those in the GINA step 1–3 group. Conversely, the never-smoker/current and ex-smoker ratio which was performed by Fisher's exact test ($P=0.002$, data not shown), daily dose of inhaled and oral corticosteroids ($P<0.001$ and $P=0.014$, respectively), and serum TNC concentrations ($P=0.002$) were significantly higher in the GINA step 4+5 group compared with the GINA step 1–3 group (Table 1).

Association of serum periostin and TNC levels with subject characteristics in asthmatic patients

We next examined whether serum periostin and TNC levels in asthmatic patients were associated with subject characteristics. Serum periostin levels were positively correlated with age ($r_s=0.261$, $P=0.003$), age at asthma onset ($r_s=0.283$, $P=0.001$), ACT score ($r_s=0.24$, $P=0.007$), FeNO levels ($r_s=0.319$, $P<0.001$), peripheral blood eosinophil counts ($r_s=0.36$, $P<0.001$), and the Th2-high to Th2-low ratio ($r_s=0.195$, $P=0.029$) (Table 2). Although serum periostin levels were negatively correlated with the daily dose of inhaled corticosteroids (ICS) ($r_s=-0.194$, $P=0.029$) and the percentages of GINA treatment steps 4+5 ($r_s=-0.224$, $P=0.012$), periostin levels were also negatively correlated with airflow limitation, including FEV_1 ($r_s=-0.203$, $P=0.023$), the mid-maximal flow rate (MMF) ($r_s=-0.25$, $P=0.005$), and percent predicted MMF (%MMF) ($r_s=-0.195$, $P=0.028$). Moreover, in the GINA step 4+5 group, serum periostin levels were positively correlated with age ($r_s=0.29$, $P=0.009$), age at asthma onset ($r_s=0.316$, $P=0.004$), FeNO levels ($r_s=0.226$, $P=0.016$), peripheral blood eosinophil counts ($r_s=0.398$, $P<0.001$), and the Th2-high to Th2-low ratio ($r_s=0.241$, $P=0.03$), but were negatively correlated with FVC ($r_s=-0.29$, $P=0.009$), FEV_1 ($r_s=-0.295$, $P=0.008$) and MMF ($r_s=-0.286$, $P=0.01$) (Additional file 1: Table S1). Serum TNC levels were positively correlated with the percentages of GINA treatment steps

4+5 ($r_s=0.274$, $P=0.002$), daily dose of ICS ($r_s=0.206$, $P=0.02$), peripheral blood neutrophil counts ($r_s=0.189$, $P=0.034$), and serum total IgE levels ($r_s=0.259$, $P=0.003$) (Table 2). These results suggest that serum periostin and TNC levels were associated with distinct subject characteristics.

Comparison of serum periostin and TNC levels between two subgroups according to asthma severity and Th2-related variables

We then divided the 126 patients into two subgroups by five different ways: according to asthma severity (mild to moderate asthma and severe asthma), the Th2-high and Th2-low subgroups based on both serum IgE levels and a peripheral blood eosinophil counts, the high and low IgE subgroups based on serum IgE levels, the high and low eosinophil subgroups based on peripheral blood eosinophil counts, and the high and low FeNO subgroups based on FeNO levels (Fig. 1 and Additional file 2: Table S2). Serum periostin levels were significantly higher in patients with mild to moderate asthma ($P=0.01$), Th2-high ($P=0.029$), high peripheral blood eosinophil counts ($\geq 0.14 \times 10^9$ cells/L) ($P=0.01$), and high FeNO levels (≥ 50 ppb) ($P<0.001$) [Fig. 1a and Additional file 2: Table S2]. Serum TNC levels were significantly higher in patients with severe asthma ($P=0.012$) and high serum total IgE levels (≥ 100 IU/mL) ($P=0.026$) (Fig. 1b and Additional file 2: Table S2). These results suggest that serum periostin and TNC levels were associated with different characteristics of asthma disease severity and Th2-related variables. Moreover, not only serum periostin but also serum TNC might have potential use as novel biomarkers for asthma.

Characteristics of patients with both high serum TNC levels and high serum periostin or IgE levels

We evaluated whether the combination of serum periostin and TNC levels were more reliable than a single biomarker approach. Receiver operating characteristic curve analysis was used to determine the optimal cut-off value of serum TNC level to discriminate the GINA step 4+5 group from the GINA step 1–3 group, with the area under the curve of 0.665 (95% CI 0.57–0.76) (Fig. 2a). A serum TNC level of 37.16 ng/mL was the best cut-off value for the optimal potential effectiveness of serum TNC using Youden's index [37]. There were no correlation between serum periostin and TNC levels ($r_s=0.111$, $P=0.216$) (Fig. 2b). We then divided the 126 patients into four subgroups according to the cut-off values for serum TNC (37.16 ng/mL) and serum periostin (95 ng/mL) (Fig. 2b, Table 3 and Additional file 3: Table S3) [19]. In patients with high serum TNC and periostin levels, the percentages of GINA treatment steps 4+5 ($P=0.042$), percentages of patients with aspirin-exacerbated

Table 2 Correlation coefficients for the association of serum periostin and TNC levels with subject characteristics in asthmatic patients

	Periostin		TNC	
	r_s	P value	r_s	P value
Sex (male)	−0.033	0.711	−0.025	0.780
Age (years)	0.261	0.003*	−0.074	0.410
Age at asthma onset (years)	0.283	0.001*	−0.019	0.831
Duration of asthma (years)	−0.165	0.066	0.019	0.833
BMI (kg/m²)	−0.071	0.428	0.029	0.749
Pack-year smoking history (pack year)	0.014	0.878	−0.032	0.722
GINA step 4 + 5	−0.224	0.012*	0.274	0.002*
AERD	0.119	0.186	0.132	0.142
Atopic dermatitis	−0.016	0.857	0.003	0.969
Allergic rhinitis	−0.041	0.651	−0.027	0.763
Chronic sinusitis	0.088	0.329	0.026	0.771
Daily dose of ICS (FP equivalent dose, µg)	−0.194	0.029*	0.206	0.020*
Daily dose of OCS (PSL equivalent dose, mg)	−0.068	0.446	0.096	0.286
ACT score, n = 125	0.240	0.007*	−0.108	0.232
FeNO (ppb)	0.319	<0.001*	0.057	0.529
Peripheral neutrophils (cells/µL)	−0.124	0.168	0.189	0.034*
Peripheral eosinophils (cells/µL)	0.360	<0.001*	0.063	0.486
Serum IgE (IU/mL)	0.110	0.221	0.259	0.003*
Th2-high	0.195	0.029*	0.046	0.609
FVC (L)	−0.167	0.061	−0.056	0.536
%FVC (predicted, %)	−0.047	0.604	−0.104	0.246
FEV₁ (L)	−0.167	0.061	−0.099	0.271
%FEV₁ (predicted, %)	−0.203	0.023*	−0.042	0.642
FEV₁/FVC ratio (%)	−0.084	0.349	−0.149	0.096
PEF (L/s)	−0.146	0.103	−0.057	0.524
%PEF (predicted, %)	−0.024	0.786	−0.103	0.252
MMF (L)	−0.250	0.005*	−0.058	0.522
%MMF (predicted, %)	−0.195	0.028*	−0.140	0.118

ACT asthma control test, *AERD* aspirin-exacerbated respiratory disease, *BMI* body mass index, *FeNO* fractional exhaled nitric oxide, *FEV1* forced expiratory volume in 1 s, *FP* fluticasone propionate, *FVC* forced vital capacity, *GINA* Global Initiative for Asthma, *ICS* inhaled corticosteroid, *IgE* immunoglobulin E, *MMF* mid-maximal flow rate, *OCS* oral corticosteroids, *PEF* peak expiratory flow, *PSL* prednisolone, *Th2* T-helper cell type 2, *TNC* tenascin-C

*$P < 0.05$

respiratory disease (AERD) ($P = 0.004$), daily dose of ICS ($P = 0.045$), and peripheral blood eosinophil ($P = 0.005$) and neutrophil counts ($P = 0.032$) were significantly higher, whereas FVC ($P = 0.01$), %FVC ($P = 0.019$), FEV₁ ($P = 0.014$), PEF ($P = 0.045$), MMF ($P = 0.045$), and %MMF ($P = 0.042$) were significantly lower as compared with patients in the other subpopulations (Table 3). These data suggest that the combination of serum periostin and TNC had the ability to reflect asthma severity and airflow limitation in asthmatic patients.

We next evaluated whether the combination of serum TNC and total IgE levels were more reliable than a single biomarker approach, as described above for periostin. We also divided the 126 patients into four subgroups according to the cut-off values for serum TNC (37.16 ng/mL) and serum total IgE levels (100 IU/mL) (Table 4 and Additional file 4: Table S4). The percentages of GINA treatment steps 4 + 5 ($P = 0.023$), percentages of patients with Th2-high ($P = 0.003$), and peripheral blood neutrophil counts ($P = 0.002$) were significantly higher, whereas %FVC ($P = 0.005$), %FEV₁ ($P < 0.001$), percent predicted PEF ($P = 0.033$), and %MMF ($P = 0.01$) were significantly lower in patients with high serum TNC and total IgE levels as compared with patients in the other subpopulations (Table 4). These data suggest that the combination of serum TNC and IgE also had the ability to reflect asthma severity and airflow limitation in asthmatic patients.

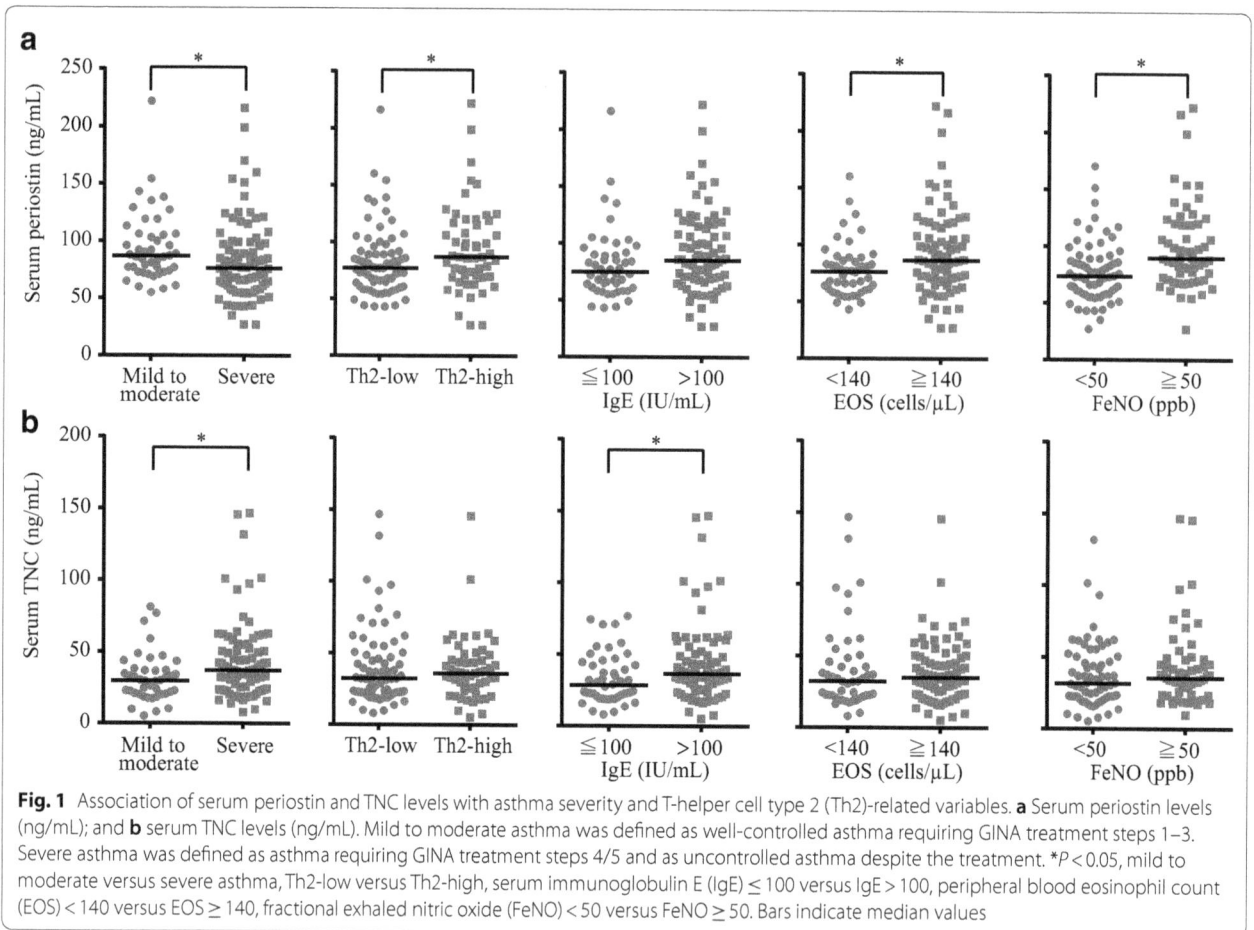

Fig. 1 Association of serum periostin and TNC levels with asthma severity and T-helper cell type 2 (Th2)-related variables. **a** Serum periostin levels (ng/mL); and **b** serum TNC levels (ng/mL). Mild to moderate asthma was defined as well-controlled asthma requiring GINA treatment steps 1–3. Severe asthma was defined as asthma requiring GINA treatment steps 4/5 and as uncontrolled asthma despite the treatment. *$P < 0.05$, mild to moderate versus severe asthma, Th2-low versus Th2-high, serum immunoglobulin E (IgE) ≤ 100 versus IgE > 100, peripheral blood eosinophil count (EOS) < 140 versus EOS ≥ 140, fractional exhaled nitric oxide (FeNO) < 50 versus FeNO ≥ 50. Bars indicate median values

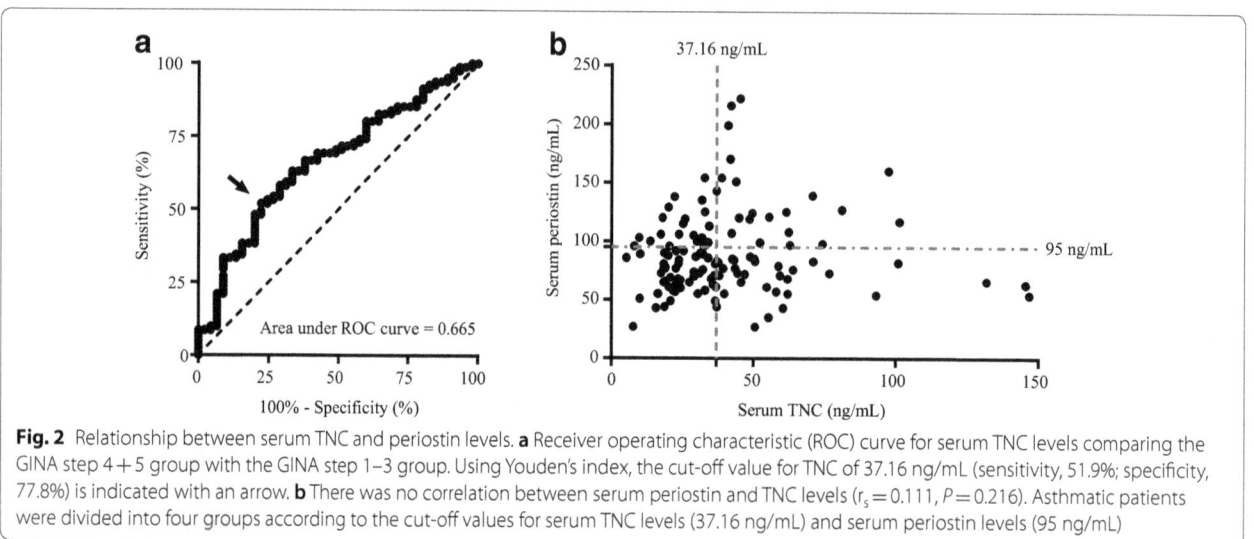

Fig. 2 Relationship between serum TNC and periostin levels. **a** Receiver operating characteristic (ROC) curve for serum TNC levels comparing the GINA step 4 + 5 group with the GINA step 1–3 group. Using Youden's index, the cut-off value for TNC of 37.16 ng/mL (sensitivity, 51.9%; specificity, 77.8%) is indicated with an arrow. **b** There was no correlation between serum periostin and TNC levels ($r_s = 0.111$, $P = 0.216$). Asthmatic patients were divided into four groups according to the cut-off values for serum TNC levels (37.16 ng/mL) and serum periostin levels (95 ng/mL)

Serum TNC levels and the therapeutic effect of omalizumab for patients with severe asthma

Twenty-one (16.7%) asthmatic patients had been treated with omalizumab, a recombinant humanized anti-IgE monoclonal antibody for severe asthma, prior to enrolling in this study. Serum TNC levels in omalizumab-treated patients were significantly higher than those in patients not treated with omalizumab (52.72 ± 31.71 ng/

Table 3 Characteristics that are statistically different between patients with high serum TNC and high serum periostin levels and others

	High TNC > 37.16 High periostin > 95 A (n = 20)	Low TNC < 37.16 High periostin > 95 B (n = 21)	High TNC > 37.16 Low periostin < 95 C (n = 32)	Low TNC < 37.16 Low periostin < 95 D (n = 53)	P value for multigroup analysis[†]	Groups B, C and D E (n = 106)	P value between groups A and E[‡]
GINA step 4 + 5, n (%)	17 (85.0)	7 (33.3)	25 (78.1)	32 (60.4)	0.001*	64 (60.4)	0.042*
AERD, n (%)	6 (30.0)	0 (0.0)	1 (3.1)	5 (9.4)	0.004*	6 (5.7)	0.004*
Daily dose of ICS (FP equivalent dose, µg)	735.00 ± 346.83	392.86 ± 346.51	629.69 ± 349.39	575.47 ± 407.10	0.021*	555.66 ± 384.91	0.045*
FeNO (ppb)	65.30 ± 46.36	65.87 ± 34.04	54.51 ± 52.86	47.21 ± 39.25	0.033*	53.11 ± 43.12	0.208
Peripheral neutrophils (cells/µL)	4588.06 ± 1452.31	3496.31 ± 1052.69	4216.49 ± 1600.66	3900.12 ± 1535.39	0.037*	3915.63 ± 1482.52	0.032*
Peripheral eosinophils (cells/µL)	423.03 ± 315.58	354.16 ± 243.56	223.62 ± 224.07	191.55 ± 159.50	0.001*	233.44 ± 206.28	0.005*
Serum periostin (ng/mL)	138.65 ± 37.94	114.33 ± 17.18	67.81 ± 15.66	69.81 ± 14.82	< 0.001*	78.03 ± 23.81	< 0.001*
Serum TNC (ng/mL)	57.93 ± 18.62	25.42 ± 8.56	62.44 ± 29.95	24.25 ± 7.94	< 0.001*	36.01 ± 24.80	< 0.001*
FVC (L)	2.72 ± 0.93	3.17 ± 0.86	3.38 ± 0.89	3.34 ± 0.98	0.063	3.32 ± 0.93	0.010*
%FVC (predicted, %)	96.10 ± 9.38	103.77 ± 16.30	102.95 ± 16.61	105.47 ± 17.57	0.118	104.37 ± 16.92	0.019*
FEV$_1$ (L)	1.99 ± 0.80	2.28 ± 0.59	2.47 ± 0.83	2.52 ± 0.80	0.062	2.46 ± 0.77	0.014*
PEF (L/s)	6.39 ± 2.00	6.92 ± 1.42	7.46 ± 2.35	7.54 ± 2.05	0.142	7.39 ± 2.04	0.045*
MMF (L)	1.51 ± 1.01	1.64 ± 0.69	1.99 ± 1.07	2.21 ± 1.14	NS	2.03 ± 1.06	0.045*
%MMF (predicted, %)	48.14 ± 24.36	54.37 ± 20.36	56.33 ± 26.21	66.39 ± 30.28	NS	60.97 ± 27.67	0.042*

Data are presented as the mean ± standard deviation unless otherwise indicated

ACT asthma control test, AERD aspirin-exacerbated respiratory disease, BMI body mass index, FeNO fractional exhaled nitric oxide, FEV1 forced expiratory volume in 1 s, FP fluticasone propionate, FVC forced vital capacity, GINA Global Initiative for Asthma, ICS inhaled corticosteroid, IgE immunoglobulin E, MMF mid-maximal flow rate, OCS oral corticosteroids, PEF peak expiratory flow, PSL prednisolone, Th2 T-helper cell type 2, TNC tenascin-C, NS not significant

*P < 0.05

[†] Multigroup analysis performed by Chi square test, One-way ANOVA and Kruskal–Wallis test as appropriate

[‡] Comparisons performed by Student's t test, the Mann–Whitney U test, and Fisher's exact test as appropriate

mL versus 36.84 ± 22.94 ng/mL; $P = 0.014$), which corresponded to previously shown results that serum TNC levels were correlated with asthma severity and the daily dose of ICS. The mean duration of omalizumab treatment and median age were 26.89 ± 17.15 months (range 0.93–66.23 months) and 53 years (range 20–86 years), respectively.

Finally, we investigated whether serum TNC levels were associated with the effect of omalizumab treatment. The 21 patients were divided into two subgroups according to change in FEV$_1$ of more or less than 12% of baseline, i.e., the ratio of FEV$_1$ at enrollment after treatment to baseline FEV$_1$ before treatment. Only serum TNC levels showed a significant difference between the two subgroups among evaluated subject characteristics (Additional file 5: Table S5). Serum TNC levels were significantly higher in the subgroup with an improvement in FEV$_1$ of ≥ 12% than that in the subgroup with improvement

in FEV$_1$ of < 12% (Fig. 3). Moreover, all of the patients with an improvement in FEV$_1$ of ≥ 12% were included in the subgroup with high serum TNC levels (> 37.16 ng/mL) and serum periostin was not associated with the omalizumab-related improvement subgroup (Additional file 6: Table S6 and data not shown).

Discussion

The results of the present study confirm previous reports by showing that serum TNC concentrations in patients with asthma were associated with disease severity [29]. Furthermore, to our knowledge, this is the first study to show that serum TNC levels in asthmatic patients are associated with clinical features of asthma and that using both the combination of serum TNC and periostin levels and the combination of serum TNC and total IgE levels in a multiple-marker approach might be a more useful biomarker for asthma. The present

Table 4 Characteristics that are statistically different between patients with high serum TNC and high serum IgE levels and others

	High TNC > 37.16 High IgE > 100 A (n = 36)	Low TNC < 37.16 High IgE > 100 B (n = 42)	High TNC > 37.16 Low IgE < 100 C (n = 16)	Low TNC < 37.16 Low IgE < 100 D (n = 32)	P value for multigroup analysis[†]	Groups B, C and D E (n = 90)	P value between groups A and E[‡]
GINA step 4 + 5, n (%)	29 (80.6)	18 (42.9)	13 (81.3)	21 (65.6)	0.002*	52 (57.8)	0.023*
Peripheral neutrophils (cells/μL)	4593.71 ± 1656.42	3823.77 ± 1249.02	3832.20 ± 1117.89	3735.33 ± 1637.25	0.018*	3793.82 ± 1365.61	0.002*
Peripheral eosinophils (cells/μL)	338.37 ± 302.52	287.01 ± 206.42	214.70 ± 194.18	172.96 ± 172.63	0.027*	233.60 ± 197.73	0.170
Serum IgE (IU/mL)	1120.92 ± 2424.39	831.76 ± 1733.44	46.26 ± 28.61	51.09 ± 25.59	<0.001*	414.55 ± 1240.42	<0.001*
Th2-high, n (%)	23 (63.9)	30 (71.4)	0 (0.0)	0 (0.0)	<0.001*	30 (33.3)	0.003*
Serum TNC (ng/mL)	63.77 ± 29.77	26.04 ± 8.42	53.79 ± 12.95	22.65 ± 7.29	<0.001*	29.77 ± 14.42	<0.001*
%FVC (predicted, %)	97.08 ± 12.80	105.44 ± 16.51	107.59 ± 16.01	104.40 ± 18.16	NS	105.45 ± 16.88	0.005*
%FEV$_1$ (predicted, %)	82.77 ± 15.57	94.92 ± 16.70	95.69 ± 19.99	92.69 ± 20.27	0.005*	94.26 ± 18.45	<0.001*
%PEF (predicted, %)	96.95 ± 19.02	103.93 ± 19.00	107.31 ± 24.44	107.53 ± 23.42	0.124	105.81 ± 21.48	0.033*
%MMF (predicted, %)	48.56 ± 20.87	63.05 ± 24.47	63.56 ± 32.29	62.88 ± 32.92	0.083	63.08 ± 28.79	0.010*

Data are presented as the mean ± standard deviation unless otherwise indicated

ACT asthma control test, AERD aspirin-exacerbated respiratory disease, BMI body mass index, FeNO fractional exhaled nitric oxide, FEV1 forced expiratory volume in 1 s, FP fluticasone propionate, FVC forced vital capacity, GINA Global Initiative for Asthma, ICS inhaled corticosteroid, IgE immunoglobulin E, MMF mid-maximal flow rate, OCS oral corticosteroids, PEF peak expiratory flow, PSL prednisolone, Th2 T-helper cell type 2, TNC tenascin-C, NS not significant

*$P < 0.05$

†Multigroup analysis performed by Chi square test, One-way ANOVA and Kruskal–Wallis test as appropriate

‡Comparisons performed by Student's t test, the Mann–Whitney U test, and Fisher's exact test as appropriate

study demonstrated that peripheral blood eosinophil counts and total serum IgE levels were associated with serum periostin and TNC levels, respectively. Moreover, disease severity, percentages of patients with AERD, and airflow limitation were associated with patients with high serum TNC and periostin levels as compared with patients in the other subpopulations, suggesting that both periostin and TNC might serve as biomarkers of asthma. It was reported that the gene expression of periostin and TNC in bronchial epithelial cells is upregulated by Th2 cytokines, including IL-4 and IL-13, and that the secretion of periostin and TNC in lung fibroblasts is also induced by both IL-4 and IL-13 [6, 10, 11]. Both periostin and TNC bind to each other and also co-localize in subepithelial fibrosis in asthmatic patients [6]. Although the production of both extracellular matrix proteins is induced by IL-4 and IL-13, it is interesting to note that different features were observed between serum periostin and TNC levels in asthmatic patients in the present study. IgE synthesis is also regulated by IL-4 and IL-13 [38, 39]. Previous report demonstrates that IgE in the bronchoalveolar lavage fluid are

significantly decreased in ovalbumin-induced asthma mice model using TNC-deficient mice and that addition of exogenous TNC to mouse spleen lymphocytes stimulates IgE secretion [28]. These data suggests that TNC has a potential of IgE synthesis. On the other hand, there are two reports using different periostin-deficient mice. One report shows that allergen-induced increases in serum IgE and airways hyperresponsiveness are exaggerated in periostin-deficient mice challenged with inhaled Aspergillus fumigatus antigen [40]. Another report using periostin-deficient mice and anti-periostin neutralizing antibody shows that periostin is required for IgE synthesis and airways hyperresponsiveness in mice challenged with inhaled aeroallergen, house dust mite [41]. These results suggest that periostin and TNC may have different function for IgE synthesis and may reflect their different features. Because both serum periostin and TNC levels were not correlation and had different features, the combination of serum TNC and periostin levels in a multiple-marker approach might be more useful biomarkers reflecting asthma severity including airflow limitation than a single biomarker approach.

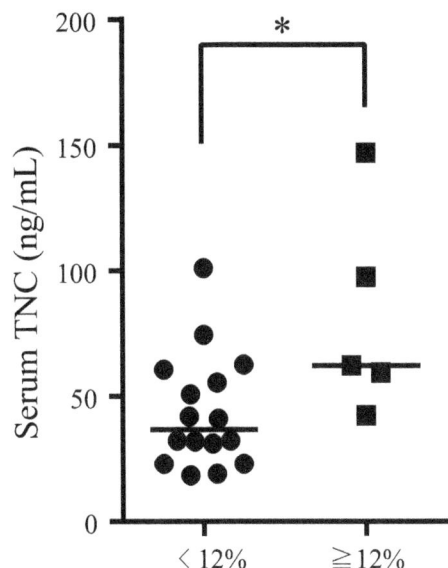

Fig. 3 Serum TNC levels and the therapeutic effect of omalizumab for patients with severe asthma. Serum TNC levels were significantly higher in the subgroup with an improvement in forced expiratory volume in 1 s (FEV$_1$) of ≥ 12% than that in the subgroup with improvement in FEV$_1$ of < 12%. *$P < 0.05$

TNC is a matricellular protein that is highly expressed during wound healing and tissue remodeling processes in chronic inflammation, including asthma [24, 42–44]. The results of the present study demonstrated that serum TNC levels were not correlated with airflow limitation despite a correlation with asthma severity and high serum IgE levels, even when the asthma was severe. However, this study suggested that serum TNC levels may reflect disease severity in asthma and may be an indicator of airflow limitation in asthmatic patients with high serum periostin levels or high serum total IgE levels. Moreover, serum TNC levels were associated with peripheral blood neutrophil counts in the especially periostin-high subgroup or IgE-high subgroup, suggesting that serum TNC levels may reflect not only type 2 airway inflammation but also neutrophilic airway inflammation.

High serum TNC levels have already some application as biomarker. Increased levels of serum TNC might be useful in liver fibrosis [45], inflammatory bowel diseases [46, 47], cardiovascular diseases [48–51], and refractory asthma [29]. Serum TNC levels in patients with inflammatory bowel disease correlate with disease severity [46], and infliximab therapy response in patients with ulcerative colitis is associated with decreased levels of serum TNC [47]. In patients with dilated cardiomyopathy, high serum TNC levels might indicate the severity of heart failure, left ventricular (LV) dysfunction and remodeling [48–50]. Moreover,

previous report on acute myocardial infarction (AMI) shows that serum TNC levels in patients with AMI is significantly elevated, peaks at day 5, and then gradually decreases, and suggests that serum TNC levels might be useful in predicting LV remodeling and prognosis after AMI [51]. These applications and the results of present study suggests that serum TNC might be a novel marker reflecting active structural remodeling in fibrosis, inflammatory bowel diseases, cardiovascular diseases, and asthma.

In previous studies, the serum periostin level had potential as a single biomarker to predict eosinophilic airway inflammation and risk of a decline in FEV$_1$ in asthmatic patients and was associated with late onset, high eosinophil counts, AERD, and chronic sinusitis [15–17, 19–21, 52]. Our results confirmed that high serum periostin levels were correlated with late onset and high peripheral blood eosinophil counts, but demonstrated that high serum periostin levels were not correlated with AERD and chronic sinusitis. However, the percentages of patients with AERD among patients with high serum TNC and periostin levels were higher than those in other subgroups, and serum periostin levels were correlated with AERD in the high serum TNC subgroup (data not shown). Furthermore, previous reports suggested that high serum periostin is associated with asthma severity [17, 18]. The present study showed that serum periostin levels were correlated with airflow limitation and showed a better correlation with airflow limitation in patients with severe asthma and high serum TNC levels. However, the present study also showed an inverse correlation between serum periostin and asthma disease severity, i.e., patients with mild to moderate asthma had high serum periostin levels. The reason for the discrepancy between serum periostin levels and asthma severity was not clear in the current study. This discrepancy may be related to dominant low FeNO levels in patients with severe asthma. Nevertheless, the findings of this unique subpopulation may lead to discrepant results between previous studies and the current study.

Omalizumab, a recombinant humanized monoclonal antibody against human IgE, has important benefits as an add-on therapy for patients with inadequately controlled severe persistent asthma who have a significant unmet need [53–56]. However, not all patients with inadequately controlled asthma respond to omalizumab and predictors of response to this biological therapy are limited [57]. It has been reported that serum IgE levels and antigen-specific IgE could not predict the response to omalizumab [58–60]. The EXTRA omalizumab study suggested the potential of three biomarkers of Th2-driven inflammation, including FeNO levels, peripheral blood eosinophil counts, and serum periostin levels, as predictors of the response to omalizumab to reduce the incidence of severe exacerbation [57]. In the present study, we demonstrated that the omalizumab-related improvement in FEV_1 of at least 12% was associated with high serum TNC levels, indicating that patients with high serum TNC levels may achieve a greater benefit from omalizumab therapy.

There were several important limitations to this study. First, the lack of data of healthy subjects is a limitation. Second, for data on omalizumab treatment (Additional file 5: Table S5), serum TNC levels were evaluated after approximately 2 years from starting omalizumab treatment, blood samples were collected at different time points after starting treatment, and the sample size was small. Therefore, the data for omalizumab treatment should be considered preliminary. Further studies are needed to investigate whether serum TNC levels and/or the combination of serum TNC and periostin levels can serve as more useful biomarkers in asthmatic patients and whether it has the potential as a biomarker to predict the therapeutic efficacy of omalizumab for severe asthmatic patients.

Conclusions

We have provided the first report that serum TNC levels in asthmatic patients were associated with clinical features of asthma and that the combination of serum TNC and periostin levels or the combination of serum TNC and total IgE levels were more useful for asthma than a single biomarker approach, suggesting that serum TNC can serve as a novel biomarker for asthma. Additional studies are needed to investigate whether serum TNC levels and/or combination with other markers are more useful biomarkers in asthmatic patients.

Additional files

Additional file 1: Table S1. Correlation coefficients for the association of serum periostin and TNC levels with subject characteristics, stratified by GINA steps.

Additional file 2: Table S2. The statistical significance and confidence intervals for serum periostin and TNC levels with asthma severity and Th2-related variables.

Additional file 3: Table S3. Characteristics of patients divided into four groups according to serum TNC and periostin levels.

Additional file 4: Table S4. Characteristics of patients divided into four groups according to serum TNC and IgE levels.

Additional file 5: Table S5. Characteristics of omalizumab-treated patients.

Additional file 6: Table S6. Omalizumab-treated patients to divide into 4 groups according to serum TNC and Periostin levels.

Abbreviations

ACT: asthma control test; AERD: aspirin-exacerbated respiratory disease; BMI: body mass index; ELISA: enzyme-linked immunosorbent assay; FeNO: fractional exhaled nitric oxide; FEV_1: forced expiratory volume in 1 s; FP: fluticasone propionate; FVC: forced vital capacity; GINA: Global Initiative for Asthma; ICS: inhaled corticosteroid; IgE: immunoglobulin E; IL: interleukin; MMF: mid-maximal flow rate; OCS: oral corticosteroids; PEF: peak expiratory flow; PSL: prednisolone; Th2: T-helper cell type 2; TNC: tenascin-C.

Authors' contributions

YA, NH, RA, and KT participated in the design of the study and drafted the manuscript. YA, NH, SH, AI, YK, YI, KM, FM, JI, JO, KT, HA, RA and KI contributed to data collection. YA, NH, and SH performed the statistical analysis and interpretation of the results. All authors read and approved the final manuscript.

Author details

[1] Department of Respiratory Medicine, Juntendo University Faculty of Medicine and Graduate School of Medicine, 3-1-3 Hongo, Bunkyo-ku, Tokyo 113-8431, Japan. [2] Department of Respiratory Medicine, Iizuka Hospital, Fukuoka, Japan. [3] Research Institute for Diseases of Old Ages, Juntendo University Faculty of Medicine and Graduate School of Medicine, Tokyo, Japan. [4] Atopy (Allergy) Research Center, Juntendo University Faculty of Medicine and Graduate School of Medicine, Tokyo, Japan. [5] Shino-Test Corporation, Sagamihara, Japan. [6] Department of Immunology, Juntendo University Faculty of Medicine and Graduate School of Medicine, Tokyo, Japan. [7] Division of Medical Biochemistry, Department of Biomolecular Sciences, Saga Medical School, Saga, Japan.

Acknowledgements

Not applicable.

Competing interests

KI reports grants from Shino-test Co. Ltd. during the conduct of the study; grants from AstraZeneca, outside the submitted work. In addition, KI has a patent effective only in Japan licensed. JO is an employee of Shino-Test Co. Ltd. The rest of the authors declare that they have no competing interests.

Funding

This work was supported in part by JSPS KAKENHI Grant Number 25461167.

References

1. Bai TR, Knight DA. Structural changes in the airways in asthma: observations and consequences. Clin Sci (Lond). 2005;108(6):463–77.
2. Nakano Y, Muller NL, King GG, Niimi A, Kalloger SE, Mishima M, et al. Quantitative assessment of airway remodeling using high-resolution CT. Chest. 2002;122(6 Suppl):271S–5S.
3. Lotvall J, Akdis CA, Bacharier LB, Bjermer L, Casale TB, Custovic A, et al. Asthma endotypes: a new approach to classification of disease entities within the asthma syndrome. J Allergy Clin Immunol. 2011;127(2):355–60.
4. Vignola AM, Kips J, Bousquet J. Tissue remodeling as a feature of persistent asthma. J Allergy Clin Immunol. 2000;105(6 Pt 1):1041–53.
5. Phipps S, Benyahia F, Ou TT, Barkans J, Robinson DS, Kay AB. Acute allergen-induced airway remodeling in atopic asthma. Am J Respir Cell Mol Biol. 2004;31(6):626–32.

6. Takayama G, Arima K, Kanaji T, Toda S, Tanaka H, Shoji S, et al. Periostin: a novel component of subepithelial fibrosis of bronchial asthma downstream of IL-4 and IL-13 signals. J Allergy Clin Immunol. 2006;118(1):98–104.

7. Wenzel SE. Asthma phenotypes: the evolution from clinical to molecular approaches. Nat Med. 2012;18(5):716–25.

8. Lambrecht BN, Hammad H. The immunology of asthma. Nat Immunol. 2015;16(1):45–56.

9. Lee JH, Kaminski N, Dolganov G, Grunig G, Koth L, Solomon C, et al. Interleukin-13 induces dramatically different transcriptional programs in three human airway cell types. Am J Respir Cell Mol Biol. 2001;25(4):474–85.

10. Yuyama N, Davies DE, Akaiwa M, Matsui K, Hamasaki Y, Suminami Y, et al. Analysis of novel disease-related genes in bronchial asthma. Cytokine. 2002;19(6):287–96.

11. Matsuda A, Hirota T, Akahoshi M, Shimizu M, Tamari M, Miyatake A, et al. Coding SNP in tenascin-C Fn-III-D domain associates with adult asthma. Hum Mol Genet. 2005;14(19):2779–86.

12. Woodruff PG, Boushey HA, Dolganov GM, Barker CS, Yang YH, Donnelly S, et al. Genome-wide profiling identifies epithelial cell genes associated with asthma and with treatment response to corticosteroids. Proc Natl Acad Sci USA. 2007;104(40):15858–63.

13. Woodruff PG, Modrek B, Choy DF, Jia G, Abbas AR, Ellwanger A, et al. T-helper type 2-driven inflammation defines major subphenotypes of asthma. Am J Respir Crit Care Med. 2009;180(5):388–95.

14. Blanchard C, Mingler MK, McBride M, Putnam PE, Collins MH, Chang G, et al. Periostin facilitates eosinophil tissue infiltration in allergic lung and esophageal responses. Mucosal Immunol. 2008;1(4):289–96.

15. Jia G, Erickson RW, Choy DF, Mosesova S, Wu LC, Solberg OD, et al. Periostin is a systemic biomarker of eosinophilic airway inflammation in asthmatic patients. J Allergy Clin Immunol. 2012;130(3):647–654.e10.

16. Wagener AH, de Nijs SB, Lutter R, Sousa AR, Weersink EJ, Bel EH, et al. External validation of blood eosinophils, FE(NO) and serum periostin as surrogates for sputum eosinophils in asthma. Thorax. 2015;70(2):115–20.

17. Kim MA, Izuhara K, Ohta S, Ono J, Yoon MK, Ban GY, et al. Association of serum periostin with aspirin-exacerbated respiratory disease. Ann Allergy Asthma Immunol. 2014;113(3):314–20.

18. Nagasaki T, Matsumoto H, Kanemitsu Y, Izuhara K, Tohda Y, Horiguchi T, et al. Using exhaled nitric oxide and serum periostin as a composite marker to identify severe/steroid-insensitive asthma. Am J Respir Crit Care Med. 2014;190(12):1449–52.

19. Kanemitsu Y, Matsumoto H, Izuhara K, Tohda Y, Kita H, Horiguchi T, et al. Increased periostin associates with greater airflow limitation in patients receiving inhaled corticosteroids. J Allergy Clin Immunol. 2013;132(2):305–312.e3.

20. Kanemitsu Y, Ito I, Niimi A, Izuhara K, Ohta S, Ono J, et al. Osteopontin and periostin are associated with a 20-year decline of pulmonary function in patients with asthma. Am J Respir Crit Care Med. 2014;190(4):472–4.

21. Nagasaki T, Matsumoto H, Kanemitsu Y, Izuhara K, Tohda Y, Kita H, et al. Integrating longitudinal information on pulmonary function and inflammation using asthma phenotypes. J Allergy Clin Immunol. 2014;133(5):1474–7, 1477.e1-2.

22. Jones FS, Jones PL. The tenascin family of ECM glycoproteins: structure, function, and regulation during embryonic development and tissue remodeling. Dev Dyn. 2000;218(2):235–59.

23. Kaarteenaho-Wiik R, Kinnula V, Herva R, Paakko P, Pollanen R, Soini Y. Distribution and mRNA expression of tenascin-C in developing human lung. Am J Respir Cell Mol Biol. 2001;25(3):341–6.

24. Laitinen A, Altraja A, Kampe M, Linden M, Virtanen I, Laitinen LA. Tenascin is increased in airway basement membrane of asthmatics and decreased by an inhaled steroid. Am J Respir Crit Care Med. 1997;156(3 Pt 1):951–8.

25. Flood-Page P, Menzies-Gow A, Phipps S, Ying S, Wangoo A, Ludwig MS, et al. Anti-IL-5 treatment reduces deposition of ECM proteins in the bronchial subepithelial basement membrane of mild atopic asthmatics. J Clin Invest. 2003;112(7):1029–36.

26. Torrego A, Hew M, Oates T, Sukkar M, Fan Chung K. Expression and activation of TGF-beta isoforms in acute allergen-induced remodelling in asthma. Thorax. 2007;62(4):307–13.

27. Karjalainen EM, Lindqvist A, Laitinen LA, Kava T, Altraja A, Halme M, et al. Airway inflammation and basement membrane tenascin

28. Nakahara H, Gabazza EC, Fujimoto H, Nishii Y, D'Alessandro-Gabazza CN, Bruno NE, et al. Deficiency of tenascin C attenuates allergen-induced bronchial asthma in the mouse. Eur J Immunol. 2006;36(12):3334–45.

29. Alam R, Good J, Rollins D, Verma M, Chu H, Pham TH, et al. Airway and serum biochemical correlates of refractory neutrophilic asthma. J Allergy Clin Immunol. 2017;140(4):1004–1014.e13.

30. Global Initiative for Asthma (GINA). Global strategy for asthma management and prevention. 2016. http://www.ginasthma.org/. Accessed 15 Nov 2012.

31. Global Initiative for Chronic Obstructive Lung Disease (GOLD). Global strategy for diagnosis,management, and prevention of COPD. 2016. http://www.goldcopd.org/. Accessed 15 Nov 2012.

32. Okamoto M, Hoshino T, Kitasato Y, Sakazaki Y, Kawayama T, Fujimoto K, et al. Periostin, a matrix protein, is a novel biomarker for idiopathic interstitial pneumonias. Eur Respir J. 2011;37(5):1119–27.

33. Page TH, Charles PJ, Piccinini AM, Nicolaidou V, Taylor PC, Midwood KS. Raised circulating tenascin-C in rheumatoid arthritis. Arthritis Res Ther. 2012;14(6):R260.

34. Vicens-Zygmunt V, Estany S, Colom A, Montes-Worboys A, Machahua C, Sanabria AJ, et al. Fibroblast viability and phenotypic changes within glycated stiffened three-dimensional collagen matrices. Respir Res. 2015;16:82.

35. Corren J, Lemanske RF, Hanania NA, Korenblat PE, Parsey MV, Arron JR, et al. Lebrikizumab treatment in adults with asthma. N Engl J Med. 2011;365(12):1088–98.

36. Thomson NC, Chaudhuri R, Spears M, Haughney J, McSharry C. Serum periostin in smokers and never smokers with asthma. Respir Med. 2015;109(6):708–15.

37. Youden WJ. Index for rating diagnostic tests. Cancer. 1950;3(1):32–5.

38. Gour N, Wills-Karp M. IL-4 and IL-13 signaling in allergic airway disease. Cytokine. 2015;75(1):68–78.

39. Ingram JL, Kraft M. IL-13 in asthma and allergic disease: asthma phenotypes and targeted therapies. J Allergy Clin Immunol. 2012;130(4):829–42 (quiz 43–44).

40. Gordon ED, Sidhu SS, Wang ZE, Woodruff PG, Yuan S, Solon MC, et al. A protective role for periostin and TGF-beta in IgE-mediated allergy and airway hyperresponsiveness. Clin Exp Allergy. 2012;42(1):144–55.

41. Bentley JK, Chen Q, Hong JY, Popova AP, Lei J, Moore BB, et al. Periostin is required for maximal airways inflammation and hyperresponsiveness in mice. J Allergy Clin Immunol. 2014;134(6):1433–42.

42. Orend G, Chiquet-Ehrismann R. Tenascin-C induced signaling in cancer. Cancer Lett. 2006;244(2):143–63.

43. Midwood KS, Orend G. The role of tenascin-C in tissue injury and tumorigenesis. J Cell Commun Signal. 2009;3(3–4):287–310.

44. Katoh D, Nagaharu K, Shimojo N, Hanamura N, Yamashita M, Kozuka Y, et al. Binding of alphavbeta1 and alphavbeta6 integrins to tenascin-C induces epithelial-mesenchymal transition-like change of breast cancer cells. Oncogenesis. 2013;2:e65.

45. Lieber CS, Weiss DG, Paronetto F, Veterans Affairs Cooperative Study G. Value of fibrosis markers for staging liver fibrosis in patients with precirrhotic alcoholic liver disease. Alcohol Clin Exp Res. 2008;32(6):1031–9.

46. Riedl S, Tandara A, Reinshagen M, Hinz U, Faissner A, Bodenmuller H, et al. Serum tenascin-C is an indicator of inflammatory bowel disease activity. Int J Colorectal Dis. 2001;16(5):285–91.

47. Magnusson MK, Strid H, Isaksson S, Bajor A, Lasson A, Ung KA, et al. Response to infliximab therapy in ulcerative colitis is associated with decreased monocyte activation, reduced CCL2 expression and downregulation of Tenascin C. J Crohns Colitis. 2015;9(1):56–65.

48. Imanaka-Yoshida K. Tenascin-C in cardiovascular tissue remodeling: from development to inflammation and repair. Circ J. 2012;76(11):2513–20.

49. Terasaki F, Okamoto H, Onishi K, Sato A, Shimomura H, Tsukada B, et al. Higher serum tenascin-C levels reflect the severity of heart failure, left ventricular dysfunction and remodeling in patients with dilated cardiomyopathy. Circ J. 2007;71(3):327–30.

50. Tsukada B, Terasaki F, Shimomura H, Otsuka K, Otsuka K, Katashima T, et al. High prevalence of chronic myocarditis in dilated cardiomyopathy referred for left ventriculoplasty: expression of tenascin C as a possible marker for inflammation. Hum Pathol. 2009;40(7):1015–22.

51. Sato A, Aonuma K, Imanaka-Yoshida K, Yoshida T, Isobe M, Kawase D, et al. Serum tenascin-C might be a novel predictor of left ventricular remodeling and prognosis after acute myocardial infarction. J Am Coll Cardiol. 2006;47(11):2319–25.

52. Matsusaka M, Kabata H, Fukunaga K, Suzuki Y, Masaki K, Mochimaru T, et al. Phenotype of asthma related with high serum periostin levels. Allergol Int. 2015;64(2):175–80.

53. Corren J, Casale TB, Lanier B, Buhl R, Holgate S, Jimenez P. Safety and tolerability of omalizumab. Clin Exp Allergy. 2009;39(6):788–97.

54. Bousquet J, Cabrera P, Berkman N, Buhl R, Holgate S, Wenzel S, et al. The effect of treatment with omalizumab, an anti-IgE antibody, on asthma exacerbations and emergency medical visits in patients with severe persistent asthma. Allergy. 2005;60(3):302–8.

55. Bousquet J, Siergiejko Z, Swiebocka E, Humbert M, Rabe KF, Smith N, et al. Persistency of response to omalizumab therapy in severe allergic (IgE-mediated) asthma. Allergy. 2011;66(5):671–8.

56. Hanania NA, Alpan O, Hamilos DL, Condemi JJ, Reyes-Rivera I, Zhu J, et al. Omalizumab in severe allergic asthma inadequately controlled with standard therapy: a randomized trial. Ann Intern Med. 2011;154(9):573–82.

57. Hanania NA, Wenzel S, Rosen K, Hsieh HJ, Mosesova S, Choy DF, et al. Exploring the effects of omalizumab in allergic asthma: an analysis of biomarkers in the EXTRA study. Am J Respir Crit Care Med. 2013;187(8):804–11.

58. Bousquet J, Wenzel S, Holgate S, Lumry W, Freeman P, Fox H. Predicting response to omalizumab, an anti-IgE antibody, in patients with allergic asthma. Chest. 2004;125(4):1378–86.

59. Bousquet J, Rabe K, Humbert M, Chung KF, Berger W, Fox H, et al. Predicting and evaluating response to omalizumab in patients with severe allergic asthma. Respir Med. 2007;101(7):1483–92.

60. Wahn U, Martin C, Freeman P, Blogg M, Jimenez P. Relationship between pretreatment specific IgE and the response to omalizumab therapy. Allergy. 2009;64(12):1780–7.

Permissions

The contributors of this book come from diverse backgrounds, making this book a truly international effort. This book will bring forth new frontiers with its revolutionizing research information and detailed analysis of the nascent developments around the world.

We would like to thank all the contributing authors for lending their expertise to make the book truly unique. They have played a crucial role in the development of this book. Without their invaluable contributions this book wouldn't have been possible. They have made vital efforts to compile up to date information on the varied aspects of this subject to make this book a valuable addition to the collection of many professionals and students.

This book was conceptualized with the vision of imparting up-to-date information and advanced data in this field. To ensure the same, a matchless editorial board was set up. Every individual on the board went through rigorous rounds of assessment to prove their worth. After which they invested a large part of their time researching and compiling the most relevant data for our readers.

The editorial board has been involved in producing this book since its inception. They have spent rigorous hours researching and exploring the diverse topics which have resulted in the successful publishing of this book. They have passed on their knowledge of decades through this book. To expedite this challenging task, the publisher supported the team at every step. A small team of assistant editors was also appointed to further simplify the editing procedure and attain best results for the readers.

Apart from the editorial board, the designing team has also invested a significant amount of their time in understanding the subject and creating the most relevant covers. They scrutinized every image to scout for the most suitable representation of the subject and create an appropriate cover for the book.

The publishing team has been an ardent support to the editorial, designing and production team. Their endless efforts to recruit the best for this project, has resulted in the accomplishment of this book. They are a veteran in the field of academics and their pool of knowledge is as vast as their experience in printing. Their expertise and guidance has proved useful at every step. Their uncompromising quality standards have made this book an exceptional effort. Their encouragement from time to time has been an inspiration for everyone.

The publisher and the editorial board hope that this book will prove to be a valuable piece of knowledge for researchers, students, practitioners and scholars across the globe.

List of Contributors

Leah T. Stiemsma and Stuart E. Turvey
Department of Microbiology & Immunology, University of British Columbia, Vancouver, BC, Canada
BC Children's Hospital, Vancouver, BC, Canada

Stuart E. Turvey
Department of Pediatrics, University of British Columbia, Vancouver, BC, Canada

Stuart E. Turvey
Department of Pediatrics, BC Children's Hospital, 950 West 28th Avenue, Vancouver, BC V5Z 4H4, Canada

Jie Gao and Feng Wu
Department of Respiratory Medicine, The Third People's Hospital, Guangzhou Medical College, 1# Xuebei Ave., Huizhou 516002, Guangdong, China

William F. S. Sellers
Broadgate House, 22 Broadgate, Great Easton, Leicestershire LE16 8SH, UK

Qing Miao, Yan Wang, Yong-ge Liu, Yi-xin Ren, Hui Guan, Zhen Li, Wei Xu and Li Xiang
Department of Allergy, Beijing Children's Hospital, Capital Medical School, No. 56 Nanlishi Road, Xicheng District, Beijing 100045, China

Ahmed Ahmed
Department of Pediatrics, University of Ottawa, Ottawa, ON, Canada

Amir Hakim
National Heart and Lung Institute, Imperial College, London, UK

Allan Becker
Section of Allergy and Clinical Immunology, Department of Pediatrics and Child Health, University of Manitoba, Winnipeg, MB, Canada

Bobby Lanier
Texas Allergy Experts, Fort Worth, TX, USA

Afia Aziz-Ur-Rehman, Angira Dasgupta, Melanie Kjarsgaard, Frederick E. Hargreave and Parameswaran Nair
Department of Medicine, McMaster University and St Joseph's Healthcare Hamilton, Hamilton, ON, Canada

Parameswaran Nair
Firestone Institute for Respiratory Health, St. Joseph's Healthcare, 50 Charlton Avenue East, Hamilton, ON L8N 4A6, Canada

Hye Jung Park, Min Kwang Byun, Hyung Jung Kim and Chul Min Ahn
Department of Internal Medicine, Gangnam Severance Hospital, Yonsei University College of Medicine, 211 Eonju-ro Gangnam-gu, Seoul 135-720, South Korea

Chin Kook Rhee and Kyungjoo Kim
Division of Pulmonary, Allergy and Critical Care Medicine, Department of Internal Medicine, Seoul St Mary's Hospital, College of Medicine, The Catholic University of Korea, Seoul, South Korea

Bo Yeon Kim
Healthcare Review and Assessment Committee, Health Insurance Review & Assessment Service, Seoul, South Korea

Hye Won Bae
Division of Quality Assessment Management, Health Insurance Review & Assessment Service, Seoul, South Korea

Kwang-Ha Yoo
Division of Pulmonary, Allergy and Critical Care Medicine, Department of Internal Medicine, Konkuk University School of Medicine, Seoul, South Korea

Matthew Wiest, Katherine Upchurch, Wenjie Yin, Jerome Ellis, Yaming Xue, HyeMee Joo and SangKon Oh
Baylor Institute for Immunology Research, 3434 Live Oak St., Dallas, TX 75204, USA

Matthew Wiest, Katherine Upchurch, Wenjie Yin, HyeMee Joo and SangKon Oh
Institute for Biomedical Studies, Baylor University, Waco, TX, USA

Mark Millard
Martha Foster Lung Care Center, Baylor University Medical Center, Dallas, TX, USA

Hongyu Wang, Melanie Kjarsgaard, Terence Ho and Parameswaran Nair
Firestone Institute for Respiratory Health, St. Joseph's Healthcare, 50 Charlton Avenue East, Hamilton, ON L8N 4A6, Canada

Hongyu Wang, Melanie Kjarsgaard, Terence Ho and Parameswaran Nair
Department of Medicine, McMaster University, Hamilton, ON, Canada

John D. Brannan
John Hunter Hospital, Newcastle, NSW, Australia

S. M. Snelder and G. J. Braunstahl
Franciscus Gasthuis & Vlietland, Kleiweg 500, 3045 PM Rotterdam, The Netherlands

E. J. M. Weersink
Academisch Medisch Centrum, Amsterdam, The Netherlands

Manali Mukherjee, Sruthi Thomas, Douglas Miller, Melanie Kjarsgaard, Roma Sehmi, Nader Khalidi and Parameswaran Nair
Department of Medicine, McMaster University & St. Joseph's Healthcare, Hamilton, ON, Canada

Hui Fang Lim
Department of Respiratory Medicine, National University of Singapore, Singapore, Singapore

Bruce Tan
Department of Otolaryngology, Northwestern University, Feinberg School of Medicine, Chicago, IL, USA

Manali Mukherjee, Sruthi Thomas, Melanie Kjarsgaard and Parameswaran Nair
Firestone Institute for Respiratory Health, 50 Charlton Avenue East, Hamilton, ON L8N 4A6, Canada

Hyekyun Rhee and Annette Grape
University of Rochester School of Nursing, 601 Elmwood Ave. Box SON, Rochester, NY 14642, USA

Tanzy Love and Donald Harrington
Department of Biostatistics and Computational Biology, University of Rochester Medical Center, 601 Elmwood Ave., Rochester, NY 14642, USA

Taiji Watanabe, Kazuyuki Chibana, Taichi Shiobara, Rinna Tei, Ryosuke Koike, Yusuke Nakamura, Ryo Arai, Yukiko Horigane, Yasuo Shimizu, Akihiro Takemasa and Yoshiki Ishii
Department of Pulmonary Medicine and Clinical Immunology, Dokkyo Medical University School of Medicine, Tochigi, Japan

Takeshi Fukuda
Dokkyo Medical University School of Medicine, 880 Kitakobayashi Mibumachi, Shimotsugagun, Tochigi 321-0293, Japan

Sally E. Wenzel
Pulmonary Allergy and Critical Care Medicine, Department of Medicine, University of Pittsburgh, 3459 Fifth Ave., Pittsburgh, PA 15213, USA

Hyekyun Rhee and Jennifer Mammen
University of Rochester, School of Nursing, 601 Elmwood Avenue, Box SON, Rochester, NY 14642, USA

Michael Belyea
Arizona State University, College of Nursing and Health Innovation, 500 N. 3rd Street, Phoenix, AZ 85004, USA

A. Grosso, E. Gini, F. Albicini1, C. Tirelli, I. Cerveri and A. G. Corsico
Division of Respiratory Diseases, IRCCS "San Matteo" Hospital Foundation, University of Pavia, Vaile C. Golgi 19, 27100 Pavia, Italy

F. Locatelli
Unit of Epidemiology and Medical Statistics, Department of Diagnostics and Public Health, University of Verona, Verona, Italy

C. R. Laratta and D. Vethanayagam
Pulmonary Research Group, Department of Medicine, University of Alberta, Edmonton, AB, Canada

K. Williams and M. Ulanova
Medical Sciences Division, Northern Ontario School of Medicine, Lakehead University Campus, Thunder Bay, ON, Canada

H. Vliagoftis
Division of Pulmonary Medicine, Department of Medicine, University of Alberta, Room 3-105 Clinical Sciences Building, 11350 83 Avenue, Edmonton, AB T6G 2G3, Canada

Suzanne Murray and Sara Labbé
AXDEV Group Inc., 210-8, Place du Commerce, Brossard, QC J4W 3H2, Canada

Alan Kaplan
Department of Family and Community Medicine, University of Toronto, 500 University Ave, Toronto, ON M5G 1V7, Canada

Kristine Petrasko
Winnipeg Regional Health Authority, Winnipeg, MB R2R 2S8, Canada

Susan Waserman
Division of Clinical Immunology and Allergy, McMaster University, 1280 Main St West, HSC 3V49, Hamilton, ON L8S 4K1, Canada

Jianghong Wei, Libing Ma, Jiying Wang, Qing Xu, Meixi Chen, Ming Jiang, Miao Luo, Jingjie Wu, Weiwei She, Shuyuan Chu and Biwen Mo
Department of Respiratory and Critical Care Medicine, Affiliated Hospital of Guilin Medical University, Guilin 541001, Guangxi, China

Shuyuan Chu and Biwen Mo
Laboratory of Respiratory Diseases, Affiliated Hospital of Guilin Medical University, Guilin 541001, Guangxi, China

Yao-Tung Wang
Division of Pulmonary Medicine, Department of Internal Medicine, Chung Shan Medical University Hospital, Taichung, Taiwan

Yao-Tung Wang and Hsu-Chung Liu
School of Medicine, Chung Shan Medical University, Taichung, Taiwan

Hsu-Chung Liu
Division of Chest Medicine, Department of Internal Medicine, Cheng Ching Hospital, Taichung, Taiwan

Hsu-Chung Liu, Yen-Ching Lee, Tung-Chou Tsai and Chuan-Mu Chen
Department of Life Sciences, College of Life Sciences, National Chung Hsing University, No. 250, Kuo-Kuang Road, Taichung 402, Taiwan

Hui-Chen Chen
Department of Microbiology and Immunology, School of Medicine, China Medical University, Taichung, Taiwan

Hsiao-Ling Chen
Department of Bioresources, Da-Yeh University, Changhwa, Taiwan

Hueng-Chuen Fan
Department of Pediatrics, Tungs' Taichung Metroharbor Hospital, No. 699, Sec. 8, Taiwan Blvd., Wuchi, Taichung 435, Taiwan
Department of Medical Research, Tungs' Taichung Metroharbor Hospital, No. 699, Sec. 8, Taiwan Blvd., Wuchi, Taichung 435, Taiwan
Department of Rehabilitation, Jen-Teh Junior College of Medicine, Nursing and Management, Miaoli, Taiwan

Chuan-Mu Chen
The iEGG and Animal Biotechnology Center, National Chung Hsing University, Taichung, Taiwan
Rong Hsing Research Center for Translational Medicine, National Chung Hsing University, Taichung, Taiwan

Jaclyn Quirt and Harold Kim
McMaster University, Hamilton, ON, Canada

Kyla J. Hildebrand
University of British Columbia, Vancouver, BC, Canada

Jorge Mazza and Harold Kim
Western University, London, ON, Canada

Francisco Noya
McGill University, Montreal, QC, Canada

Mina Yasuda, Norihiro Harada, Sonoko Harada, Ayako Ishimori, Yoko Katsura, Yukinari Itoigawa, Kei Matsuno, Fumihiko Makino, Jun Ito, Kazunori Tobino, Ryo Atsuta and Kazuhisa Takahashi
Department of Respiratory Medicine, Juntendo University Faculty of Medicine and Graduate School of Medicine, 3-1-3 Hongo, Bunkyo-ku,Tokyo 113-8431, Japan

Mina Yasuda and Kazunori Tobino
Department of Respiratory Medicine, Iizuka Hospital, Fukuoka, Japan

Norihiro Harada, Kei Matsuno, Jun Ito and Kazuhisa Takahashi
Research Institute for Diseases of Old Ages, Juntendo University Faculty of Medicine and Graduate School of Medicine, Tokyo, Japan

Norihiro Harada and Sonoko Harada
Atopy (Allergy) Research Center, Juntendo University Faculty of Medicine and Graduate School of Medicine, Tokyo, Japan

Junya Ono
Shino-Test Corporation, Sagamihara, Japan

Hisaya Akiba
Department of Immunology, Juntendo University Faculty of Medicine and Graduate School of Medicine, Tokyo, Japan

Kenji Izuhara
Division of Medical Biochemistry, Department of Biomolecular Sciences, Saga Medical School, Saga, Japan

Index

www.ingramcontent.com/pod-product-compliance
Lightning Source LLC
Chambersburg PA
CBHW082014190326
41458CB00010B/3180